Balanced Ligamentous Tension in Osteopathic Practice

of related interest

An Inner Approach to Cranial Osteopathy
Timothy Marris
Forewords by Liz Hayden and Hollis King
ISBN 978 1 91342 637 8
eISBN 978 1 91342 638 5

Osteopathy for the Over 50s
Maintaining Function and Treating Dysfunction
Nicette Sergueef and Kenneth Nelson
ISBN 978 1 90914 109 4

Osteopathic and Chiropractic
Techniques for Manual Therapists
A Comprehensive Guide to Spinal and
Peripheral Manipulations
Jimmy Michael, Giles Gyer and Ricky Davis
ISBN 978 1 84819 326 0
eISBN 978 0 85701 281 4

The Five Osteopathic Models
Rationale, Application, Integration – From an
Evidence-Based to a Person-Centered Osteopathy
Ray Hruby, Paolo Tozzi, Christian
Lunghi and Giampiero Fusco
ISBN 978 1 90914 168 1
eISBN 978 1 90914 169 8

BALANCED LIGAMENTOUS TENSION IN OSTEOPATHIC PRACTICE

Susan Turner

Forewords by Renzo Molinari and Rachel Brooks

Illustrated by Heloise Niamh O'Donoghue

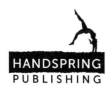

HANDSPRING
PUBLISHING

First published in Great Britain in 2024 by Handspring Publishing, an imprint of Jessica Kingsley Publishers
Part of John Murray Press

1

A CIP catalogue record for this title is available from the British Library and the Library of Congress

ISBN 978 1 91342 639 2
eISBN 978 1 83997 628 5

Printed and bound in Great Britain by CPI Group

Jessica Kingsley Publishers' policy is to use papers that are natural, renewable and recyclable
products and made from wood grown in sustainable forests. The logging and manufacturing
processes are expected to conform to the environmental regulations of the country of origin.

Handspring Publishing
Carmelite House
50 Victoria Embankment
London EC4Y 0DZ

www.handspringpublishing.com

John Murray Press
Part of Hodder & Stoughton Limited
An Hachette UK Company

'No force that can safely be brought to bear upon the living human body is as powerful for the correction of strains of the skeletal machinery as the forces and powers within the patient's mechanisms.'

W.G. Sutherland DO

The therapeutic approach described in this book originates in what W.G. Sutherland DO learned as a student from osteopathy's founder, Dr Andrew Taylor Still. Dr Sutherland practised this all his life, alongside his better known work on the development of cranial osteopathy. His close friend and student Anne Wales DO, in turn, instructed the author and contributors. They have been teaching this approach for nearly three decades, both in the UK and internationally, and also training other teaching faculties to pass on this important part of the osteopathic legacy. The BLT principle has immense clinical value, guiding the practitioner to engage with great precision the innate healing potential within the living body as a whole. All the procedures described in this book work from the perspective of creating the environment where the inherent forces of health can come to bear most effectively.

Contents

THERAPEUTIC ENGAGEMENT

Foreword by Renzo Molinari

I feel humbled and privileged to have been asked to introduce Susan Turner's book covering the Balanced Ligamentous Tension approach. The word 'approach' is used intentionally as BLT represents a lot more than techniques.

Stephen Paulus DO gave a clear explanation: 'The Osteopathic approach to healthcare is not based upon performing sequential manipulative techniques, but in expressing the philosophy of Osteopathy in a clinical context' ('Core principles of Osteopathy'; *IJOM*, 5th November 2012). This book is the exact expression of this statement. BLT presents the real meaning of our art and science: the body's structure is the medium through which osteopaths engage and access the Intelligent Organisation and Inner Intelligence of the human system as a whole. Both the manual contact and the presence of the practitioner facilitate the expression of the inherent Potency of the patient's body. William Garner Sutherland wrote that this Intelligence with a capital 'I' is at work within the human system and of all life.

When I first met Sue Turner in the 1980s, I already had some experience of indirect approaches as taught by some French osteopaths in the late 1970s. As described in the writings of H.V. Hoover and W.G. Sutherland, the application of these techniques took pulmonary breathing into account. As stated by Hoover, 'A given lesion occurs at a certain point in the respiratory cycle and in a certain position' ('The use of respiratory movements as an aide in the correction of osteopathic spinal lesions'; *AOA Journal 45*, N3, 1945).

It was through meeting Sue that I came across the teachings of Anne Wales DO and her ideas on Osteopathic Dynamics, as described in an early article, 'Osteopathic Dynamics' (*AAO Yearbook*, 1946), where she referred to the necessity for the practitioner to take into account 'the analysis of the dynamic aspects of the living organism'. The integration of Sutherland's teachings brought another dimension to osteopathy for me, as does the principle of BLT, described here by Sue and her contributors.

Sue is a precious person in our profession. She is a living embodiment of osteopathy, not only for her extraordinary contribution to the teaching of undergraduate and postgraduate students, her dedication to her patients and to the principles and philosophy of osteopathy, but also for the human qualities she has developed and which she transmits. I firmly believe that every practitioner who wants to help patients to find their way to optimal health should develop these indispensable qualities; the first was already highlighted by Andrew Taylor Still:

Humility: we are dealing with a multidimensional patient of immense complexity and it is presumptuous to believe we can completely understand this level of complexity.

Empathetic Awareness as described by Anthony Chila DO.

Non-judgemental Presence that allows the patient to establish a real treatment partnership with the practitioner.

These qualities in a practitioner, if real and sincere, will allow the patient in treatment to switch from the predominance of an overactive neocortical brain mode to a more archaic brain activity that engages the self-regulating and healing factors. Thomas Dummer DO, founder of the European School of Osteopathy, often emphasised in his lectures that techniques are not as important as the way you are when you are applying them.

This book is important as it not only presents every technique and how to apply it with precision and detail, but most importantly, it is really a legacy offered by Sue Turner and her contributors to future generations of osteopaths; enabling them to be in direct contact with the original lineage of the BLT approach, through the philosophy and the extraordinary understanding of the human being, developed by William G. Sutherland and Anne Wales.

This book comes at a turning point in our history: osteopathy is expanding very quickly and progresses towards recognition and regulation in many countries. It is crucially important that the historical and traditional approaches are kept intact and pure, so that the founding principles and initial philosophy will remain the core of osteopathy.

Professor Renzo Molinari DO
FESO MROF GOsC (UK)
Principal of the Molinari Institute of Health (UK)

Foreword by Rachel Brooks

I have been eagerly awaiting this book since Sue Turner first spoke to me about the project in 2017 when we were both teaching at a conference dedicated to the teachings of Anne Wales DO. Having known and respected Sue as a colleague for almost 30 years, I wholeheartedly encouraged her to proceed with the project as I knew her to be quite qualified to take on the task. Now, today, I remain eager to have this book available for many reasons, including:

- Balanced ligamentous tension (BLT) is a very valuable osteopathic treatment approach.
- It is both important and exciting to have an additional vehicle that preserves the teachings of Dr Anne Wales.
- This work by Sue Turner and her collaborators shares their insightful perspectives on using BLT, having taught this approach for many years in many countries.

BLT is a great osteopathic treatment approach, in part, because even a beginning practitioner can achieve good and helpful results using it. Then as one's skills develop, BLT treatment becomes even more effective with the potential to have at times quite profound results for the person being treated. Even the most experienced practitioner using BLT will find it an avenue into a continually deepening understanding of health, healing and osteopathy.

Dr Wales dedicated a great deal of her many decades of teaching to passing on with precision the BLT approach for treating the body that Dr Sutherland had taught her. And many of those who studied with Anne have been dedicated to passing on with precision the BLT approach they learned from her. Osteopathy has a long tradition of being passed on from hand to hand, and this lineage is vital to both the individual practitioner and the osteopathic profession as a whole. Sadly, all too often and quickly, the wisdom and skills of great practitioners fade from practice once they pass from view. It takes a deliberate effort to keep the work of those who have gone before us alive. I am so grateful to Sue Turner for taking on the challenge of passing on the teaching that Anne Wales chose to pass on to her.

Regarding this passing on of teachings from our osteopathic elders, an interesting reality became apparent at that 2017 conference dedicated to Dr Anne Wales. The conference was presented by the Sutherland Cranial Teaching Foundation and there were probably 15 or more of us who were presenting there. Every one of us teaching there had the privilege of having been engaged in a meaningful relationship with Anne. Before the conference began, the faculty gathered so each of us could share with the others the techniques we had chosen to present and demonstrate how we would have the participants perform them at the treatment tables.

As each faculty member began to show how they had learned their BLT technique from Anne, it quickly became clear that there was far more variation in 'what we had learned from Anne' than any of us expected. There was some consternation about these discrepancies, but in the end, to me, it revealed a truth about how any teaching is naturally modified as it is passed down through a lineage. It seemed several factors contributed to the inconsistency we observed. One factor was that Anne did indeed teach different approaches to the same technique; another factor was the variability in what we *remembered* about what Anne had taught us 12 to 30 years before; and maybe most importantly, there was how we each, as individuals, carried forward what she had taught us.

Anne taught what she knew freely with the wish that the work she had received from Dr Sutherland would be passed on to those that would follow her. Many practitioners who studied with her lived in or near New England and had the opportunity to study with her over a long period of time. Gratefully, I was able to spend ten years studying with Anne, while others were with her for many more years than that. Sue Turner, along with her colleagues from England, had more limited time with her, but Anne was keen for them to receive her teaching and carry it on. In the 1990s she instructed them to take what she was teaching them and go and work it out for themselves. And that is what they did.

The information in *Balanced Ligamentous Tension in Osteopathic Practice* comes from knowledge and experience gained in teaching BLT courses for nearly 30 years in 15 countries. My congratulations and thanks go to Sue Turner, Kok Weng Lim, Zenna Zwierzchowska and Lynn Haller for sharing their work.

Rachel Brooks MD
Editor of Three Great Teachers of
Osteopathy: Lessons We Learned from
Drs Becker, Fulford, and Wales

Acknowledgements

This book is written in deep gratitude to Anne Wales DO for the enormous generosity of all she has shared, which has enriched both the professional and personal lives of all of us who have had the pleasure of learning from her.

I also wish to heartily thank all those osteopathic colleagues who have given their encouragement and support through their insightful feedback and discussion of the text, especially Eva Mockel, Hugh Ettlinger and Rachel Brooks, and also Mary Monro, Donald Hankinson, Taj Deoora, Flurina Thali and Jessica Busen Smith.

Deep appreciation also to Katharina Hoffmann, Fesih Alpagu, Richard Eayrs and Ian Sadler for their work on the videos and photography and to Claudia Knox, Christoph Hasse, Jessica Busen Smith and Vijay Netto for generously giving of their time to act as models; special thanks also to Heloise O'Donoghue for her diligence in undertaking the anatomical illustrations.

Thanks also to Professor Frank Willard, Professor Jane Carreiro DO and Graham Scarr, both for their thought-provoking influence on our understanding and for permission to use pictures from their collections.

I wish to thank Gabriella Colangelo for sharing the hospitality of her home as an inspiring writing retreat. Thanks to Jason Haxton, Christine Gran and Anna Gruhlherr of the Kirksville Museum of Osteopathic Medicine and also to John Lewis for their help in finding source material pertaining to A.T. Still.

A debt of gratitude also to all the colleagues and students who have inspired our understanding with their spirit of enquiry. Among these are our fellow teachers of the Sutherland Cranial College of Osteopathy, the European School of Osteopathy, Fondazione di Osteopatia Pediatrica, Italy and the confraternity of the Andrew Still Sutherland Study Group, USA. Special appreciation also to Orianne Evans and Ana Bennett for the fruitful exchanges of our study meetings. A special acknowledgement is due to our beloved colleagues Piers Chandler and Christian Chemin, who played an essential part in the development of our courses through all they wholeheartedly gave before they died in 2021 and 2022.

Gratitude to Rachel Brooks for the gift she has given to all of us exploring W.G. Sutherland's approach by publishing the books of Rollin Becker DO, *Life in Motion* and *The Stillness of Life*, which are an endless source of inspiration. Likewise, her work with Anne Wales DO to assist in the editing of Sutherland's *Contributions of Thought* and *Teachings in the Science of Osteopathy* has provided an invaluable resource.

Thanks to Mary Law and Katie Forsythe from Handspring/JKP for their patience and positive support through the stages of writing and publication of this book.

And last but not least, heartfelt thanks to my co-authors, Kok Weng Lim, Zenna Zwierzchowska and Lynn Haller for their generosity of spirit and dedicated work towards this publication and the journey of shared discovery we have travelled together over many years.

About the Author and Contributors

SUSAN TURNER MA, DO, PGCE, FSCCO, POD

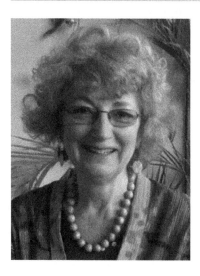

Sue Turner has been practising osteopathy since graduating from the European School of Osteopathy (ESO) in 1979, where she also taught for 26 years. Her special interest has always been in the osteopathic approach of W.G. Sutherland which led her to explore and teach cranial and paediatric osteopathy and to study Balanced Ligamentous Tension with Anne Wales DO in the late 1980s and 1990s. Since that time, she has taught in 16 countries, helping to establish a BLT teaching faculty in the UK, Germany, Italy and Spain.

She is a founder member and fellow of the Sutherland Cranial College and was also part of the founding team of the Osteopathic Centre for Children (OCC) UK. She is on the faculty of the Associazione OCC, Italy and the Molinari Institute of Health. She pioneered osteopathic education in Russia through the international faculty of the ESO between 1998 and 2012 and contributed to the *Textbook of Paediatric Osteopathy* (Mockel and Mitha 2008).

The sharing of what she has learned from her teachers, colleagues, patients and students remains an important part of her professional life.

LYNN HALLER BA, DO, POD, FSCCO

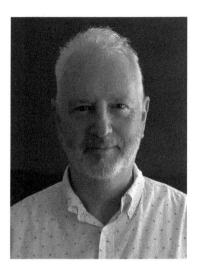

Lynn Haller graduated from the European School of Osteopathy (ESO) in 1987. In his osteopathic practice in North London, he treats patients with a wide variety of conditions and his special interest is in paediatric osteopathy in which he holds a postgraduate diploma. He worked, for 17 years, in a multidisciplinary obstetric team attached to the birth unit at St John and Elizabeth's Hospital in London, in the prenatal and postnatal osteopathic care of mother and baby.

Through the SCTF he benefitted from the teaching of Drs Rollin Becker and John Harakal and especially Dr Anne Wales. He has been a teaching fellow of the Sutherland Cranial College of Osteopathy (SCCO) for 30 years and has taught osteopathic medicine, paediatric osteopathy and BLT in the UK, Germany, Sweden, Ireland, Italy, Poland and Spain.

KOK WENG LIM DO, MSC(OST), FSCCO

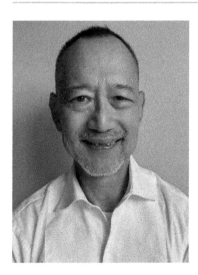

Kok Weng Lim is a graduate of the British School of Osteopathy (BSO) and also the European School of Osteopathy (ESO) and the University of Greenwich where he completed his postgraduate training. He has a special interest in paediatric osteopathy and has co-authored two books on paediatric osteopathy and published a paper on infantile colic.

He has worked and taught at the Osteopathic Centre for Children since its inception in 1991. He is on the faculty of various osteopathic educational institutions both in the UK and in Europe, including the international faculty at the ESO, the Sutherland Cranial College of Osteopathy (SCCO), Wiener Schule für Osteopathie, Barcelona School of Osteopathy, Panta Rhei in the Netherlands and osteopathic institutions in St Petersburg and Moscow. For the past eight years he has also worked in a hospital neonatal unit in London, providing osteopathic care.

ZENNA ZWIERZCHOWSKA MA, DO, FSCCO

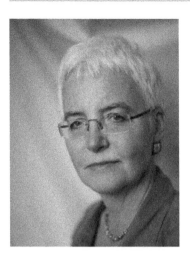

Zenna has been in osteopathic practice in North London, treating patients of all ages, since graduating from the European School of Osteopathy (ESO) in 1985. Through the Sutherland Cranial Teaching Foundation (SCTF), the most significant influence on her osteopathic work has come from Dr Anne Wales, but also Dr Robert Fulford and Dr Rollin Becker. She is a longstanding and committed faculty member of the Sutherland Cranial College of Osteopathy (SCCO) and has pioneered the teaching of Dr Sutherland's approach to the body as a whole (BLT) in the UK, Germany, Sweden, France, Poland, Italy and Spain.

Abbreviations

AAO American Academy of Osteopathy

AIIS Anterior inferior iliac spine

ALSL Anterior longitudinal spinal ligament

A/P Antero-posterior

ASIS Anterior superior iliac spine

ASO American School of Osteopathy, Kirksville, Missouri

ASS fulcrum Automatic shifting suspension (Sutherland) fulcrum

BLT Balanced ligamentous tension

BMT Balanced membranous tension

BSO British School of Osteopathy (now UCO)

COT *Contributions of Thought* by W.G. Sutherland (1961/1998), A.L. Wales and A.S. Sutherland (eds), Sutherland Cranial Teaching Foundation

CPG Control pattern generator

CV4 Compression of the 4th ventricle, a cranial technique of W.G. Sutherland

ECM Extracellular matrix

ESO European School of Osteopathy

GALT Gastrointestinal-associated lymphatic tissue

GERD Gastro-oesophageal reflux

GIT Gastrointestinal tract

IBD Inflammatory bowel disease

IoM Interosseous membrane

LC Longus colli

LIM *Life in Motion* by Rollin Becker (1997), R.E. Brooks (ed.), Stillness Press

LS Lumbo-sacral

MALT Mucosa-associated lymphatic tissue

OA Occipito-atlantal

OCA Osteopathic Cranial Academy, USA

PCL Posterior cruciate ligament

PLSL Posterior longitudinal spinal ligament

PRM Primary respiratory mechanism

PSIS Posterior superior iliac spine

PTF Pretracheal fascia

PVF Prevertebral fascia

RTM Reciprocal tension membrane

SCCO Sutherland Cranial College of Osteopathy, UK, Germany and Spain

SCTF Sutherland Cranial Teaching Foundation, USA and Australia

SI Sacroiliac

SOL *The Stillness of Life* by Rollin Becker (2000), R.E. Brooks (ed.), Stillness Press

TLF Thoracolumbar fascia

TSO *Teachings in the Science of Osteopathy* by W.G. Sutherland (1990), A.L. Wales (ed.), Sutherland Cranial Teaching Foundation

UCO University College of Osteopathy

ZO Zona orbicularis of hip joint

Clarification of Some Key Terms

W.G. SUTHERLAND'S HYPOTHESIS OF THE CRANIOSACRAL MECHANISM

This is also referred to as the 'involuntary' or 'primary respiratory' mechanism (PRM). Sutherland described an inherent biphasic rhythmic motion of the central nervous system and fluctuation of the cerebrospinal fluid (Jiang-Xie *et al.* 2024), together with a very fine degree of motion of the cranial bones, sacrum and intracranial and intraspinal dural membranes.

This motion is considered primary, in contrast to the response of these tissues to thoracic respiration, and so is referred to as the 'primary respiratory mechanism'. As with thoracic respiration, primary respiration exhibits inhalation and exhalation phases. Total body shape change occurs during primary inhalation with axial shortening and widening, and during primary exhalation with lengthening and narrowing. Additionally, during the inhalation and exhalation phases, the midline bones of the cranium and sacrum rotate around transverse axes into flexion and extension respectively. During primary inhalation and exhalation all paired bones and structures also externally and internally rotate respectively.

Reading these shape changes under the hands is an important component of osteopathic diagnosis. Sutherland's ideas may be extended to include all fascias and connective tissues, not just dura. Also included is the entire nervous system, not just the central nervous system, and similarly, all interstitial fluids outside of the cranium. There is also a bioelectrical field component to this model.

THE TIDE

Sutherland originally used this term to describe the inherent fluctuation of the cerebrospinal fluid, likening its quality to the ebb and flow of the tide of the ocean.

The Tide describes a biphasic palpatory sense of potency (or energy) expressing longitudinally through the midline, three-dimensionally and bilaterally through the limbs and paired structures of the body. The quality of the fluctuation of the Tide can be included implicitly in the diagnosis of balanced tension (see Chapter 1 for more details on the point of balanced tension). The potency in the Tide can also be directed to specific structures in treatment.

The term 'Tide' has also come to refer more widely to an expression of primary respiration, not only within the living body, but also throughout the natural world.

RECIPROCAL TENSION MEMBRANE (RTM)

This term describes a function of the falx cerebri and tentorium cerebelli around the straight sinus, and came to include the spinal dura with its sacral attachment. The 'three sickles' of the falx and tentorium attach to all the bones of the neurocranium and are under constant and equally distributed 'reciprocal tension'. This means that if any one of the RTM's osseous attachments from cranium to sacrum is fixed, or either intraosseously or suturally strained, every other part of the dural continuum will be affected.

The cranial bones develop within an embryological mesenchymal 'sac', of which the falx cerebri, tentorium cerebelli and falx cerebelli are the infoldings. This means that the cranial bones move reciprocally with the primary respiratory motion of the RTM. Balanced membranous tension (BMT) engages the same principle for resolving cranial strains as BLT for the joints of the body, albeit on a finer scale.

THE SUTHERLAND FULCRUM

This describes an 'automatic shifting suspension fulcrum' functionally located towards the anterior end of the straight (cranial venous) sinus, where the falx cerebri adjoins the tentorium cerebelli. Sutherland so emphasised its importance that his students persuaded him to call it the 'Sutherland' fulcrum.

This is seen as the functional area around which the involuntary biphasic motion of the cranial and spinal dural continuum (RTM) operates. Including the wider field, it acts as a fulcrum for the expression of primary respiratory motion through the whole connective tissue matrix of the body. Referring to this, Dr Anne Wales likened the body to 'a mobile on a fulcrum'.

This *suspension fulcrum* is at a point of balanced tension for the reciprocal tension membrane poised *between* the longitudinal falx cerebri and bilateral tentorium cerebelli. Its location *automatically shifts* slightly on the straight sinus with each rhythmic shape change of the RTM in flexion (widening) and extension (narrowing).

In 1989, a group of British osteopaths spent a week at Bar Harbor in Maine, USA with the members of Dr Wales' study group. We were invited to visit the dissection lab of Professor Frank Willard at the University of New England, College of Osteopathic Medicine. The supraocciput of one of the cadavers had been removed, making it possible to rhythmically move the area of the Sutherland fulcrum by placing a finger under the anterior end of the straight sinus. Those present were amazed to feel the sacrum and whole body, including the periphery, moving in synchrony with this induced movement of the fulcrum. This confirmed to us what a strategic place this indeed is in the organisation of the entire body.

NUT AND BOLT

The analogy of the relationship between a nut and bolt is referred to frequently in the text. In normal use, a nut is turned around a bolt. In many of the procedures described in this book, however, this is reversed, so that the operator holds the bolt while the patient turns the nut. Here the often peripheral part, e.g., the limb, is held steady while the patient turns the proximal part or trunk.

Examples of this are seen in the standing iliosacral and seated hip and rib procedures.

This is in contrast to more familiar osteopathic approaches where the central part, e.g., the trunk, is stabilised by the patient supine on the table, while the operator moves the limbs, ribs or ilia. This is also seen in the lateral disengagement of the ribs, ilia and hip as described in the text.

REFERENCE

Jiang-Xie, L.F., Drieu, A., Bhasiin, K. *et al.* (2024) Neuronal dynamics direct cerebrospinal fluid perfusion and brain clearance. *Nature* 627, 157–164.

Some Key Figures in Osteopathic History Referred to in the Text

ROLLIN BECKER (1910–1996)

Rollin Becker DO was immersed in osteopathy from an early age, as his father, Arthur Becker DO, was a dedicated osteopath and served on Dr Still's faculty at the American School of Osteopathy (ASO). He and his younger brother, Alan, both studied with Dr Sutherland and became members of his cranial faculty. Rollin Becker, like Anne Wales, had a close relationship with William Sutherland and was greatly respected for the depth of his wisdom and his understanding of this work.

VIRGIL HALLADAY (DATES UNKNOWN)

Virgil Halladay DO was professor of anatomy at the ASO in Kirksville and the Des Moines Still College of Osteopathy. He is the author of *Applied Anatomy of the Spine.* This was based on his own laboratory dissections and presented a dynamic view of functional anatomy from the point of view of the osteopathic physician. In his lectures and demonstrations of applied anatomy and osteopathic technique, he used his own dissection models of the spine, ribcage and pelvis which left only the skeleton, discs and ligaments in situ. The ligaments and discs had been preserved in a way that would maintain their flexibility, enabling him to illustrate the movements of the spine and pelvis. His exhibit at the American Osteopathic Association Convention of 1919 greatly impressed William Sutherland. Sutherland's handling of the exhibit confirmed his earlier experience of the importance of the ligaments in articular function. The understanding he gained changed his views on pelvic diagnosis and inspired him to devise some of the pelvic techniques described in Chapter 3.

JOHN MARTIN LITTLEJOHN (1865–1947)

Dr J.M. Littlejohn was born in Glasgow, the son of a presbyterian minister. He was ordained in 1886, studied Law and Medicine at Glasgow University and, after attending Columbia University in New York, became president of Amity College in Iowa in 1895. Having always had a weak constitution, in 1895 he was treated by Dr Still who successfully resolved his recurrent neck haemorrhages. He joined the ASO in 1898 as both a student and lecturer where he taught William Sutherland physiology. He went on to found the American School of Osteopathy in Chicago in 1900, returning to London in 1914. There he opened an osteopathic practice, treating people traumatised by the First World War. He founded the British School of Osteopathy (BSO) in 1917. His student, John Wernham, continued to teach his approach until his passing and it is still taught by the Institute of Classical Osteopathy, UK.

ANDREW TAYLOR STILL (1828–1917)

Dr A.T. Still, the founder of osteopathy, grew up in a settler family and was the son of a Methodist preacher. In his youth he lived with, and learned the language of, the Shaunee people with whom his father worked as a missionary. He worked as an army surgeon in the American Civil War, and his later search for a drugless approach to medicine was driven by a deep personal tragedy when all but one of his children died of spinal meningitis. His explorations and yearning to help humanity led him, in 1874, to 'become aware of the science of osteopathy' and obtain extraordinary results in the treatment of his patients.

He founded the ASO in 1892. As the reputation of osteopathy grew, the school also grew enormously (especially after 1900) from a two-room building with a student body of 5 women and 16 men. Fortunately for William Sutherland who trained there from 1898 to 1900, Dr Still was still closely supervising the classes and guiding his students at that time.

WILLIAM GARNER SUTHERLAND (1873–1954)

William Sutherland DO attended the American School of Osteopathy between 1898 and 1900, where, through Dr Still, he was inspired to begin a lifetime's exploration of the cranium and the self-correcting powers within the living body. Although he was exploring the cranial concept from his student days onwards, he did not begin teaching formal training courses in cranial osteopathy until after 1944. The principles applied in BLT formed the basis for treating the finer membranous-articular mechanism of the cranium.

Introduction

SUSAN TURNER

HOW THIS BOOK CAME TO BE

Dr Anne Wales first came to my awareness in 1981 at the British School of Osteopathy (BSO) postgraduate Sutherland Cranial Teaching Foundation (SCTF) course in osteopathy in the cranial field. I was struck then by the warmth, empathy and respect she expressed for the very young in her lecture on treating children. Her advice was to 'give them a chance to take a good look at you before you treat them so that they can make up their minds about you'.

In 1988 I had the pleasure of being introduced by James Jealous DO to Dr Wales' study group which was then in its third year. I was again impressed with the way she constantly related the anatomy under her hands to physiology and her thought-provoking one-liners such as: 'Unwellness is an undesirable change of space. Our aim is to change the geometry of the space; spaces large and small', or 'The pelvis can be seen as the centre of a tripod with the third leg turned upwards as the spine'.

It had long been a mystery to me as to why, at least in Britain, there was no guidance or awareness of Sutherland's treatment principles as applied to the body, while his work on the cranium was being so widely taught. Over the years since 1988 I had seen Dr Anne Wales demonstrate his 'general approach' and experienced directly its beneficial results under her hands. When asked, she confirmed that we were indeed missing an important part of his teaching. She related how in 1947, at a meeting with his students who were ever eager to do more study of the cranium, Dr Sutherland told them that they had done enough on the head for the time being. He was going to use that seminar to show them how he had 'been working since 1900' on completing his Kirksville training with Dr A.T. Still. He told them that he did not want them to become so centred on the head that they forgot the rest of the body. He felt that they were in danger of becoming the inverse of the rest of the osteopathic profession at the time, who treated the body as if it had no head. He stressed that the cranial concept is osteopathy and nothing more (Wales 1996). That seminar was transcribed and photographed by Howard Lippincott DO and is reproduced in the appendix to *Teachings in the Science of Osteopathy* (Sutherland 1990) and the American Academy of Osteopathy (AAO) 1949 Year Book.

When I asked if she could recommend a member of her study group to lead a course on Sutherland's 'general approach', Dr Wales suggested that I could gather up a few people to spend time with her and she would prepare us to teach it ourselves. 'Come over with a video recorder,' she said. 'It will take me five days to unload.' In 1995, at her invitation, a small group of British osteopaths who were then teaching at the European School of Osteopathy (ESO) and the Sutherland

Cranial College of Osteopathy (SCCO) visited her home in Massachusetts, armed with a video recorder, for five days of intensive teaching. The agreement was that we would do our best to pass on what she was sharing with us. This led to further five-day sessions, visits, phone calls and correspondence over the following years, until her passing in 2005 at the age of 101.

Those first sessions began when she was in her 90s, but her energy seemed boundless, exceeding that of us 'youngsters'. Although she described our gathering as 'a social occasion', she would teach us for seven hours with only one short break. Her infectious passion for the work, and the clarity, precision and openness with which she taught, made learning with her a true pleasure. We were aware of how great a privilege it was that she was so generously sharing her knowledge, born of 70 years' immersion in osteopathy. She and her husband, Chester Handy, had been committed students and close friends of Will Sutherland. He, in turn, had been a dedicated student of Dr Andrew Taylor Still, osteopathy's founder. The principles that she was imparting to us had been passed from hand to hand directly from the primary source.

In the 28 years that have followed, members of our group have taught four- and five-day courses in Sutherland's 'general approach' in 15 countries, and annually through the SCCO in the UK and Germany. Where possible, we work with a ratio of one tutor to four students to create the best conditions for embodying the necessary perceptual and manual skills. Since the mid-1990s this has also been part of the undergraduate curriculum of the ESO. Over these years of teaching and practice we have been gradually developing an understanding of what appears to help or hinder learning and effectiveness in treatment. We have learned from each other, from our students and from our patients, and this learning ever continues.

It may appear, on first view, that this is a manual of techniques. We do describe techniques, but the main purpose of this book is the exploration of the principle whereby the body's inherent therapeutic potency can be engaged through balanced tension in the ligamentous-articular, membranous-articular or fascial mechanisms. Individual 'techniques' are simply handholds that are adapted to the unique anatomy and applied physiology of individual areas. The same principle of engaging the 'forces and powers within the patient's mechanisms' is applied throughout. It is hoped that the reader will enjoy making discoveries beyond what is described here, through reading the language of the tissues and discerning what is required to meet and match the therapeutic potential within them.

Dr Wales emphasised that every treatment is an exploration into the unknown. No two patients are ever the same, nor are two sessions the same in any one patient. While precision and accuracy are essential, moment-to-moment guidance comes from the living response in the tissues under our hands.

THE LIFE OF ANNE WALES (1904–2005)

Anne Wales was born in Rhode Island, USA and began her osteopathic training at the American School of Osteopathy (ASO) in Kirksville in 1922, completing it at the Kansas City School in 1926. In her internship she worked in maternity with mothers and infants and, among other conditions, she treated pneumonia with osteopathy before the discovery of antibiotics or vitamin C. In 1933 she spearheaded the founding of the Osteopathic Hospital in Rhode Island, which the community wholeheartedly supported with time and donations despite the financial hardships of the great depression.

In 1942, Drs Anne Wales and Chester Handy

attended a lecture by William Sutherland DO on Osteopathy in the Cranial Field. Although she already had 20 years of osteopathic experience, what he had to say made her 'head spin'. They both decided that this was the work to which they wanted to dedicate their lives.

In 1943 they attended Dr Sutherland's first course, out of which he developed his teaching programme with Anne and Chester as active members of his faculty. They also assisted in laying the foundations for the Osteopathic Cranial Academy (OCA) and the Sutherland Cranial Teaching Foundation (SCTF) which continue to offer courses to this day.

In 1952 Drs Wales and Handy established a free osteopathic clinic for disabled children and their siblings in Providence, Rhode Island, which ran until 1964. Dr Wales was also instrumental in starting a nursery school for children with learning difficulties and worked at the state level to develop legislative guidelines to support the care of children with congenital disorders. This led to the funding and establishment of three schools for disabled and Deaf children in Rhode Island.

Dr Will Sutherland and his wife, Adah, were close friends of Anne and Chester and enjoyed holidays together, sharing ideas and discoveries. After Will's passing in 1954, Anne worked with Adah to collect his works, completing their task in the early 1960s. Their manuscript eventually became the book *Contributions of Thought* (1967 and 1998), a compilation of Sutherland's ideas and clinical experiences from 1914 to 1954. In her late 80s she edited *Teachings in the Science of Osteopathy* (1990). This book was based upon Sutherland's recorded lectures from 1949 to 1951, which she managed to rescue only just in time, as the tapes were deteriorating and becoming unintelligible. She also published many articles and papers in the *Journal of the Osteopathic Cranial Association* (JOCA) and in the *Journal of the American Osteopathic Association.* She received many honours during her life for her contributions to the osteopathic profession.

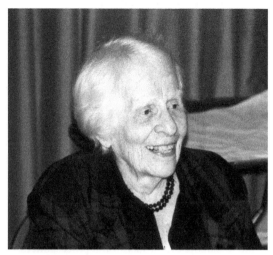

Anne Wales DO.
Used with permission of Michael Burruano DO.

Dr Wales made her first attempt to retire in 1981 at the age of 77. However, the last two decades of her life became very full as she became engaged with teaching the new colleagues and students who sought her out, many of whom became her friends. During this period, she directed the Andrew Still-Sutherland Study Group and taught both in America and Europe. She insisted that, as she was retired, she would only treat students, colleagues, family and friends. This still kept her very busy! She retained her youthful spirit until her departure at the age of 101. What she has given to the development of osteopathy and to making available the teachings of Drs Still and Sutherland is immeasurable.

With thanks to Michael Burruano DO
and Jane Carreiro DO for their
contribution to this biography.

HISTORY OF BLT

'The technique he presented to us is a reflection of the clear vision of our founder.'

(Lippincott 1949)

W.G. Sutherland is best known for his development of osteopathy in the cranial field, following encouragement from his teacher and osteopathy's founder, A.T. Still, to 'dig on' in his study of the cranium (Speece *et al.* 2009, p. 12). His application of Still's principles to the rest of the body is less widely known, but it is an essential part of the osteopathic heritage and is also key to understanding the whole-body context of cranial osteopathy. This book aims to make this approach more accessible to osteopathic students and practitioners.

The following excerpt from *Contributions of Thought* describes a fundamental principle which W.G. Sutherland learned as a student under the hands of A.T. Still, when he had a surprising experience of the body's self-correcting mechanism at work.

'In technique we endeavour to follow Dr Still's methods. That is getting to the point of release with no jerking and then allowing the natural agencies to return the bones to their normal relations and positions.'

What are the natural agencies? The ligaments, not the muscles are the natural agencies for the purpose of correcting the relations and positions of joints.

Dr Still's application of the technique is the gentle exaggeration of the lesion that allows the natural agencies to draw the bones into place.

Dr Still has taken my hand into his and allowed me to feel the lesion as it was being exaggerated and then as the natural agencies pulled the bones into place.

There is reason for applying that technique in the cranial mechanism. The difference between spinal technique and cranial technique is like the difference between an automobile mechanic and watchmaker.

We do not force anything into place in the reduction of a lesion. We have something more potent than our own forces working always in the patient towards the normal.

What are the natural agencies in the cranium? The brain, the cerebrospinal fluid and the reciprocal tension membrane.' (Sutherland 1998, COT p. 160)

The many points for consideration in this passage are explored below.

'The gentle exaggeration of the lesion'

We have here an image of young Will Sutherland at work in the student clinic, with his hands perhaps around the knee joint of a seated patient. Along comes Dr Still and places his large hands over those of his student who experiences, with astonishment, an innate self-correcting potency within the articular structure. That seminal moment, no doubt, influenced the course of his life's professional journey. Out of this simple principle of 'the gentle exaggeration of the lesion' to a point where all the forces acting on the joint are held in a neutral, but potent, state of equally balanced tension, he later came to realise that the same indirect action, on a finer scale, was as effective in the resolution of membranous-articular strains within the cranium.

The ligaments, not the muscles, as 'natural agencies' of self-correction

Another aspect of his surprise was an awareness that in the 'musculoskeletal system' it is actually the ligaments that are the dynamic agencies of correction of the joints rather than the muscles. He surmised that this self-correcting mechanism must be of an *involuntary nature*, i.e., independent of the voluntary control enacted by the neuromusculoskeletal system.

'Ligamentous-articular mechanisms' and 'membranous-articular mechanisms'

Realising that 'the ligaments...are the natural agencies for correcting the relations and positions of joints', he came to refer to the gross joints of the body as '*ligamentous*-articular mechanisms', and the fine sutures of the cranium as '*membranous*-articular mechanisms'. By placing the words 'ligamentous' and 'membranous' before 'articular' in each case, Sutherland was emphasising that, to his perception, the ligaments and membranes were *primary* and the bones functionally secondary in the organisation of the joints.

In 'balanced ligamentous tension', an injured joint is held and the ligaments guided to a place of equally balanced tension from which the correction can then unfold. In a similar way but on a different scale, 'balanced membranous tension' (BMT) uses the dural membrane for the correction of osseous strains of the cranium and sacrum.

In 1919, after 19 years in practice, Sutherland's sense of the key role of the ligaments was confirmed at the AOA Convention in Chicago. Here, he had the opportunity to handle Virgil Halladay's seated dissection of the spine, pelvis and ribcage which left only the bones and ligaments in situ. The ligaments had been treated so as to keep them pliable, enabling Sutherland to manually explore their relationship to articular movement. Through this he was inspired to revise his ideas on pelvic diagnosis and devise several of the pelvic techniques described in Chapter 3 (Sutherland 1998, COT p. 132).

BLT as a therapeutic principle

The corrective procedure using 'the gentle exaggeration of the lesion' involves enabling the ligaments to find a position of *equally balanced tension* around the *displaced* fulcrum of the strained joint. In the words of Anne Wales, 'If we position the bones so that the ligaments are relieved of the strain then the bones can move spontaneously back to their correct position. Astonishing!' (Wales 1978).

'We have something more potent than our own forces working always in the patient towards the normal'

Rollin Becker DO emphasised the importance of listening deeply to body physiology and allowing it to teach us to develop a sense of knowing touch:

> 'Dr Still and Dr Sutherland were students. They spent their entire lives studying the science of osteopathy. They consented to be used by the fundamental laws that are within each body physiology. They learned to know and use the rules of health as they apply within us, and it is these rules of health that are sought in any dysfunction, disease or trauma for which the patient is seeking service. Dr Still and Dr Sutherland studied every single mechanism within body physiology as it applied to a given patient, and they were taught by each individual case, the appropriate diagnostic and treatment programme. They were taught by that which the body itself was trying to do.' (Becker 2001, LIM)

This way of working necessitates becoming receptive to the wisdom of the inner teacher-physician within the living mechanism of the patient.

Historical background of 'Indirect' or 'Exaggeration' technique

'In technique we endeavour to follow Dr Still's methods. That is, getting to the point of release with no jerking and then allowing the natural agencies to return the bones to their normal relations and positions.'

In the mind of the public, osteopathy is associated with high velocity low amplitude thrust technique (HVT or HVLA) for realignment of articular strains. From the accounts of his students, it appears that Dr Still used HVLA rather rarely. There are strong indications that the balanced tension approach taught by W.G. Sutherland applies the same principles as those practised by A.T. Still, and also that this preceded HVLA. This is reflected in the following anecdotes and written records below:

'At a course given by the Dallas Osteopathic Study Group in the late 1980s, Brian Knight DO recalled the delight of his elderly male patient at being treated with ligamentous articular strain technique, as this was the same way as he had been treated by A.T. Still as a young man.' (Speece *et al.* 2009, p. 11)

'Dr Jenny Chase DO who was a student of A.T. Still, graduating in 1912, was interviewed in 1980 by Gerry Dickey DO at the Kirksville College of Osteopathic Medicine. Having experienced Dr Still's treatment, she described how gentle he was and told Dr Dickey, off camera, that the person who treated most like him, of any osteopath she had known, was Dr Sutherland.' (Cranial Letter 2022)

Edythe Ashmore DO, a professor of osteopathic mechanics at the ASO and also a student of A.T. Still, wrote:

'General Rules: The articulating surfaces must retrace the path they took in their displacement. It has been well said that it requires but a little force at exactly the right angle to produce a lesion, and conversely that a little force applied in exactly the right direction will reduce a subluxation. There are two methods commonly employed by osteopaths in the correction of lesions, the older of which is the traction method, the later the direct method of thrust.' (Ashmore 1915)

In terms of terminology, she stated: 'The word "direct" is preferred for the reason that the imitators of osteopathy have given to the word "thrust" an objectionable meaning of harshness.' The 'traction' method refers to what we now call 'balanced ligamentous tension' or 'ligamentous articular strain technique', although approximation or leverage are also used to awaken self-organising activity.

Ashmore continues:

'Those who employ the traction method secure the relaxation of the tissues about the articulation by what has been termed "exaggeration of the lesion", a motion in the direction of the forcible movement which produced the lesion, as if its purpose were to increase the deformity. C.P. McConnell states that this disengages the tissues that are holding the parts in the abnormal position. The exaggeration is held, traction made upon the joint, replacement initiated and then completed by reversal of the forces.' (Ashmore 1915)

Arthur Hildreth DO, a student and close friend of Dr Still and principal of the ASO in the early 1900s, describes the 'old doctor' also using approximation:

'If he stood on the right side of the body, he would use his right hand as a fulcrum on the neck, and with his left hand on top of the head he would press down on the head, thus throwing the vertebrae closer together and relaxing the muscles. When he felt that these muscles were completely relaxed, he would gently rotate the head with his left hand, holding the fingers of the right hand on the exact vertebrae he wished to correct.' (Hildreth 1942)

Howard Lippincott confirms Edythe Ashmore's statement that Dr Still's gentle method preceded the 'direct' or HVT approach:

'It is evident that Dr Still treated his patients carefully, with due consideration for the delicacy and the welfare of the tissues beneath his fingers. It is also evident that he imparted to the students who came under his supervision, this wholesome respect for the tissues, structures and their functioning.' (Lippincott 1949)

He continues:

'Then, after the turn of the century, it became popular with many of the vigorous and enthusiastic young doctors to treat with vigour and enthusiasm. They developed techniques that would produce a 'pop' regardless of the force required to produce it.'

The reason for the change after 1900 is that this is when the ASO expanded enormously, and it would have been hard-pushed to meet the demand for enough experienced teachers to give students the individual instruction they needed. Edythe Ashmore, writing in 1915, commented that the 'older', indirect method was more difficult to teach than the direct method

and therefore even discouraged it from being taught to students (Speece *et al.* 2009, p. 17). This was a big departure from William Sutherland's time of training (1898–1900) when classes were smaller and Dr Still closely supervised the teaching. Lippincott writes: 'The principles that were taught had to conform exactly to his concept. Dr Sutherland made good use of every opportunity to learn and understand them and has adhered closely in his thinking and practice to Dr Still's principles' (Lippincott 1949).

A.T. Still wanted his students to understand osteopathic principles and the mechanisms and anatomy of the body, rather than techniques, so that they would each develop individual and unique ways of treating. This is the way W.G. Sutherland learned from him. Our wish is to support the reader to develop the 'thinking, seeing, feeling, knowing fingers' that discover new ways of applying the principles described according to the conditions present in each patient.

INTRODUCTION TO THE VIDEO DEMONSTRATIONS

Chapters 1–17 contain additional video clips that support some of the practical procedures described, indicated by ⊙ in the text. Video clips can be accessed via the web link and QR code found at the end of each of these chapters.

This video series is offered with the intent to assist the translation of the written word into practical application, acknowledging that this is not an easy process for many people. The clips accompany the procedures described in the text with the exception of those which are very simple and easier to follow.

These demonstrations should not be seen as definitive, since each osteopath will find his or her own adaptation, taking into account the morphology and therapeutic needs of each patient.

Adhering to the principles demonstrated to the author and contributors by W.G. Sutherland's

close friend and student Anne L. Wales DO, we have stayed as faithful as possible to what she showed us. However, this is inevitably filtered through individual experience, and just as she modified her approach to each individual patient, we also have adapted some of the procedures, based on what we have found easiest and most effective, both in treatment and for the purposes of teaching.

No book or video demonstration can ever replace the hand-to-hand tuition from others who have embodied this approach, and patience is needed to 'make it your own'. This series is intended as a support for the ongoing lifelong process of gaining confidence, effectiveness and proprioceptive sensing for the benefit of both patients in need of help and the evolution of the practitioner.

REFERENCES

Ashmore, E. (1915) *Osteopathic Mechanics: A Textbook.* Kirksville, MO: The Journal Printing Company; p. 72.

Becker, R.E. (2001) *Life in Motion: The Osteopathic Vision of Rollin E. Becker, DO,* 3rd edition. R.E. Brooks MD (ed.). Portland, OR: Stillness Press; pp. 148–9.

Hildreth, A.G. (1942) *The Lengthening Shadow of Dr. Andrew Taylor Still,* 2nd edition. Paw Paw, MI: A.G. Hildreth & A.E. Van Vleck; p. 195.

Lippincott, H.E. (1949) *The Osteopathic Technique of Wm G. Sutherland DO.* Yearbook of the Academy of Applied Osteopathy.

Speece, C.A., Crow, W.T., Simmons, S.L. (2009) *Ligamentous Articular Strain,* 2nd edition. Seattle, WA: Eastland Press; pp. 11, 12 & 17.

Sutherland, W.G. (1990) *Teachings in the Science of Osteopathy.* A.L. Wales (ed.). Fort Worth, TX: Sutherland Cranial Teaching Foundation, Inc./Rudra Press; pp. 233–84.

Sutherland, W.G. (1998) *Contributions of Thought,* 2nd edition. A.L. Wales and A.S. Sutherland (eds). Fort Worth, TX: Sutherland Cranial Teaching Foundation, Inc.; pp. 132 & 160.

The Cranial Letter (2022). Vol 75, No 3. Accessed August 2023 at: https://cranialacademy.org/wp-content/uploads/2022/12/The_Cranial_Letter_Vol-75_No-3_2022_HR.pdf.

Wales, A.L. (1978) Video: A Demonstration of Balanced Ligamentous Tension. Sutherland Cranial Teaching Foundation, Inc.

Wales, A.L. (1996) Personal communication.

CHAPTER 1

Foundations of Balanced Ligamentous Tension

SUSAN TURNER

PART 1: WHAT IS BLT?

'When all the ligaments around a strained joint are enabled to find a state of equally balanced tension in relation to each other, there is a point at which these forces all converge. This point of "balanced ligamentous tension" acts as a fulcrum around which the inherent self-corrective forces are activated to reverse and so correct the articular strain.'

(Carrciro 2003)

This description of the process of balanced

ligamentous tension (BLT) challenges the often-held habitual view of the operator as active and the patient as passive. It also illustrates the potency of the homoeostatic forces continuously at work in the living body's articular system. Working with this principle requires an understanding of the living anatomy under our hands, which in A.T. Still's definition also includes physiology, histology and chemistry (Still 1899). The following offers suggestions for locating and activating a state of BLT for therapeutic change.

LIGAMENTOUS FUNCTION, NORMAL AND STRAINED

Each joint is enclosed in a serous sac with the ligaments binding the bones together, while also maintaining the joint space, by holding the articular surfaces apart in a frictionless state (Xu *et al*. 2022). In normal articular alignment, the ligaments that proprioceptively guide, support, protect and centre a joint remain in *a state of equally balanced tension in relation to each other throughout any normal movement.* That is to say that they remain in an automatically shifting, but constant, state of BLT. Although ligaments neither stretch nor become slack, nor do they

possess the same contractile qualities as muscles, they constantly accommodate the shape changes between the articular surfaces.

In a position of strain resulting from injury however, the articular surfaces become misaligned, so that the joint is less free to adapt to continual functional demands. The ligaments will then be in unequal tension in relation to each other, tight on one side, loose or torsioned on the other, and the whole joint mechanism will be in 'ligamentous-articular strain'. The distribution of tension through the three-dimensional joint space will then be altered so that the fulcrum, around which the joint moves, will be displaced or 'off centre'. This tends to result in diminished freedom of movement, tightness, locking or instability. However, although all the ligaments in a strained joint are potentially compromised (Lippincott 1949, TSO p. 234), they adapt to the joint distortion by attempting to find a new position of balanced tension to create stability. If the ligaments are damaged, scarred or the articulation has been forced beyond physiological limits, this adaptive capacity may be disrupted.

POINT OF BALANCE

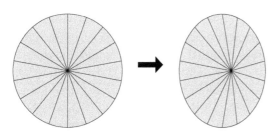

Figure 1.1 Diagrams of a balanced and displaced joint fulcrum.

The new compensatory pattern will tend to reflect the position that the joint took up in the original injury, although not to its extreme extent. The fulcrum for the new ligamentous balance, adopted by the strained joint, will correspondingly be towards the direction of original displacement. This is seen, for example, in an inversion sprain of the ankle, which often remains slightly inverted, caught between the extreme position of the injury and the body's attempt to 'spring back' towards normal. The persisting osseous misalignment, which puts

the ligaments in an unbalanced relationship with each other, renders the joint unstable and prone to repeated similar injury. Once realigned, however, the equalised tone of the ligaments in relation to each other will tend to stabilise the joint, relieving the stresses on them and optimising ligamentous healing.

Balance

The concept of balance is illustrated by the image of old-fashioned weighing scales, where two metal trays are suspended from a pivot on the central beam. When the weight within the trays is equal, the pivot on the beam, suspending the trays, will be central. If they are of unequal weight, in order to find balance, the pivot fulcrum would have to move laterally along the beam for the trays to be at the same level horizontally.

There is an analogy here with the centred balance fulcrum of a ligamentous-articular or membranous-articular mechanism when aligned, and the compensatory balance point for a joint or suture in strain.

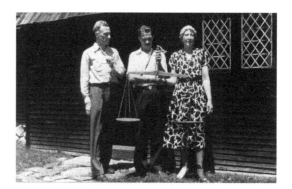

Figure 1.2 Balance scales with Sutherland's students Howard and Rebecca Lippincott DO. *Used with permission of Michael Burruano DO.*

ENGAGING BLT THERAPEUTICALLY

As a bio-tensegrity system, a living ligamentous articular mechanism expresses nonlinear self-stabilising properties that predispose it to

returning to its original shape once the force retained within it is released. This is enabled both by its geometrical arrangement and via an interaction with the nervous system, which enables the active regulation of the spacing and pressure between joint surfaces (Levin 2017) (see Part 4: Tensegrity). Living systems are primed for self-organisation.

It is this self-organising nature of the living system that, in Sutherland's words, makes it possible to 'work with the forces within the patient that manifest the healing process'. And in the words of Anne Wales, 'If we position the bones in relation to each other, so that the ligaments are relieved of the strain, then the bones can move spontaneously back to their correct position. Astonishing!' (Wales 1978).

The point of balanced ligamentous (or membranous) tension is defined as the point where all forces acting on a joint are balanced equally in all directions. In a strained articulation this is where all components of the 'lesion' balance each other in a neutral state. This is also where there is minimum resistance to the inherent self-corrective potency at work in the living body. The 'off-centre' compensatory balance point, then, will be the place of least strain within the distortion, where the potent physiological forces for correction of the dysfunction are most accessible in treatment.

To use this principle therapeutically, therefore, if the bones of a restricted joint are placed precisely in their position of distortion, paradoxically, the strain is taken out of the ligaments as the tension between them equalises. The point where all the conflicting forces balance each other functions as a fulcrum around which the ligaments are activated to guide the bones back into alignment, where free articular movement is restored. As Anne Wales observed, 'The point of balanced ligamentous tension is where physiology comes alive.' To engage the therapeutic potential of a strained joint, it is necessary first then to perceive, accept and support it as we find it and then seek that point where 'physiology comes alive'.

SUMMARY

The operator positions the bones of a strained or misaligned joint so that the tension between the ligaments is as balanced as it would be if that joint were in its normal state. The articular surfaces will often be shifted towards the direction that caused the injury. *The ligamentous mechanism may be further activated by either approximating or distracting the joint to the precise degree where the tone, tension and quality of the tissues are 'matched'.* This position is maintained and supported until the power within the balanced ligamentous articular mechanism moves the bones to their normal alignment. Having set up the balance point, the operator continues to observe as the work of readjustment is taken over by the homoeostatic forces within the patient's body. In Anne Wales' words again, 'Once in contact, we become observers of the state of things as they are.'

Approximation or distraction are often used to activate the ligaments. Drawing the bones together shifts the fulcrum around which joint action takes place, activating and freeing the ligaments to seek a new fulcrum of balanced tension, around which the bones are moved back into alignment. Subtle and precise traction may also be applied and maintained until ligamentous action amplifies. Another important activating force is the patient's natural breathing which is constantly moving the connective tissue continuum of the entire body. Where needed, the active postural or respiratory cooperation of the patient can be engaged.

At the point of balance, it is important to be patient, to trust and wait without hurry, to allow whatever changes the system needs to make without interference.

THE PROCESS OF APPLYING BLT

Example: BLT of a finger joint

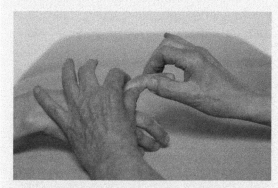

Figure 1.3 BLT of finger joint on a live model.

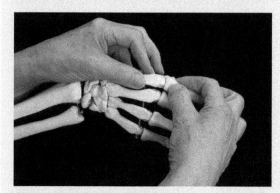

Figure 1.4 Handhold for BLT of a finger joint on skeleton.

1. MOTION TESTING FOR DIAGNOSIS

Diagnosis as a first step involves observation and interpretation of all components of a strain pattern. Under listening hands, diagnosis often leads to treatment and continues to clarify throughout the treatment process.

HANDHOLD

Taking an interphalangeal joint as an example, hold each bone between your index finger and thumb on either side of the joint. Systematically test ease of motion within the range of flexion/extension, torsion, sidebending and shearing. Be sure to take the joint back to neutral between each movement.

Torsion, for instance, is revealed by gently and slowly rotating the distal phalanx on the proximal. If there is a strain, it will move more easily in one direction than the other. For precision in diagnosis, it is important to respect the very first hint of resistance. The position of balance for each component of movement will be towards the position of ease, which is normally also the direction towards which the joint is strained.

2. POSITIONING THE JOINT IN ITS STATE OF BALANCE

Place the joint in its position of ease or neutral, starting with the most obvious component of the strain; for example, having found the easy point between flexion and extension, continue to hold this position and sensitively add in the neutral point for any other previously discerned component, e.g., torsion, sidebending etc.

In this way, a composite state of ligamentous balance is found. *Include in your awareness the three-dimensional shape that the joint takes up between its surfaces.*

The 'gentle exaggeration of the lesion' of which Sutherland spoke (Sutherland 1998, COT p. 160) refers to supporting the strain pattern only up to the point where the ligaments and joint capsule find reciprocal balance. This does not involve any motion barrier as it is the point of least resistance; the tissues appear to seek it, moving there most easily.

3. LIGAMENTOUS ACTIVATION AND ENGAGEMENT

Using slight approximation or distraction of the joint to match the compressive or tensional forces held in the joint acts to disengage the articular surfaces. This shifts the fulcrum around which joint action takes place to awaken inherent therapeutic ligamentous activity. It is sometimes combined with leverage.

Using approximation: *While holding the joint in its position of balanced tension (neutral), approximate it by gently and precisely bringing the distal and proximal bones towards each other until there is a sense that the ligaments are 'coming alive'. This is subtly adjusted to seek the point where they feel most alive.*

Using distraction: If approximation fails to evoke a response, distraction may be required.

Holding the joint in its position of balanced tension within its strained position, introduce gentle, precise and sustained traction, matching the tension between the proximal and distal joint surfaces to the point where the ligaments begin to enliven.

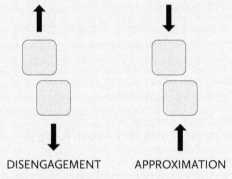

DISENGAGEMENT   APPROXIMATION

Figure 1.5 Disengagement and approximation.

4. THE INHERENT FORCES GO TO WORK

After an active, 'searching' phase, ligamentous activity becomes still, poised at the point of balanced tension. *Simply hold this position until the ligaments begin to recentre the bones.* Sometimes the bones follow a surprising path before realigning. The patient may spontaneously take a deep breath at this point.

Varying qualities of the balance point: The point of balanced tension may express itself differently according to what the patient's system requires in that area at that time. Sometimes it is a simple momentary sense of quiet, ease and opening, from which therapeutic realignment unfolds. At other times the neutral point has a quality of deep stillness and potent poise. This may feel like a window opening into a deeper space or dimension from which a quality like 'fresh air' and renewal flows through the tissues. It is important to trust that what is happening is appropriate, rather than holding specific expectations.

5. END POINT OF BLT TREATMENT

This may also manifest in various ways. Sometimes it is a simple, local structural realignment which is all that is needed. Sometimes the local reorganisation may be perceived in distant parts or in the body as a whole. Realignment of a joint is often accompanied by a palpable sense of increased spaciousness, warmth and rhythmic flow, in addition to freer mobility. This may, in part, be explained by improved flow in the extracellular matrix (ECM) as it shifts from the gel to the sol phase, promoting cellular fluid interchange.

6. RETESTING

Retest the joint as in the initial diagnosis and compare the range of movement.

Take note also of any qualitative changes that signify the return of a healthier tissue state.

The primary respiratory mechanism (PRM; see craniosacral mechanism in Key Terms) can often be felt during, and especially after, treatment as subtle tissue breathing, rhythmic axial lengthening and shortening and three-dimensional expansion and contraction.

Exceptions to the use of 'exaggeration'

As described above, in the majority of cases, an indirect approach using initiation by either approximation or disengagement is combined with exaggeration up to the balance point. In the ribs, hands and feet this is often effectively combined with leverage. There are occasions, however, when a direct approach appears to work more effectively. This is especially so when a patient is ill or inherent energy is low. Whereas the indirect approach carries the part in the direction that caused the injury, a direct approach may be used by first taking the joint into ease, and then simply holding the displaced part towards normal position, to evoke a dynamic ligamentous or membranous response.

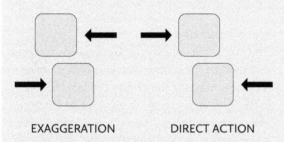

EXAGGERATION   DIRECT ACTION

Figure 1.6 Diagrams of exaggeration and direct action.

Many of the indirect procedures to be described can also be sensitively adapted to direct action where appropriate. An example is when engaging the fibula in relation to the interosseous membrane (IoM). A direct approach is also sometimes indicated for both individual vertebral strains and vertebral groups, especially in juvenile functional scoliosis. Another notable situation where direct action is recommended is when addressing compression of the condylar parts of the infant occiput. This is because of the importance of creating space in and around the foramen magnum, to avoid risk of compromising it further.

In instances of acute recent injury in which exaggeration increases pain, another type of *direct action* may be appropriate. In this situation, where two bones are positionally strained in relation to each other, the operator can hold the distal of the two bones (the 'bolt'), while the patient actively moves the proximal bone (the 'nut') slowly towards normal apposition (see Key Terms). This is often more comfortable and less likely to induce further strain on the ligaments than the operator directly moving the distal bone (Lippincott 1949, TSO p. 235). Examples of this are the standing iliosacral manoeuvre and the lap technique for the sacrum.

All treatment principles, e.g., exaggeration, direct action, disengagement, opposite physiological motion, etc., are equally useable in any situation, often in combination. These all reflect the innate therapeutic principles that the living body uses in its self-correcting process. The choice of approach is directed by the body itself, according to which evokes the most robust physiological response.

OTHER INHERENT FORCE APPROACHES

There are a variety of indirect approaches in osteopathy, each having their own focus. BLT differs from fascial unwinding and functional technique, which also use the patient's inherent forces. Fascial unwinding uses exaggeration of the strain up to the indirect motion barrier rather than a point of balance. Functional technique engages the muscle spindles rather than the ligaments so that the range of motion within which it works is normally wider than the close range involved in BLT. 'Reconstructed A.T. Still technique' (Van Buskirk 2006) has some features in common with BLT, but in Still technique the final articulatory movement plays a stronger role.

PART 2: ESSENTIAL ELEMENTS OF THE APPLICATION OF BLT

'The powers within the patient's body are more potent and accurate than any force that can safely be brought to bear from outside.'

(Wales 1996)

The process of BLT is less about 'doing' than being receptive to the response and living action of the tissues at each stage. This moment-to-moment 'conversation' is ideally part of every osteopathic manoeuvre and is not limited to Sutherland's approach.

This part will explore some of the essential elements in applying BLT to help the practitioner to achieve the most profound and durable result for the patient. It will present some ways of avoiding the frustration that can sometimes limit the outcome.

When treating a patient with this approach there are times when the dynamic ligamentous-articular response seems to have suddenly disappeared, or even worse, seems not to have engaged at all. This can be due to a complicating factor such as lack of therapeutic potency in the patient. However, often what is needed is for something to readjust within the osteopath. Here are some suggestions for an inner checklist:

- Engaging one's whole body: Working with BLT involves the engagement of the operator's whole body and not only the hands. It is helpful to think of 'listening' with one's back or with all the connective tissues or bioelectrical field around the body. This supports our own proprioceptive awareness of movement and position in space, to include the body of the patient. This is not only for a better understanding of the patient but also for practitioner self-care.

- Consciously 'dwelling' in our connective tissue network, as the crucible for the body's fluid systems, fosters a sense of connection with the ground. This can help release the operator from the tyranny of the busy mind, bringing a sense of receptivity, relaxed breathing and inner stillness. In turn, this can help open the pathways to haptic sensing, to receive palpatory information in a more efficient and comfortable way than 'probing' with too much forebrain curiosity.

- If we use predominantly muscular engagement, we will primarily meet a response in the patient's *voluntary musculoskeletal* system. Where applicable, the sensitive use of our own weight and of gravity is likely to evoke an optimum response in the patient's *involuntary* and proprioceptive ligamentous-articular system. This involves either leaning towards the involved structure to precisely approximate the tissues, or leaning slightly away when balanced tension by distraction is required.

GROUNDING

The ligamentous articular system is an involuntary mechanism in the sense that it functions independently of the voluntary control of the neuromusculoskeletal system. In order for the *voluntary musculoskeletal* system to quieten enough to allow the *involuntary ligamentous articular* mechanism to become predominant, the patient must feel unwaveringly supported by the stability of the operator during treatment. This means that the osteopath must be well grounded, feet well-planted, steady as a mountain and connected to the centre of the earth. Also crucial is a commitment to maintaining consistent support until the completion of the manoeuvre when the patient once again takes back postural control.

It can happen that the operator begins in a steady and grounded way, but then becomes so fascinated by the processes at work under the hands that the centre of gravity shifts upwards to his or her shoulders and head. This can have the frustrating effect of suppressing the palpatory sensitivity and engagement of the osteopath's hands with the patient's tissues. Deprived of support, a protective response will then be evoked in the patient's voluntary musculoskeletal system which overrides and suppresses the therapeutic ligamentous response. This may give the patient a subtle sense of physiological betrayal. If this happens, it is a reminder to check one's centre of gravity and reconnect with the support from the ground.

THE USE OF FULCRA

In this approach, the osteopath's hands need to remain sensory (afferent) throughout each procedure, reading subtle moment-to-moment changes in the three-dimensional joint space between the articular surfaces. This continues until spontaneous realignment is complete and rhythmic vibrancy is perceived, re-perfusing the tissues.

To keep the manual proprioceptive pathways attuned, it is helpful to use the forearms (more often than the elbows) as fulcra, to provide leverage for activating proprioception in the hands (Becker 2001, LIM pp. 184–202). A fulcrum provides an activating force, transmitted from the kinetic potential (potency) in the still point at one end of a long lever (forearm or elbow) to generate power or heightened proprioceptivity at the other (hand) end.

To engage fulcrum support in treating a supine patient, the osteopath sits well-grounded beside the patient, with forearms on the table and hands on, or under, the part of the body to be addressed. Leaning forward slightly from the lumbar spine, the amount of weight transmitted through the operator's forearm fulcra is adjusted to the precise degree needed to match the tone and tension in the patient's tissues. This moment of matching is perceived as a sense of enlivening in the ligaments, which Rollin Becker referred to as their 'going shopping', in a search for refinement of the point of balanced tension. Use of the forearm fulcra enhances proprioceptive attunement in the hands, enabling them to remain relaxed enough to adapt to, and perceptually engage with, the tissues. There may be a sense of the hands acting as 'antennae', while the tissue changes are 'read' and interpreted from the fulcra (Becker 1989) (see Chapter 2).

To find the point where the ligamentous-articular mechanism feels most alive, it is helpful initially to put more leaning force than necessary onto the treatment table through the forearm or elbow fulcra, so that you know what is more than enough. Then lighten up and use too little fulcrum engagement. Between too much and too little is the point where your fulcrum force most precisely matches the tone quality and tension of the tissues you are engaging. This is where the tissue response will be most enlivened, dynamic and therapeutically active. Forearm fulcrum engagement should be maintained through the ligamentous 'shopping' phase and balance point until realignment.

If the operator is standing for the procedure, the fulcra can be established, for example, by including a wider stance, leaning against the treatment table or keeping the elbows against the sides of one's own body etc. The toning of the forearm flexor digitorum profundus muscles can also be used as a fulcrum.

Although a fulcrum is commonly defined as the point on which a lever turns, another definition of osteopathic relevance is offered by Dennis Burke DO, as 'an agent through which the vital powers are exercised' (Burke 2022). The fulcrum can be the elbow, the forearm and, beyond that, our hearts or simply our therapeutic presence. When we acknowledge the emotional aspect of the patient, strains in the fluids and the fragility of the CNS, 'matching tension' is not necessarily physical, and the fulcrum is not necessarily a place or a point (Lim 2023) (see Chapter 18).

The concept of the fulcrum may be extended still further. Walter Russell, a friend of William Sutherland, spoke of the balanced Stillness of the spiritual universe as the foundation of the Motion of the material universe. He saw this as underlying the nature of everything in existence, including the essential nature of the human being (Russell 1994).

HONOURING THE BALANCE POINT

It is important to remain present and receptive at the point of balance. If we become impatient and seek to 'hurry it up', we may block the subtle therapeutic changes at work in the stillness. If we wait as if we had all day, the shift to the resolution phase tends to happen without delay. However, discerning whether a moment of stillness is a balance point or simply that the mechanism is being blocked by the operator's intensity can be confusing. Inwardly asking of oneself 'If I expect nothing, what is happening here?' can open, refresh and relax perception and also free the patient's process.

At the balance point there can sometimes be a tendency to feel as if one has done the necessary work in arriving there and that we can just let our minds wander while we await the release. Our ongoing presence, however, is an important and integral part of allowing the patient's physiology to make its greatest response. In this regard, the operator is like an ally.

The potency for therapeutic change that is held at the balance point is analogous to the kinetic potential energy contained in the pause at the end of a pendulum swing, from which a new cycle of motion is generated. In BLT, the point of stillness should be appreciated and enjoyed as a moment of pure presence, uncluttered by expectation.

Before Rollin Becker entered the room to greet a patient he would often inwardly say, in preparation, 'Thank you for giving me the opportunity to watch you heal yourself' (Brooks 2003). This same phrase as a mantra, at the stillness of the balance point, allows a sense of timelessness where a space within and 'behind' the physical dimension may emerge as a *knowing*, which requires the operator to simply trust.

In a letter to Sutherland, Becker described the BLT process as guided, not only by Intelligence, but also by an innate, directed, therapeutic force in the living body:

> 'A membranous-articular strain or ligamentous articular strain suddenly releases its tension as a form of clay when it enters the spaces and takes on reciprocal tension that has Intent, Purpose and Meaning. In its new releasing patterns, it goes back to the original position of strain and dissolves.' (Becker 2000, SOL pp. 190–191)

The words '*Intent, Purpose and Meaning*' are a powerful affirmation of the forces at work in the living system, supporting the practitioner's intent and purpose in the service of the patient.

CONSIDERING THE 'SPACES BETWEEN'

Dr Wales recalled Dr Sutherland saying to her about a student, when teaching on a course, 'I can't get him to understand that we are not so much treating the structure as the space' (Wales 1988). In his later years, Sutherland contemplated the importance of looking at the 'spaces between'. This included 'reading between the lines' of Still's writings to sense his deeper meaning, and considering the minute spaces between the grains of sand composing a rock, knowing that the rock would eventually become sand again.

He wrote of the pause-rest between the shutter opening of a camera, making a picture possible. He described the value of looking at the minute spaces in the body, as if looking through a 'mental microscope', for example, acknowledging the space between the trigeminal nerve and its dural sleeve, and the minute pivot space between the articular surfaces of the sacroiliac joint (SI; Sutherland 1998, COT pp. 254–256, 261). Acknowledgement of the subperiosteal layer of metabolic water is helpful in the treatment of intraosseous strains as described in Chapter 17.

It is possible that Sutherland was offering a clue here to opening palpatory pathways and deeper perception. Just as when we look at a miniature painting the brain transforms that small image into a landscape, acknowledging the minute spaces of the body can act as a magnifying glass to reveal unforeseen detail. Considering the three-dimensional space *between* structures involves the right side of the brain where non-linear and intuitive faculties of consciousness are more accessible. This is in contrast to the logical, linear and verbal left side of the brain with which it is complementary (McGilchrist 2019). It also happens that looking at a structure indirectly (here consider the space between the bones composing a joint) allows an opening of peripheral awareness to offer unexpected insights.

Anne Wales often referred to the value of acknowledging the space between our hands, to sense the relationship between the container and its contents. The skeleton, for instance, may be used as a 'handle' through which to engage with the spatial environment of the contained organs. This is most obvious in the thorax, pelvis or cranium but is applicable everywhere, hence her saying, 'Unwellness is an undesirable shape of space. Our aim is to change the geometry of the space' (Wales 1988).

Applying this to BLT, it is helpful to consider the 3D shape and quality of the joint space as the ligaments seek the precision of the balance point. When treating the spine, for example, taking the shape of the disc into the picture facilitates engagement with the whole segmental relationship as a dynamic unit. Likewise, the meningeal spaces, suspending the spinal cord within the fluid spinal canal, may be lightly held in the mental picture and included in the field of balance.

BEING OPEN TO THE UNEXPECTED

There are many variations of response in the process of BLT. Sometimes, for instance, just as the ligamentous articular mechanism appears to be emerging from the stillness of the balance point towards resolution of the strain, an alternating fluid fluctuation starts flowing back and forth through the joint. When this happens, it appears to indicate the need for resolution of a complex pattern of an old injury. This fluid activity will normally resolve into a new point of balance once it has 'done its work' before the joint mechanism opens and realigns.

There are occasions when engaging ligamentous balance primarily is not the most appropriate or effective approach. One such situation is in the active inflammatory stage of osteochondrosis, e.g., in Osgood-Schlatter disease of the knee, when it is difficult to engage ligamentous activity. In this situation it is often more helpful to think in terms of 'balanced tissue tension' or 'balanced fluid tension' to engage with the ECM of the bone and joint tissues. The aim here, through active listening, is to awaken the potency in the fluid space between the cells, until a sense of fluid interchange returns.

THINGS THAT HELP AND THINGS THAT GET IN THE WAY

Perceiving and engaging without trying too hard

A common cause of frustration arises when the operator is trying too hard so that his or her will or anxiety overrides the intelligent therapeutic tissue response. This creates tension in the operator's hands so that the sense of proprioception and therapeutic engagement is lost.

It is helpful in this situation to take a deep breath, drop the shoulders and relax, letting go of expectations or interpretations and starting afresh. It may be helpful to remember Rollin Becker's reminder that the real physician is within the patient and the osteopath is the assistant.

The acknowledgement that 'We have something more potent than our own agencies working always in the patient towards the normal' (Sutherland 1998, COT p. 160) may change the osteopath's relationship to the process, allowing him or her to become the assistant of the patient's inner physician. Dr Becker's advice 'The body is smarter than you are. Learn to learn from it' places the operator also in the position of a student (Becker 2001, LIM p. 11). These statements reflect an experience that, becoming receptive to the Intelligence of the self-renewing life potency within the patient, can bring clarity. Empathetic resonance and entrainment between osteopath and patient can provide a conduit for the diagnostic and therapeutic information that the patient's system needs you to perceive (Dove 2003).

Asking silent questions such as 'How do you need to be held?' or 'If I were this person or this area, how would I need to be held?' can have the effect of spontaneously readjusting the way we sit within ourselves and our bodies. It can then seem to the operator as if his or her own body and hands receive a directive from the patient's body to give either more spaciousness or more support; we may notice subtle changes in our own posture as if being adjusted by the patient's system, guiding us to find the meeting point.

Acceptance and trust without judgement

BLT begins by accepting the 'osteopathic lesion' as the body's best adaptation to an area in difficulty. It therefore involves acceptance rather than judgement, meeting the strain pattern in the patient's body as we find it. The osteopath and patient are partners in a shared objective, to work together towards the patient's wellbeing (Klug 1975). Both are supported by the wisdom and potency of Life in that we are all part of Nature. Trust in this resource is fundamental.

Rollin Becker advised that the most important step in learning to understand and use living health mechanisms is to 'accept the Living Mechanism in you and the patient', acknowledging that 'Life is always seeking to express health'. He emphasised the importance of surrender and of accepting that what the body is telling us is *true*, as we learn to feel and read what the primary physician, within both ourselves and the patient, is doing to deliver health from within (Becker 2001, LIM p. 11).

At the point of balanced tension, therefore, a truer resolution of the strain often arises from waiting with trust in whatever way it unfolds, than giving in to the temptation to exert will.

Remaining present without getting distracted

As stated above, remaining quietly present is fundamental to effectiveness and the patient's system senses when we lose presence. When the three-dimensional joint capsule and its ligaments begin to enliven, it is easy to become fascinated by changes happening elsewhere in the fascial continuum of the body. One may also be tempted to lose focus on the ligaments and become distracted by the muscles. While it is clear that any local change involves the connective tissue continuum of the whole body, it is important to remain openly attentive to what is going on under our hands. One's peripheral awareness may note distant changes but this should not dissipate an unwavering commitment to the area being addressed.

Because no-one is the same every day, it will sometimes be more difficult to stay attuned than at other times. What is important is to do one's best, however that 'best' is on a particular day. It is often surprising how the patient's system can respond to the operator's sincere intent even on days that feel more 'uphill'.

Ligaments are primary, bones are secondary

It can be helpful to reverse a habitual view of bones as solid and think of them as 'fluid' structures on a microscopic level, directed by the ligaments as the active agents for guiding articular alignment. In other words, 'The bones go where they are told' (see Part 3: Why ligaments?).

WHEN THE PSYCHE HOLDS THE PHYSICAL PATTERN

There are times, in practising BLT, when it becomes apparent that painful emotions or past trauma are bound into a patient's physical being. These may need to be acknowledged, either silently through the hands and heart, or in words, before a physical strain pattern is able to rebalance and integrate. The reciprocal influence of psyche and soma is discussed in Chapter 18 and Chapter 19.

'SETTING THE STAGE' AND WHAT FOLLOWS

Anne Wales used to speak of osteopathic treatment as simply 'setting the stage' for the body to be better able to make further significant changes in the period that follows. The living forces are continuously seeking to deliver balance and healing and the aim of osteopathic treatment is to release what may be obstructing that ongoing process. In this way, the treatment can be seen as a beginning.

There may be a readjustment phase in the following days to integrate the changes that have taken place during a session and this is not always comfortable. As the tissues realign and release their contracted state, they also rehydrate, sometimes resulting in temporary discomfort. This need not be a cause for alarm and the outcome is normally positive.

To avoid unnecessary treatment reactions, however, Anne Wales recommended checking that the occipito-atlantal relationship is balanced and settled at the end of the session (see Chapter 2, Part 2: Transitional areas). This is because this area will have responded proprioceptively to any shifts that have happened elsewhere in the body during the treatment.

TREATING THE PATIENT IN THE MOMENT

Throughout this book, there will be much focus on how to accomplish various technical procedures using BLT, and this is of course important information. However, the descriptions are not 'techniques' to be followed to the letter but applied principles, from which to meet the patient and the tissues in the moment. This means bringing the tissues under the hands to a place of balance in whatever way possible, often in unexpected ways. Central to this work is the importance of never losing sight of the knowledge that the depth of the therapeutic benefit is directly related to your presence, perception and attunement to the living forces.

PART 3: WHY LIGAMENTS?

'The ligaments, not the muscles, are the natural agencies for the purpose of correcting the relations and positions of joints.'

(Sutherland 1998, COT p. 160)

What we now know about the dynamically alert and proprioceptive qualities of ligaments, Drs Sutherland and Still knew only through their palpatory skills and ability to read and engage with tissue behaviour.

Sutherland's experience as a student, of feeling 'the ligaments guide the bones back into place' with his hands under those of A.T. Still, would have been a great surprise to him. It can still be a surprise even though we now know that, though ligaments were once thought to be inactive, passive tissues, they are highly proprioceptive and complex sensory organs (Johansson *et al.* 1991; Dyhre-Poulsen and Krogsgaard 2000; Payr 1900; Rein, Hagert and Sterling-Hauf 2021). They are responsive to both local and systemic influences, guiding appropriate muscle responses to stabilise joint function in both articular health and injury.

Seeing the skeleton as a dynamic ligamentous-articular mechanism, an involuntary physiological system which informs the voluntary musculoskeletal system, involves a shift from habitual ways of seeing for most people. The importance of the motor cortex and control pattern generators (CPGs) of the neuromusculoskeletal system are not to be underestimated in providing the power and control for purposeful voluntary movement. However, the functions that support life and homoeostasis are maintained by *involuntary* activity, as seen in the cardiovascular, digestive, respiratory, renal, hepatic and autonomic nervous systems. The skeletal system is no exception, where underlying voluntary control is involuntary action, involving the continuous ligamentous and fascial responsiveness that is key to both the stability and healing of articular mechanisms.

Healthy ligaments maintain the balance between stability and mobility. They guide but also protectively limit joint motion, preventing the bones from being sidebent, twisted or pulled apart beyond their normal physiological range. So long as they are intact, they constantly adapt to the shape changes between the articular surfaces, yet maintain balanced tension between them through all normal movements. They suspend the joint surfaces in reciprocal tension to keep them in centred apposition, buffered by synovial fluid. The frictionless state of synovial joints is maintained by the crossed helical joint network, acting as 'tensegrity springs' to keep the surfaces apart (Flemons 2012).

It is significant that Sutherland referred to joints as '*ligamentous*-articular mechanisms' to emphasise the primary importance of the connective tissues in articular organisation (Sutherland 1990). The tensegrity model echoes this view in seeing all bones as sesamoids, 'islands of compression floating in a sea of tension' (Scarr 2018, p. 79).

While proprioceptive ligamentous action stimulates protective muscle response, conversely, muscle hypertonicity often normalises tone, following resolution of ligamentous articular strain. This may explain Sutherland's observation that restoring balance in a strained joint often proves more effective, over time, in resolving muscle hypertonicity or fibrosis than working directly on the muscles (Wales 1996).

SOME MECHANISMS IN BLT

In the process of placing our attention on the ligaments in treatment, their continuity with the whole joint capsule means that all components of the articular mechanism will be involved, including the related muscles and fascia. The mechanoreceptors which innervate them are probably all engaged at the point of balance. As an example, when the radioulnar IoM is brought into balanced tension, the whole forearm articular mechanism is engaged with all associated tissues participating in reorganisation.

Neural, mechanical and vascular pathways all participate in the resolution of a joint strain in the application of BLT. When treating in this way it appears that the first perceivable therapeutic change is a local, neurally mediated shift in tissue density and fluid interchange, which then permits an improved range of motion. There is undoubtedly a neurological component involving different classes of mechanoreceptors which are distributed through capsule, ligament, fascia and muscles. These can be unmyelinated (fast) or can be simply free nerve endings (interstitial muscle receptors). They convey proprioception to the central nervous system (CNS) which then effects autonomic changes such as local regulation of blood flow to the tissues as well as active regulation of pressure and spacing in the joint (Levin *et al.* 2017; Scarr 2018, p. 85). Sensory information from the ligaments, joint capsule and fascia enables complex reflex patterns in the spinal cord and brainstem to exchange information between different parts of the system, supplementing supraspinal control (Turvey and Fonseca 2014).

The propriospinal tract coordinates function by linking different parts of the body, communicating over short and long distances and integrating the CPGs. These mechanisms may together explain why patients often feel distant parts of the body responding during treatment (Laliberte *et al.* 2019; Pocratsky *et al.* 2020).

However, although reflex systems supplement supraspinal control by initiating muscle contraction, even the fastest monosynaptic reflex responses involve a time delay and do not account for the immediacy of the body's ability to respond to unexpected changes (Brown and Loeb 2000; Kiely and Collins 2016; Scarr 2018, p. 85). And yet, tensegrity systems such as the connective tissue network of the living body are naturally self-organising, as seen when a ligamentous-articular mechanism spontaneously corrects around a balance fulcrum: 'Closed chain geometries show how multiple structures can be organised in a way that enables them to respond instantaneously with mechanoreceptors providing information that feeds into the nervous system and enables the amount of pressure or spacing between the joints to be actively regulated' (Levin *et al.* 2017). 'The movement of a single modular joint is then more than just a local event but one that involves the entire body through its heterarchical connections' (Scarr 2018, p. 85; see also Ribeiro and Oliveira 2011).

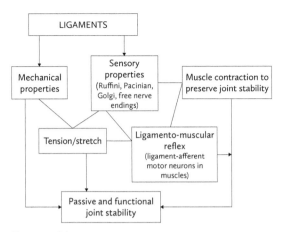

Figure 1.7 Ligaments as a sensory organ.
Adapted from Johansson, H., Sjölander, P. and Sojka, P. (1991) A sensory role for the cruciate ligaments. Clinical Orthopaedics and Related Research 268, 161–178.

This is an important point in terms of postural control and balance in relation to gravity. The effect of BLT on a joint seems to result in the integration of postural reflexes over a wide area. This can be true of any joint but is perhaps especially noticeable in treatment of the spine, the foot or the RTM (see Key Terms).

LIGAMENTOUS COMPOSITION

From an embryological point of view, bone, fascia, tendons and all connective tissues share a mesenchymal origin, the endoskeleton being the last to form within the connective tissue sea.

Ligaments are longitudinally arranged modifications of the dense irregular connective tissue forming deep fascia. The pericardium, periosteum, dura mater, perichondrium, dermis of the skin and perimyceum of muscles are all examples of deep fascia. This consists of randomly arranged collagen fibre bundles with very little extracellular ground substance, in which fibroblasts are the most common cells. In ligaments and tendons the collagen fibres become organised in a parallel arrangement, according to the developmental and ongoing stress exerted on them (Kessel and Kardon 1979). Fibroblasts maintain the ECM and may enable cell-to-cell communication (Hauser *et al*. 2013).

Collagen comprises 75 per cent of the dry weight of ligaments, together with proteoglycans, elastin and glycoproteins. Collagen fibres are arranged in bundles of smaller parallel fibrils aligned with the long axis of the ligament. A cross-linked pattern and undulation, known as *crimping*, gives great strength and capacity to resist both loading and tension. This provides the resiliency, shock absorption and internal springiness essential to the stabilising and proprioceptive function of ligaments. Under normal load, crimping allows the ligament to elongate without structural damage (Hauser *et al*. 2013).

The *viscoelastic properties* of ligaments provide joint homoeostasis through the interaction of collagens, proteoglycans, water and proteins. These work together with the crimped collagen to increase ligamentous tolerance to loading. As the collagen fibres lengthen and un-crimp under tension, the fibres straighten so that the ligament stiffens, providing strength. However, if the ligaments are overstretched, their crimp and tensile capacity can be disrupted, leading to joint instability and further ligamentous damage. If they are chronically elongated, they can lose the ability to return to their original shape, and their laxity will make the joint prone to instability and osteoarthritis through loss of protection from abnormal force transmission through the joint (Hauser *et al.* 2013).

Mechanoreceptors with nerve endings, Pacinian corpuscles, Golgi tendon organs and Ruffini endings are essential to the sensory function of ligaments in their ability to engage *ligamento-muscular reflexes.* The proprioception and kinaesthesia these provide can activate or inhibit muscle activity as appropriate. This protective ligamento-muscular reflex, generated via sensory receptors in the ligaments, is able to prevent injury by modifying ligamentous load. An example of this is seen where inhibitory reflexes prevent foot eversion in walking by activating intrinsic local muscles.

Sensory and proprioceptive nerves are contained in the epiligament layer of vascular and cellular tissue covering each ligament. These are densest in the areas close to the bony insertion site. When strained or injured, the proprioceptive nerves initiate neurological feedback signals to activate protective muscle contraction to stabilise and protect the joint. The mechanoreceptors of the cruciate ligaments of the knee, for example, interact with afferents in the thigh muscles, especially the quadriceps and hamstrings in response to load and pre-load (Frank 2004; Johansson *et al.* 1991; Raunest *et al.* 1996). This explains the loss of quadriceps function and weakness that can result from a loss of proprioceptive feedback in cruciate ligament injury.

Relevance to palpation

The blending of ligaments with the joint capsule and periosteum provides a perceptual osteopathic entry point into the three-dimensional volume of the joint and all its components. In many cases ligaments are functionally modified parts of the joint capsule, as seen in the hip joint, just as bursae are often modified parts of the synovial cavity, as seen in the suprapatellar bursa and shoulder.

On palpation, chronically strained ligaments have a quality like 'old rope'. This possibly correlates with the straightening and loss of the internal 'spring' arrangement in the collagen. It is often pleasantly surprising, however, to observe some return of a quality of aliveness and rhythmic resiliency in all the periarticular tissues in immediate response to a successful BLT manoeuvre.

INJURY

Ligamentous injury or disequilibrium can disrupt the balance between stability and mobility. When a joint is injured or inflamed it is the ligaments that adapt to the strain and maintain it, caught between the position of original injury and the body's attempt to pull it back to normal. Since it is the ligaments that maintain a joint in a position of strain, it follows that ligamentous balance needs to be restored for it to be realigned (Frank *et al.* 1985; Lippincott 1949; Van Buskirk 1990).

In cases of true ligamentous injury, repair requires time after the stage has been set for healing by osteopathic treatment. The patient has a part to play in taking care not to reinjure the joint during the healing phase. However, ligaments also require a degree of joint motion in order to heal, and complete immobilisation has been shown to impede ligamentous repair and lead to joint degeneration. Normally, the process of ligamentous healing progresses from an initial inflammatory phase to proliferation/regeneration, and then to tissue remodelling (Hauser *et al.* 2013). Corticosteroid treatment has been shown to carry the risk of delaying healing by suppressing the essential initial inflammatory phase (Slominski and Zmijewski 2017).

In fractures, ligaments have a role beyond the crucial part they play in joint function in that their attachment to the periosteum stimulates the potential within the periosteum for bone growth and repair.

PART 4: TENSEGRITY

'Bones as "islands of compression floating in a sea of tension".'

(Scarr 2018, p. 95)

The therapeutic effect of BLT is closely related to the phenomenon of tensegrity. This term, derived from 'tension' and 'integrity' or 'tensional integrity', was first used by the architect R. Buckminster Fuller to describe the principles he saw in nature, which he applied to the construction of geodesic domes (Fuller 1961).

In a tensegrity structure, struts (compression elements) are held apart by a network of cables under tension (tensional elements). The continuity of the tensional elements provides three-dimensional support for the discontinuous compression elements. Tension and compression interact three-dimensionally in dynamic balance, enabling maximum strength, while using minimum mass and energy. This differs radically from the way traditional architecture achieved structural stability through compression only, and these principles now play a significant part in contemporary architectural design.

Fuller's student Kenneth Snelson illustrated the principle of tensegrity through his sculptures, the best known of which are the 1961 Snelson arch and the Needle Tower (Snelson 1996). These light, strong and resilient structures show how tensegrity will operate in the same way, whatever position or gravitational direction they are adapting to. If an external force is distributed through the structure, causing it to deform, it will automatically return to its original shape once the force is removed. In their efficiency and nonlinear viscoelastic properties, tensegrity structures resemble the self-stabilising mechanisms at work in living organisms.

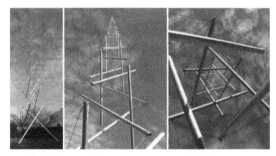

Figure 1.8 Kenneth Snelson's Needle Tower.
With permission, G. Scarr/Handspring Publishing.

BIOTENSEGRITY

The balance between compressive (centrifugal, outward-pushing) and tensional (centripetal, inward-pulling) elements is seen throughout nature, e.g., in the structure of spider's webs, viruses, blood cells and water molecules. In the living body the bones may be seen as compression elements (struts). The continuity of the soft tissues, comprised of ligaments, fascia, membrane and muscle, as tensional elements, defy gravity by providing spacing and support through balanced reciprocal tension. The dynamic tensional network, so formed, gives living organisms the capacity to continually adapt to the demands of movement, gravity and both internal and external spatial environments (Scarr 2018).

The totality of the living body's connective tissue system is a tensegrity structure at both a macro and micro level, constantly deforming and returning to its original shape. A change in one area of this dynamic unity affects the whole. As described by Donald Ingber, this principle which is visible in the gross structures of the joints and large body cavities is reflected into the intracellular and molecular levels (Ingber *et al.* 2014).

The cytoskeleton itself is a tensegrity structure wherein the microtubules act as compression elements (struts). The microfilaments and intermediate filaments, meanwhile, act as tensional elements whose contractile properties pull the plasma membrane towards the nucleus. The ECM and microtubules counter these tensional forces while adjacent cells constantly interact in isometric tension. There is continuity between the visible form and intracellular and atomic levels, and tissue deformation has been found to alter the cytoskeleton, gene behaviour and cellular metabolism. This points to the significance of normalising tissue strains (Chen and Ingber 1999; Ingber 1998).

A moment of revelation

Steven Levin, an orthopaedic surgeon and pioneer in the biotensegrity model, discovered during a surgical operation that *tightening of the cruciate ligaments of the knee moved the joint apart.* He also saw that where the ligaments are intact, it is virtually impossible to force the joint surfaces together (Levin 1999). On a subsequent occasion, when he himself was undergoing minor knee surgery, at his request, the surgeon performed some manoeuvres which confirmed that continuous spacing of 1.3 mm was present in both the patellofemoral and meniscofemoral joints. These were constant even when pressure on the foot exerted compression on the joint or when quadriceps femoris was actively contracted (Levin and Madden 2005). This suggests that the ligaments play a crucial role in enabling synovial joints to remain frictionless.

One can see that tensegrity plays a fundamental role in the functioning of the neuromusculoskeletal system. Sensory input from different interacting parts of the system, including joints, capsules, ligaments and fascia, is received and responded to in the motor cortex, brainstem and spinal cord (Scarr 2018, p. 85; Turvey and Fonseca 2014). Mechanoreceptors constantly feed information back to the nervous system which *actively* regulates the pressure and spacing in the joints (Levin *et al.* 2017). Through this interaction, the soft tissues guide the stability of the bones on either side of the joint, enabling them to move with minimum effort (Scarr 2018, p. 85). Tensegrity is, no doubt, one of the key elements in the effectiveness of a BLT approach and of osteopathy as a whole (Swanson 2013).

VIDEO FOR CHAPTER 1

Scan the QR code or visit https://www.youtube.com/playlist?list=PL3j_YuMBqigFvuthVIShyfqfKsjxQ8eSu to find a playlist of the video that accompanies this chapter.

REFERENCES

Becker, R.E. (1989) Lecture/workshop. British School of Osteopathy (BSO/UCO).

Becker, R.E. (2000) *The Stillness of Life: The Osteopathic Philosophy of Rollin E. Becker, DO*. R.E. Brooks MD (ed.). Portland, OR: Stillness Press; pp. 190-191.

Becker, R.E. (2001) *Life in Motion: The Osteopathic Vision of Rollin E. Becker, DO,* 3rd edition. R.E. Brooks MD (ed.). Portland, OR: Stillness Press; pp. 11, 184-202.

Brooks, R.E. (2003) Sutherland Cranial College of Osteopathy, Rollin Becker Memorial Lecture, London.

Brown, I.E. & Loeb, G.E. (2000) Measured and modelled properties of mammal skeleton muscle: dynamics of activation and deactivation. *Journal of Muscle Research & Cell Motility 21*, 33-47.

Burke, D.A. (2022) The President's Message. *The Cranial Letter.* Osteopathic Cranial Academy, Inc., Vol 75, No 3, p. 2.

Carreiro, J.E. (2003) *Foundations for Osteopathic Medicine,* 2nd edition. R.C. Ward (ed.). Lippincott, Williams & Wilkins/American Osteopathic Association; p. 917.

Chen, C.S. & Ingber, D.E. (1999) Tensegrity and mechanoregulation: from skeleton to cytoskeleton. *Osteoarthritis Cartilage 7* (1), 81–94.

Dove, C.I. (2003) SCCO Rollin Becker Memorial Lecture, London.

Dyhre-Poulsen, P. & Krogsgaard, M.R. (2000) Muscular reflexes elicited by electrical stimulation of the anterior cruciate ligament in humans. *J Appl Physiol 89* (6), 2191-5.

Flemons, T. (2012) Bones of Tensegrity. Accessed August 2023 at: http://intensiondesigns.ca/?s=bones+of+tensegrity.

Frank, C. (2004) Ligament structure, physiology and function. *Journal of Musculoskeletal and Neuronal Interaction 4* (2), 199–201.

Frank, C., Amiel, D., Woo, S.L., Akeson, W. (1985) Normal ligamentous properties and ligament healing. *Clinical Orthopaedics and Related Research 196,* 15–25.

Fuller, R.B. (1961) Tensegrity. *Portfolio and Art News Annual 4,* 114–148.

Hauser, R.A., Dolan, E., Phillips, H., Newlin, A., Moore, R., Woldin, B. (2013) Ligament injury and healing: review of current clinical diagnosis & therapeutics. *Open Rehabilitation Journal 6,* 1–20.

Ingber, D.E. (1998) The Architecture of Life. *Scientific American 278,* 48–57.

Ingber, D.E., Wang, N., Stamenovic, D. (2014) Tensegrity, cellular biophysics and the mechanics of living systems. *Reports on Progress in Physics 77* (4), 046603.

Johansson, H., Sjölander, P., Sojka, P. (1991) A sensory role for the cruciate ligaments. *Clinical Orthopaedics and Related Research 268,* 161–178.

Kessel, R.G. & Kardon, R.L. (1979) *Tissue and Organs.* Freeman & Co; p. 15.

Kiely, J. & Collins, D.J. (2016) Uniqueness of human running coordination: the integration of modern and ancient evolutionary innovations. *Frontiers in Psychology 7,* 262.

Klug, H. (1975) ESO, personal communication.

Laliberte, A., Goltash, S., Lalonde, N.R., Bui, T.V. (2019) Propriospinal neurons: essential elements of locomotor control in the intact and possibly injured spine. *Frontiers in Cellular Neuroscience 13,* 512.

Levin, S. (1999) Personal communication.

Levin, S.M. (2017) What puts the spring in your step? Accessed August 2023 at: http://www.researchgate.net/publication/314678997_What_puts_the_spring_in_your_step.

Levin, S.M. & Madden, M.A. (2005) In vivo observation of articular surface contact in knee joints. Accessed August 2023 at: www.biotensegrity.com.

Levin, S.M., De Solorzano, L.M., Scarr, G. (2017) The significance of closed kinematic chains to biological movement and dynamic stability. *Journal of Movement and Bodywork Therapies 21* (3), 664–672.

Lim, K.W. (2023) Personal communication.

Lippincott, H.A. (1949) The Osteopathic Technique of Wm. G. Sutherland, D.O. In: W.G. Sutherland (1990) *Teachings in the Science of Osteopathy.* A.L. Wales (ed.). Fort Worth, TX: Sutherland Cranial Teaching Foundation, Inc./Rudra Press; pp. 234, 235.

McGilchrist, I. (2019) *Master & His Emissary.* New Haven, CT: Yale University Press.

Payr, E. (1900) Der Herlige Stand der Gelinkchirurgerie. Arch. *Klin. Chir 148*; p. 404–51.

Pocratsky, A., Shepard, C.T., Morehouse, J.R., *et al.* (2020) Long ascending propriospinal neurons provide flexible, context specific control of interlimb coordination. Accessed August 2023 at: https://elifesciences.org/articles/53565.

Raunest, J., Sager, M., Bürgener, E. (1996) Proprioceptive mechanisms in the cruciate ligaments: an electromyographic study on reflex activity in thigh muscles. *The Journal of Trauma 41* (3), 488–493.

Rein, S., Hagert, E., Sterling-Hauf, T. Altered ligamento-muscular reflex patterns after stimulation of the anterior talofibular ligament in functional ankle instability. *Knee Surg Sports Traumatol Arthrosc. 29* (5), 1544–1553.

Ribeiro, F. & Oliveira, J. (2011) Factors influencing proprioception. What do they reveal? In: V. Klinka (ed.) *Biomechanics in Applications.* Accessed August 2023 at: https://www.intechopen.com/chapters/19663.

Russell, W. (1994) *The Secret of Light,* 3rd edition. Swannona, VA: University of Science and Philosophy; pp. 16–17.

Scarr, G. (2018) *Biotensegrity: The Structural Basis of Life.* Edinburgh: Handspring Publishing Ltd; pp. 79, 85 & 95.

Slominski, A.T. & Zmijewski, M.A. (2017) Glucocorticoids inhibit wound healing: novel mechanism of action. *Journal of Investigative Dermatology 137* (5), 1012–1014.

Snelson, K. (1996) Snelson on the tensegrity invention. *International Journal of Space Stuctures 11* (1 & 2), 43–48.

Still, A.T. (1899) *Philosophy of Osteopathy.* Kirksville, MO: A.T. Still; p. 16.

Sutherland, W.G. (1990) *Teachings in the Science of Osteopathy.* A.L. Wales (ed.). Fort Worth, TX: Sutherland Cranial Teaching Foundation, Inc./Rudra Press; p. 119.

Sutherland, W.G. (1998) *Contributions of Thought,* 2nd edition. A.L. Wales and A.S. Sutherland (eds). Fort Worth, TX: Sutherland Cranial Teaching Foundation Inc.; pp. 160, 254–256, 261.

Swanson, R.L. (2013) Biotensegrity: a unifying theory of biological architecture with applications to osteopathic practice, education, and research – a review and analysis. *Journal of Osteopathic Medicine 113* (1), 34–52.

Turvey, M. & Fonseca, S. (2014) A medium for haptic perception: a tensegrity hypothesis. *Journal of Motor Behaviour 46* (3), 143–187.

Van Buskirk, R.L. (1990) Nociceptive reflexes and somatic dysfunction: a model. *Journal of the American Osteopathic Association 90* (9), 792–794,797–809.

Van Buskirk, R.L. (2006) *The Still Technique Manual,* 2nd edition. AAO.

Wales, A.L. (1978) Video demonstration, SCTF.

Wales, A.L. (1988) Andrew Still Sutherland Study Group (ASSSG). Rhode Island, USA.

Wales, A.L. (1996) British tutorial group meeting. North Attleboro, MA, USA.

Xu, G., Chen, W., Yang, Z., *et al.* (2022) Finite element analysis of elbow joint stability by different flexion angles of the annular ligament. *Orthopaedic Surgery 14* (11), 2837–2844.

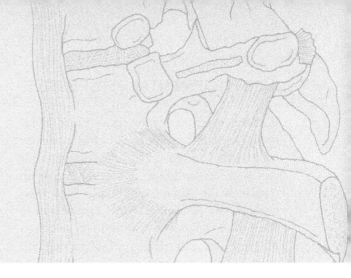

CHAPTER 2

The Spine

SUSAN TURNER

PART 1: SEGMENTAL RELATIONSHIPS

*'If I hold the vertebral bodies in a state of lig-
amentous balance, the patient's breathing is
moving the vertebral column. Pretty soon the
ligaments at the heads of the ribs and the discs,
everything the anterior longitudinal ligament is
attached to, starts to move...The anterior longitudinal ligament is the 'main street' of the whole
body, at least the trunk. It will move everything.'*

(Wales 1995)

Anne Wales' statement refers to the powerful
effect of the anterior longitudinal spinal ligament (ALSL) on the axial organisation of the
whole spinal column, rhythmically moving all
its articulations and contents with each cycle of
thoracic respiration, 24 hours a day. Its most fundamental effect on the spine is exerted through
its blending with the diaphragmatic crura, which
Dr Sutherland referred to as having 'more effect
on physiology than almost any other structure'
(Wales 1987).

A similar mutual influence between the spinal sphere and the anterior structures is exerted
through the attachment of the ALSL to the
prevertebral fascia (PVF) at T3 and between the
uterosacral ligaments and sacral periosteum (see
Chapter 5).

The significance of the ALSL in the application of BLT is not only in orientating the
operator to the front of the vertebral 'tube' being
engaged, but as a powerful activating force for
the ligaments in the state of balanced tension.
It is often the action of the crura on the whole
ALSL which shifts the joint fulcrum, enabling
the ligaments to move from the state of balance
to the reorganisation phase, where they actively
realign the joint. This illustrates Dr Sutherland's
statement that 'The powers within the patient's
body are more potent and accurate than any force
that can safely be brought to bear from outside'
(Wales 1995).

He further comments:

'In all spinal technic it is my custom to have the
patient exercise his own natural forces rather
than the application of mine. There are no
thrusts, no jerks nor the application of another
or a distant part of the body as a lever. The principle is that used and taught by Dr Still, namely,
exaggeration of the lesion to the degree of
release and then allowing the ligaments to draw
the articulations back into normal relationship.
This same method is applied in sacroiliac technic.' (Sutherland 1971)

A DEVELOPMENTAL PERSPECTIVE

Fundamental to osteopathy, the vertical orientation of the human spine is part of what defines our humanity. In Taoist, Hindu and other ancient philosophical traditions, the vertebral column represents the alignment of human consciousness between Heaven and Earth. Attunement to the flow of vital energy (Chi or Prana) through the spine is an essential part of Taoist and Hindu yogic practice.

The neurospinal axis, from cranium to sacrum, encompassing the brain and spinal cord, is the primary holder of the body's axial and segmental organisation, that makes possible the neurotrophic conversation between centre and periphery. The axial organisation of the neurospinal axis owes its original midline orientation to the 'north-south signature' of the embryological notochord. The notochord unfolds in the mesodermal layer of the embryonic plate from the 17th to the 24th day after conception (de Bree et al. 2018). It inducts the development of the vertebral bodies and intervertebral discs, as well as the midline structures of the cranial base.

These are a modification of the same primordiae that form the vertebral column (Cunningham 1984; Filler 2007; Weaver 1938). The notochord also inducts the development of the neural tube, from which the brain and spinal cord develop. Some of its cells persist in adulthood as a 'notochordal echo' at the centre of the nucleus pulposus. The presence of this energetic midline blueprint is perceptible throughout life.

Osteopaths often refer to 'unlocking a restriction between two vertebrae'. However, in treating the spine, from a developmental point of view, the nucleus pulposus *may be* regarded as a natural fulcrum for segmental motion. Each vertebral body is formed from the unification of an upper and lower half, formed from the migration of the somites of the embryological segments above and below (Christ and Wilting 1992). This is reflected in the way the ribs and spinal nerve roots orientate to the space *between* the vertebral segments, rather than to vertebrae themselves. When an intervertebral strain is corrected, therefore, *it is a harmonisation of one embryological segment with itself*. Working with this in mind brings a sense of cooperating with the potent forces of the body's essential developmental geometry and self-organisation.

INTERVERTEBRAL DISCS

It is the weight-bearing and shock-absorbing intervertebral discs that permit intersegmental movement. The ligamentous-articular mechanism of the articular processes in the neural arches protects the discs by regulating and limiting their motion. The articular processes are not themselves weight bearing, except at C1 and C2.

The strong collagenous double spiral arrangement of the annulus fibrosus around the nucleus pulposus is well-adapted for stability, movement and weight bearing, provided the fibres are equally balanced (Chu et al. 2018). When the intervertebral relationship is unbalanced, e.g., torsioned, sidebent, axially compressed or carrying a vectorial residue of sustained shearing or compressive forces, this weakens the helical support between some of the fibres of the annulus. This may result in a tear in these fibres, rendering the disc vulnerable to bulging and eventual herniation. Once herniated, if the original intervertebral strain pattern is not rebalanced, disc recovery may be slower. In such a case, a BLT approach is immensely useful for realignment and decompression in that it is gentle and engages the precision of the self-corrective forces.

From the point of view of the tensegrity model, the ability of the discs to resist lateral expansion and vertical compression is made possible by the soft tissue support supplied by the tensional elements, i.e., ligamentous network of the vertebral column and its related muscles and fascia (Scarr 2018, p. 76). Whyte (2017) further suggests that functional scoliosis has more to do with a change of soft tissue organisation than with the bones themselves. This supports the relevance of restoring ligamentous balance for realignment.

'The vertebrae then become local islands of compression within the much larger tensional network, both of which enable the spinal columns of humans and other animals to function well within both horizontal and vertical positions' (Scarr 2018, pp. 85–86). This tensegrity principle is well illustrated by the sculptor Kenneth Snelson's tensegrity Needle Tower (1968), as shown in Figure 1.8.

THE SPINAL LIGAMENTS

In addition to the proprioceptive input received from the ligaments and capsules of the facet joints, the longitudinal spinal ligaments, running from cranial base to sacrum, are essential integrators in its axial organisation. Every part mutually influences and responds to every other part, in dynamic adaptation to constant functional demands.

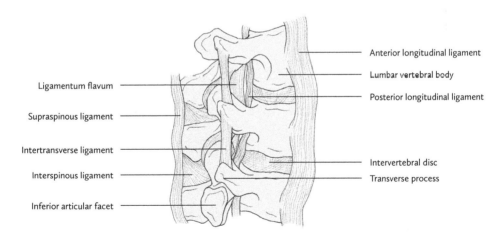

Ligamentum flavum

Supraspinous ligament

Intertransverse ligament

Interspinous ligament

Inferior articular facet

Anterior longitudinal ligament

Lumbar vertebral body

Posterior longitudinal ligament

Intervertebral disc

Transverse process

Figure 2.1 Ligaments of the lumbar spine, lateral view.

The spinal 'ligamentous stocking'

The ALSL and posterior longitudinal spinal ligament (PSLS) together form a ligamentous stocking around the vertebral bodies. The ALSL wraps the anterior surfaces of the vertebral bodies and discs from basiocciput to sacrum.

The ALSL is functionally continuous with the PLSL on the posterior surface of the vertebral bodies within the spinal canal. The PLSL is suspended from the intracranial surface of the basiocciput via the tectorial membrane which adjoins the PLSL at C2.

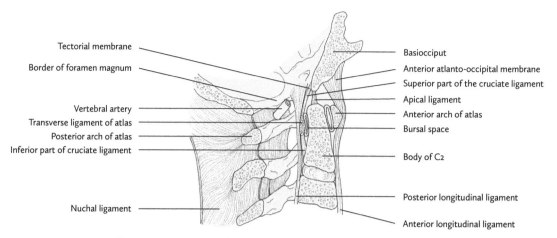

Tectorial membrane

Border of foramen magnum

Vertebral artery

Transverse ligament of atlas

Posterior arch of atlas

Inferior part of cruciate ligament

Nuchal ligament

Basiocciput

Anterior atlanto-occipital membrane

Superior part of the cruciate ligament

Apical ligament

Anterior arch of atlas

Bursal space

Body of C2

Posterior longitudinal ligament

Anterior longitudinal ligament

Figure 2.2 Ligaments of the craniocervical junction, sagittal section.

These two thickened ligamentous bands connect via the periosteum at the sides of the vertebral bodies, encompassing them between the laminae.

In the thoracic region the radiate ligaments of the rib heads blend with the ALSL.

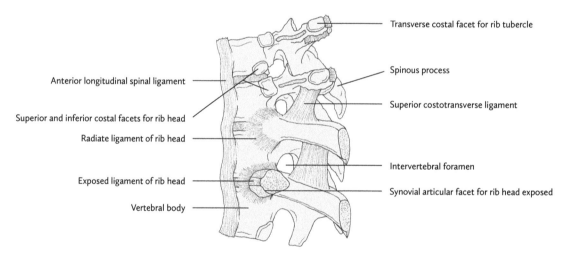

Anterior longitudinal spinal ligament

Superior and inferior costal facets for rib head

Radiate ligament of rib head

Exposed ligament of rib head

Vertebral body

Transverse costal facet for rib tubercle

Spinous process

Superior costotransverse ligament

Intervertebral foramen

Synovial articular facet for rib head exposed

Figure 2.3 Lateral view of thoracic spine and rib relationship.

Spinal ligamentous chains

The chain of supraspinous and interspinous ligaments in the lumbar and thoracic regions is homologous with the ligamentum nuchae in the neck. This originates on the superior nuchal line of the occipital squama.

The intertransverse ligaments in the thoracic and lumbar spine are homologous with the intertransverse muscles in the cervical spine.

Immediately anterior to these, the ligamentum flavum connects the laminae longitudinally and attaches to the fibrous capsules of the zygapophyseal joints. The ligamentum flavum is continuous with the periosteum of the laminae and pedicles.

The small muscles of the neck, rotatores and intertransversarii, contain a high density of collagenous tissue which suggests that they perform a strong proprioceptive function similar to ligaments (Willard 1995).

The dural tube

Another axial organiser is the dural membrane within the spinal canal, forming an 'inner tube' through the whole canal as far as the 2nd sacral segment. The dural membrane surrounds the arachnoid mater, pia mater, spinal cord, cerebrospinal fluid and brain. Dentate ligaments anchor the spinal cord to the dura mater along its length at each side. They also link the pia and arachnoid mater to the dural layers. The spinal dural tube attaches to the PLSL on the posterior surface of the vertebral bodies (Tardieu *et al.* 2016). Dissections have confirmed Sutherland's observation that the firmest attachments are at C2 and the second sacral segment (Unal and Sezgin 2021; Von Lanz 1929). The spinal dural tube is functionally continuous with the intracranial dura, forming a 'reciprocal tension membrane' (RTM; see Key Terms).

INFLUENCE OF ANTERIOR STRUCTURES ON THE SPINE

Sutherland observed that, when treating the vertebral column, it is useful to be aware of tension exerted on the ALSL by the structures ventral to it. Points where anterior structures attach firmly to the ALSL, e.g., T2–T3 and L1–L3, merit special attention (see Chapter 5).

Arteriovenous circulation

One factor illustrating the relevance of anterior influences on the spine is that respiratory excursion of the diaphragm helps to normalise vascular and lymphatic flow to and from the vertebrae and spinal cord (Sutherland 1990, TSO p. 179), by exerting rhythmic traction and release on the crural attachments to the ALSL. Together with the respiratory movement of the ribs, this pumping action counters a tendency to fluid stasis and passive congestion. In the author's experience, restoring the inherent pump supplied by diaphragmatic freedom can speed recovery in cases of acute lumbar strain. This is especially relevant in pain and injury where there is a tendency for a sufferer to limit deep breathing in an effort to control pain. A tightly held diaphragm is also a common response to any form of shock.

Good arteriovenous circulation is essential for health and repair of the vertebrae, discs and intraspinal tissues. Batson's plexus of veins, draining the spinal canal and cord, is valveless. For this reason, its flow and drainage are dependent on body movement, especially the rhythmic action of breathing. In spinal injury or acute somatic dysfunction, fluid stasis within the spinal structures is often exacerbated by local swelling, just as it is in a sprain of any joint.

Effects on spinal development

The spine of a newborn infant should form a smooth, slightly 'C' shaped curve. If on examination a flexed thoracolumbar junction is observed, this may be a response to a tight diaphragm whose crura are tugging upwards on their ALSL attachments at L2 and L3 (Wales 1995). This is a common finding following a respiratory infection or when the first breaths of life were difficult. If this restriction persists, it may interfere with the development of the normal spinal curvature.

Effects of visceroptosis

Ptosis of the abdominal viscera may cause drag on the whole anterior fascial column up to the cranial base and also on the root of the mesenteries. The mesenteric root suspends from the posterior abdominal wall, left of L2, and passes obliquely, in front of the aorta, to the right sacroiliac joint (SI). Although it does not attach directly to the vertebral column, visceroptosis may drag on the area of L3, exaggerating kypho-lordosis

(Ettlinger 2017). An engorged liver can similarly affect spinal curves via its firm attachment to the diaphragm through which it can impose weight on the thoracic fascia (see Chapters 5 and 6).

Prevertebral muscular and fascial influences

Where the cervical spine is rigid or too straight, with loss of normal cervical lordosis, a hypertonic and shortened longus colli (LC) muscle may sometimes be implicated. LC contraction may have originally been a protective response to a spinal insult, not just at a local level but even remote from the neck. In the long term, such hypertonicity may render the intervertebral discs vulnerable to degeneration. This muscle, on the anterior surface of the cervical and upper thoracic spine, originates on the transverse processes of C5–T3 and inserts into the vertebral bodies of C2–C6 and superior arch of the atlas. In the author's experience, whiplash injury may leave it contracted. When this is the case, enabling it to relax by applying gentle axial approximation between its origin and insertion may release the chronic contraction for restoration of a natural cervical lordosis.

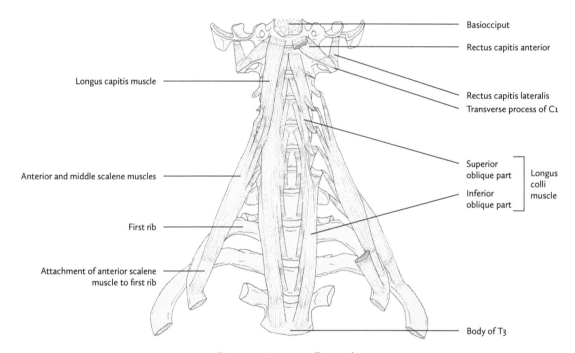

Figure 2.4 Longus colli muscle.

Where there is marked flexion and rigidity at the cervico-thoracic junction, also consider the PVF and its connections. The PVF overlies the LC muscle and extends from the undersurface of the basiocciput to T3 where it blends with the ALSL. It runs free of attachment to the vertebral bodies between its origin and insertion and encompasses the cervical spine and deep muscles of the neck like a sleeve. Sutherland likened it to a 'check ligament' for the cranial mechanism, noting its tendency to disturb the 'Sutherland fulcrum' (automatic shifting suspension fulcrum; see Key Terms) when subject to fascial drag from anterior cervical and thoracic structures. Drag on its upper thoracic attachment creates a tendency to a short flexion curve of the cervico-thoracic junction, known as 'dowager's hump' or in Sutherland's terms the 'old age centre' (Sutherland

1990, TSO p. 279). (See Chapter 5, section on anterior cervical fascial lift and manubrial lift.)

Another change, frequently due to anterior influences, is a fixed lumbar lordosis. In conjunction with the erector spinae and quadratus lumborum muscles, a fixed lumbar hyperlordosis may be predisposed or maintained by bilateral contraction of the psoas muscles which originate on the transverse processes and discs of T12–L4. Like the LC muscle, psoas major lies ventral to the vertebral column, bridging a transitional region. Both muscles exert a strong influence on the spinal curves, although when hypertonic, they tend to produce opposite effects from each other on natural lordosis in each area.

In rotational strains of the lumbar spine a possible cause may be a malalignment of the hip joint in which the iliopsoas muscle is implicated. A hypertonic obturator internus may also need to be considered as a maintaining factor in lumbar strains. (See Chapter 5, fascial lifts and Chapter 16, obturator internus and psoas.)

The 'straight spine'

Where a thoracic spine is rigid and lacking natural kyphosis, Sutherland likened this 'straight spine' to a 'flat foot', being without the shock absorption and resilience that the arches should bring (Sutherland 1990, TSO p. 250). He commented that in thoracic hyperextension, the sympathetic ganglia, blood and lymph channels relating especially to the spinal cord could be compromised through anterior ligamentous and crural tensity (Sutherland 1998, COT pp. 32–33).

In referring to 'flat foot lesions of the spine' he observed that rib heads may be anterolaterally impacted onto the hemifacets and intervertebral discs of the thoracic vertebrae to which they correspond. This can create an intersegmental 'wedge' or 'splint' that limits mobility and normal kyphosis. This is one reason why he recommended freeing the thoracic spine from any impingement by the ribs before addressing it directly (Wales 1995). The costovertebral junctions and intervertebral strains can also be treated simultaneously (see Chapter 4).

Kyphosis

The opposite problem is seen in an exaggerated thoracic kyphosis. Intrathoracic tensions, including those involving the heart and lungs and their encompassing fascia, can exert a kyphotic influence on the thoracic spine as can strains in the ribcage, clavicles and diaphragm. A common cause may be a bad cough which can leave the fan-shaped retrosternal transversus thoracis muscle in a state of residual hypertonicity (see Chapter 5, fascial lifts).

The spine, in relation to the anterior body, has been likened to a bow and bow string, the kyphotic curve representing the bow, and the anterior fascia, the bow string (Slijper 1946). In an exaggerated kyphosis the bow string of the anterior fascia may need to be released.

THORACOLUMBAR FASCIA (TLF)

Acknowledgement of the anterior fascial influences on the spine would be incomplete without consideration of the stabilising role played by the TLF (see Chapter 5). In continuity with the latissimus dorsi, gluteus maximus and hamstring muscle groups, the TLF provides posterior tone and tensegrity to the back. This counterbalances potential anterior fascial and visceral drag on the spine (Willard *et al.* 2012). The psoas and quadratus lumborum muscles are also closely associated with the middle and anterior layers of the TLF. See also Figure 5.3.

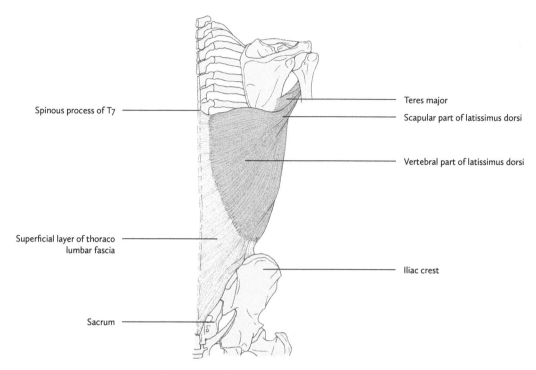

Spinous process of T7

Teres major

Scapular part of latissimus dorsi

Vertebral part of latissimus dorsi

Superficial layer of thoraco lumbar fascia

Iliac crest

Sacrum

Figure 2.5 Superficial layer of thoracolumbar fascia with latissimus dorsi.

The TLF works in concert with the diaphragm, abdominal muscles, ribcage and scalenes to straighten the spinal curves in thoracic inhalation, through the tension exerted on its attachment to the supraspinous and interspinous ligaments.

SPINAL 'SPHERES OF INFLUENCE' AND RELATIONSHIPS

Each area and segment of the spine has its own 'sphere of influence' through the afferent and efferent nerve traffic communicating with the spinal cord via the nerve roots and reflex arcs. The diagram in Figure 2.6, drawn in 1900 by J.M. Littlejohn and R.H. Dunnington (Wernham 1981), attempts to illustrate the complex somaticovisceral and viscerosomatic relationships dynamically working at each spinal level as part of an osteopathic working model. Sutherland, for example, advised checking the thoracic spine for activity of the somaticovisceral and viscerosomatic reflexes before and after treating an acute abdomen (Sutherland 1990, TSO p. 213).

The physiological significance of each vertebral level in relation to specific musculoskeletal, organic and vasomotor regions of influence has been fundamental to osteopathic thinking from its earliest beginnings. This concept was first subjected to research by Louisa Burns in the 1920s. The 'facilitated segment' model was later developed by Korr (1947) and supported by Denslow *et al.* (1947). This has now been modified by the central sensitisation model (Bogduk 1994; Fryer 2016). Central sensitisation is maintained by structural changes in the microglia, astrocytes, gap junctions and membrane excitability (Woolf 2011).

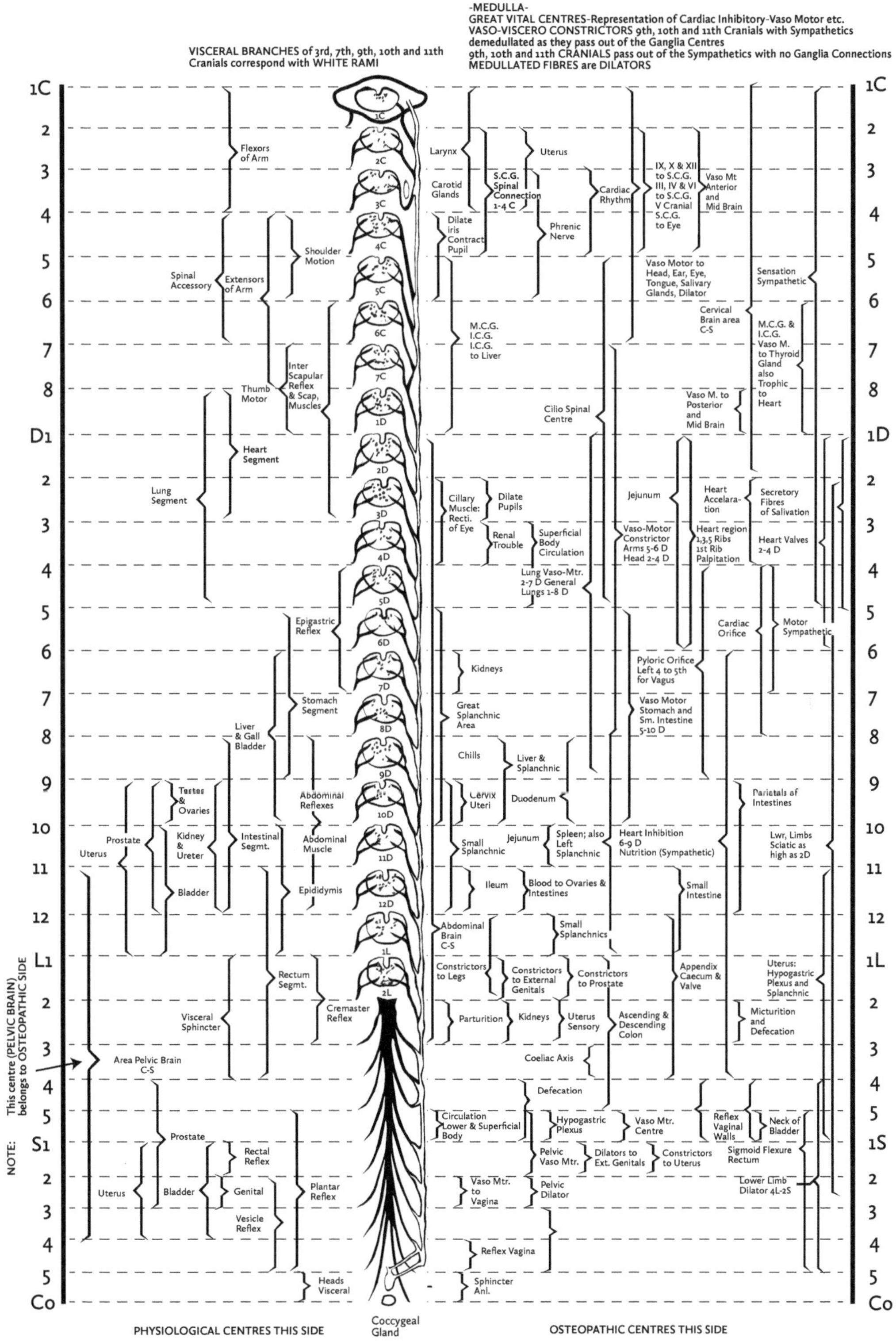

Figure 2.6 J.M. Littlejohn's chart of osteopathic centres.
With kind permission of Institute of Classical Osteopathy.

In the experience of the author, both the concepts of an association of centrally referred pain with altered axonal transport and that of the facilitated segment are equally useful in osteopathic practice.

The facilitated segment hypothesis suggests that myofascial strains produce exaggerated motor and sympathetic responses at the corresponding level in the spinal reflex arc. Altered afferent input reaching the cord, following injury, tends to lower the threshold of the spinal interneurons, leading to exaggerated sensory, motor and sympathetic outflow for the involved spinal segment(s). The research of Korr and Denslow focussed on sensory input, and although they only briefly mentioned the effect of inflamed, irritated or pathological viscera, they proposed that somatic dysfunction/facilitation of a spinal segment is maintained by sensory information, mainly from proprioceptors/muscle spindles from factors such as contracted muscle (Van Buskirk 1990).

In their experimental work Korr and Denslow observed segmental facilitation, in the acute phase, to produce cutaneous changes, e.g., increased skin resistance (sweat), temperature (blood flow) and a prolonged red reflex over paraspinal tissues. They observed facilitated segments in the acute phase to exhibit a 'doughy, boggy' quality in the paraspinal myofascial tissues. Viscerosomatic reflexes may progress to produce neuromuscular changes in segmentally related tissues, altering paraspinal muscle tone. This may show in tight or thickened paraspinal muscles and restricted articular movement, thickened subcutaneous tissues, and dryness of overlying skin.

Thus the quality of segmental movement, paraspinal muscle tone and qualities of the overlying skin can give useful supporting diagnostic pointers suggestive of both somatic and visceral function. Conversely, releasing the paraspinal and suboccipital muscles by slow, gentle inhibition appears to calm and normalise the excitation of a facilitated segment, improving segmental movement and tissue quality. This approach was frequently used by A.T. Still (Hildreth 1942).

Assessment of spinal segmental facilitation is a routine part of osteopathic diagnosis of acutely and chronically ill hospitalised patients with systemic disease in the USA. In the words of Hugh Ettlinger DO, former director of the osteopathic manipulative treatment department at St Barnabas Hospital, New York, '10 years of doing structural examinations in the acute care setting has demonstrated to this author that the great majority of cases present with significant, obvious reflex patterns which are easily recognised' (Ettlinger 2003; Cox et al. 1983).

In locating the visceral relationships to the spine, it is useful to keep in mind that all structures above the diaphragm, including heart, lungs, oesophagus and viscera of the head and neck, are innervated sympathetically by T1–T5 spinal levels. T5–T9 spinal nerve roots receive and transmit input via the greater splanchnic nerve involving spleen, stomach and pancreas. T10–T12 roots receive and transmit via the superior mesenteric ganglion and relate to the kidneys, ovaries, testes and upper ureters, fallopian tubes, small intestine and ascending and transverse colon. T12–L2 innervate the lower ureter, lower part of the fallopian tubes and lower abdominal and pelvic viscera including uterus, prostate and bladder. Spinal reflexes tend to react on the left or right according to the side of the organ involved (Ettlinger 2003).

When treating the spine, a large sphere of segmentally specific somatic and visceral relationships is constantly interacting under our hands. A spinal problem may initially appear to be purely mechanical but it is well to be alert to any possible viscero-somatic or somatico-visceral effects, especially in complex chronic conditions (Switters 2021; Te Poorten 1979). Occupational repetitive strain patterns which are continually reinforced can have far-reaching effects on both organic and somatic function, so understanding is needed, by both osteopath and patient, of the forces exerted on the body by everyday activities and past traumata.

Intervertebral joints are innervated by adjacent spinal nerves, especially their dorsal divisions and sympathetic nerves. Where a segmental reflex becomes irritated or, in the osteopathic sense, 'facilitated', the vasomotor influence exerted by those nerves diminishes the nutritive blood flow to the spinal segments (Wright 1955). The resulting diminishment of fluid perfusion to the discs can therefore adversely affect the quality of tissue health in the spinal structures themselves. Defacilitation and restoration of neurotrophic flow is one of the positive physiological outcomes of resolution of intervertebral strains, changing the osseous and soft tissue texture from dry and brittle to warm and resilient (Korr 1986).

Freeing the spinal ligamentous stocking to allow freer interchange of fluids may improve venous drainage and arterial perfusion to all the spinal tissues, including the discs and bones. In the author's experience, this improvement in tissue hydration appears to be beneficial in some cases of disc prolapse, osteochondritis, Scheuermann's disease, etc. In these situations, the vasoconstrictive effect of overactive local sympathetic activity is associated with a palpable sense of desiccation in the vertebrae and adjacent tissues.

CHRONIC PROBLEMS

Dr Wales spoke of Dr Sutherland's advice to allow time for old fibrotic spinal lesion patterns to change just a little at a time, rather than trying to break them up. This is to allow the rest of the body to adjust to the compensation and create an environment where the tissues are healthy and resilient enough to embrace change. The body will often immobilise an area where function is too impaired. Muscle contracture and fibrosis may actually be providing a supporting function through immobilisation for protection, so this situation requires patience and time (Wales 1987).

She also advised that in patients whose bodies are chronically rigid, it can be helpful to begin by working with the anterior fascia or viscera to 'give them a little lift in their sag', i.e., to initially create better balance between the anterior fascial compartments or body cavities (see Chapter 5). The resulting small improvement in tissue fluid interchange and respiratory movement will work on the skeletal tissues between sessions, preparing them for more specific work.

THERAPEUTIC ENGAGEMENT

Spinal diagnosis

Ideally the apices of the spinal curves are at C5, T4 and L3 with overall bilateral symmetry and easy vertical alignment between the transverse process of the atlas through the tarsal arches of both feet. Variations of this ideal normal lead us to examine what forces are acting on the spine, either from within it or from different areas, e.g., hips, pelvis, ribcage, anterior fascia, viscera, cranium or extremities. Provided that spinal articular relationships are functionally balanced as a whole, the body can adapt to some variation with comfort and efficiency. The primary aim is to restore function and integration.

The spine may be assessed and treated in the sitting, prone or supine position, and sidelying in late pregnancy, etc. To check for consistency, it is helpful to examine in more than one position. As stated above, it is worth noting dermal and paraspinal signs of segmental facilitation, e.g., sweating, red response and tenderness in the acute phase or dryness, rigidity and paraspinal muscle hypertonicity or hardness if chronic.

1. PALPATION OF RESPONSES TO BREATHING HANDHOLD

If examining a supine patient, it is easiest to sit at the side with finger pads under the spinous processes.

Keeping your fingers relaxed and receptive, observe how segments or groups are moved by the vertebral response to breathing as the spinous processes rhythmically spread and approximate your fingers. When the spinal curves change in inhalation and exhalation, it is revealing to note any segments or groups that resist free movement in either phase. For example, a thoracic vertebra that is fixed in extension may reveal a resistance to flexion on exhalation; a thoracic vertebra that is fixed in flexion may resist extension on inhalation.

Notice also if, in either respiratory phase, sidebending, rotation, flexion or extension become exaggerated, either in an individual segment or group.

Perception may also be enhanced by observing the spinal expression of primary respiratory motion to sense the degree to which the bones 'breathe' intraosseously.

2. MOTION TESTING FOR LIGAMENTOUS BALANCE

A strained joint will permit exaggerated motion in one direction but resist it in the opposite direction.

Permitted motion of a segmental strain can be assessed in all planes, e.g., flexion, extension, sidebending, rotation, axial compression, translation. Note which is the most obvious component.

To test for segmental motion, *encourage movement slowly, staying within the necessarily small ligamentous range. Respect the first hint of resistance rather than taking the segment into the extreme of its range.*

This will make it possible to feel the point of ease within this range of movement where ligamentous tensions are at a minimum, balanced in relation to each other.

In a strained segment this neutral point will be different from the (often central) physiological neutral of a well-balanced articular relationship. However, it is also the point where all components and vectors of the distortion reveal themselves, allowing a diagnostic process to lead into a therapeutic one. The point of BLT will act as a fulcrum around which the innate self-corrective forces are activated, enabling the ligaments to 'guide the joint home'.

The action of natural breathing upon the anterior longitudinal 'ligamentous stocking' shifts the balance fulcrum within the strained joint into the therapeutic phase of realignment.

To further test the resiliency of the spinal tissues, spring upwards (anteriorly) on the supine spine with your fingertips.

Cervical spine
Assessment

C3 to C7 is considered here which, in Sutherland's model, defines the neck proper. The occiput, C1 and C2, which are seen as the cranio-cervical junction, will be addressed in the following section on the transitional areas of the spine.

1. HANDHOLD

Sitting behind the head of the supine patient, place your hands around the back of the neck with your finger pads on the articular pillars, between the medial and lateral musculature.

2. PALPATING INHERENT MOTION

Let your hands be receptive to the movement of each segment in response to the patient's natural breathing, noting symmetry or the lack of it. Take note also of any segment that does not spontaneously move with breathing. Sense tissue quality for aliveness and resilience as your hands also 'listen' for the presence of primary respiratory motion, through the area.

3. TESTING FOR PERMITTED MOTION

Check for tendencies in each vertebra towards flexion, extension, sidebending, rotation, translation, axial compression, etc. Allow a pause between testing each side. The ligamentous range is small, so notice the first point of resistance in each range.

Example: Test for rotation of C3 on C4

1. HANDHOLD

To test for rotation, sitting behind the supine patient's head, place your right index or third finger under the articular pillar of C3, while stabilising the left articular pillar of C4 with the index or third finger of the left hand. Alternatively, a four-finger hold can be used, with bilateral contact on each segment.

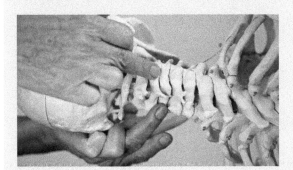

Figure 2.7 C3 on C4 handhold.

2. TESTING ROTATION

Gently encourage the articular pillar of C3 anteriorly on the right, by lifting your finger pad contact towards the ceiling. Sense the first point of resistance to easy motion and then allow the vertebra to return naturally. Compare this with ease and range of motion on the left side, now stabilising C4 on the right.

If C3 rotates more easily towards the left but is restricted towards the right, C3 would be referred to as rotated left. The neutral point for BLT would then be slightly towards left rotation.

TESTING SIDEBENDING

Stabilising the opposite articular pillar of C4, test sidebending of C3 by slowly moving its articular pillars caudad on one side and cephalad on the other. Compare the two sides. The segment will move more willingly *towards* the side of ligamentous restriction.

TESTING FLEXION

Stabilise the articular pillars of C4 bilaterally with your third fingers, while your fourth fingers encourage the articular pillars of C3 anterosuperiorly (towards the head) to find the position of ease for the capsular ligaments, noting ease of motion.

TESTING EXTENSION

With the same finger contact, bilaterally encourage the articular pillars of the inferior of the two vertebrae (C4) anterosuperiorly, i.e., cephalad, keeping the capsular ligaments in mind.

Treatment

Summary: If a segmental relationship is simply supported within its spinal 'stocking', at the 'sweet spot' of ligamentous balance, the action of natural breathing on the ALSL will tend to shift the fulcrum of balanced tension, enabling the joint to spontaneously move towards resolution of the strain. Ways of empowering this process are described below.

Example: C3 rotated left on C4

1. SUPPORTING THE POSITION OF EASE

With a finger pad of your right hand under the right articular pillar of C3, and a left finger pad stabilising the left articular pillar of C4, gently move C3 towards its left rotation, as described for diagnosis.

Note the moment-to-moment ligamentous response. *Rotate C3 only to the point of ligamentous balance. This is not to the extreme of motion or indirect barrier.*

2. THE LIGAMENTS GO TO WORK

Taking the strain out of the ligaments by matching the segmental position as you find it enables them 'to go to work'. As they explore, with your support, they may reveal previously unseen components of the strain, e.g., sidebending, rotation, axial compression, translation, vectorial impact. *Support these components as the ligamentous-articular mechanism searches for the composite balance point and all elements of the 'story' held in the joint are encompassed.* At the point of balanced tension, the ligaments are ideally as balanced around the strained joint position as they would be if the joint were in healthy alignment.

3. WAITING AND SUPPORTING
THE POINT OF BALANCE

At the stillness of the balance point, maintain your support. Be present to the ligamentous stocking and what is contained in the spaces of the segment, e.g., the meninges, spinal cord, nerves and the disc shape between the vertebral bodies. The patient's natural breathing will be working to shift the fulcrum of the joint until inherent ligamentous action releases the strain by actively realigning the bones.

It can be helpful to acknowledge the presence of the spinal cord and how it may be placed within the spinal canal. It too is suspended in a connective tissue network that includes the dentate and Hoffmann ligaments (Martinez Santos and Kalhorn 2021). It is also anchored by the filum terminale and can sometimes be tethered by the upper cervical myodural bridges. *In the upper cervical region include the transition from medulla to spinal cord in the perceptual field.* Does it feel as if the neural tissue encompassed in this space is floated, suspended and perfused with CSF?

The shape of the intervertebral foraminae can also lightly be kept in mind. They provide a conduit, not only for the spinal nerve roots, surrounded by their vasa nervorum, but also the arterial and venous vessels pertaining to the spinal cord.

4. RESOLUTION

When this happens, *continue to support the tissues in their spontaneous reversal of the strain whatever their idiosyncratic path back to resolution.*

5. RETESTING

When retesting the joint, it is natural to take it through its range of free motion, observing changes in tissue quality and mobility. Note any increase in spaciousness, texture, fluid interchange or inherent rhythmic motion, signifying the return of normal physiological activity.

For an alternative handhold that takes in the prevertebral fascial 'tube', include the antero-lateral surface of the neck with the thumbs, staying just lateral to the carotid sheath. This handhold is comfortable and can give a slightly different three-dimensional view. The fascia here may be tender when the mucous membranes are dry or inflamed in sinusitis.

Empowering the process
1. Engagement and use of forearm fulcra

The engagement of ligamentous activity is enhanced by leaning a little weight through your forearms as fulcra. This action seeks to 'match' the forces holding the pattern within the tissues, especially the ALSL, to activate innate therapeutic potency.

A suggestion by Rollin Becker DO was to *try putting, first more, then less of your weight through your fulcra. Between too much and too little fulcrum engagement, the moment when the tone and position of the tissues are matched, is indicated by a sudden increased sense of aliveness. It is as if the ligaments then actively explore for refinement of the balance point* (Becker 1989).

2. Further activation by
approximation or disctraction

To further awaken the intervertebral ligaments, *add a little axial approximation or distraction. To tune your finger proprioceptors and increase your palpatory engagement, try toning the flexor digitorum profundus muscles of your forearm.*

To engage structures that are deeper in the body, stronger forearm fulcrum application is needed than for superficial structures; for instance, more leaning into the fulcra is required to match the forces held in the ALSL than for matching the spinous processes; matching the forces held in the crura may need more still.

3. Respiratory cooperation

Thoracic inhalation tends to straighten the spinal curves while exhalation increases cervical and lumbar lordosis and thoracic kyphosis. This can be applied usefully, by the patient's active inhalation or exhalation, for augmenting and matching the flexion or extension patterns of a spinal segment or group.

A cervical extension pattern, for example, may be augmented by asking the patient to exhale as long as possible. The final inhalation assists the positional resolution of the strain. Conversely, for a cervical flexion strain, the patient may be asked to assist by holding inhalation. The reverse respiration is applied for naturally kyphotic areas, e.g., the thoracic spine.

4. Postural cooperation

The patient's postural cooperation may be enlisted to focus the balance point by bringing a larger area of the body to bear upon it:

SIDEBENDING PATTERN

If the patient is asked to raise the right shoulder towards the ear, the neck will slightly sidebend to the right and the thoracic spine will slightly sidebend towards the left. If, for instance, C3 is sidebent right, once a point of BLT is found, slight raising of the right shoulder helps to focus the balance point and amplify its potency. For clear instruction, ask the patient to *slowly raise* the right shoulder towards the ear, *just to the point of ease*, as perceived by the operator.

ROTATION PATTERN

If C3 is rotated right, the patient can assist in matching the strain by either turning the eyes to look right or slowly turning the head to the point of ease, as registered by the operator.

FLEXION OR EXTENSION PATTERN

Raising both shoulders towards the ears tends to increase lordosis (extension) in the cervical spine and increase kyphosis (flexion) in the thoracic spine. When both shoulders are lowered, all the spinal curves tend to straighten. This may be actively applied as described for the patterns above.

COMPLETION

When a sense of tissue change and reorganisation happens, the patient is asked to reverse all postural and respiratory cooperation.

Ideally the 'key lesion' holding the strain pattern of the neck is sought. Where there is a complex pattern of sequential injuries, it may be necessary to release several segments in turn. Where chronic strains have led to fibrosis, resolution of an intervertebral strain will often, over time, help to rehydrate the soft tissues enabling fibrosis to resolve.

LC muscle

Where the LC muscle is involved in stiffness and loss of cervical kyphosis, a simple manoeuvre may relax it and enable it to regain its lordosis (see Chapter 16).

Thoracic spine

Problems in the thoracic spine sometimes offer the key to those in the neck since the T4 area may be viewed as the baseline for the neck and of the whole unit of function of all that is above it, including the shoulders and arms.

Assessment

When diagnosing the thoracic spine, check rib movement and costovertebral relationships. If the ribs are impinging on the spinal demifacets this may need resolution first. The thoracic kyphosis normally spans from C5 to L3.

1. PRELIMINARY OVERVIEW

View the spinal pattern as a whole, noting in which direction the vertebrae move easily and where there is resistance, individually and as a group. Ideally, examine in different positions to see which patterns are consistent.

2. PALPATION

Sit beside the supine patient, with fingertips contacting the thoracic spinous processes, and assess the quality of inherent motion, both as a whole and segmentally. As above, note which segments are naturally moved by the patient's breathing and which are not, and how patterns are exaggerated on either respiratory phase.

The thoracic spine is where the sympathetic nervous system is most expressive and accessible, so observe signs of segmental facilitation, e.g., local sweating, bogginess, red response, hardness, for comparison before and after treatment. Acknowledge the sphere of influence of the area under your hands, with its specific visceral and somatic neural pathways. *Accept that your hands are receptive to information from the whole ligamentous stocking and associated nerves, blood vessels and organs.*

3. HANDHOLD FOR MOTION TESTING

If working from the side of the supine patient, contact adjacent spinous processes with your fingertips. Move them towards and away from you, cephalad and caudad etc., to test for ease in rotation, flexion, extension and sidebending. Keep in mind that the vertebral body will move in the opposite direction to the spinous process, whether in flexion, extension, rotation etc.

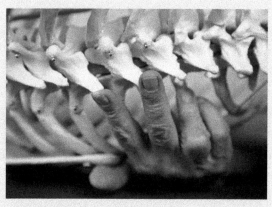

Figure 2.9 Supine thoracic finger hold on skeleton (single hand).

As the thoracic spinous processes can be unreliable for locating their corresponding vertebral body, it is sometimes preferable in the upper thoracic spine *to sit behind the supine patient's head, placing the fingertips of each hand on the transverse processes of adjacent vertebrae.* The thoracic spine is then motion tested similarly to the neck, the difference being that for the thoracic spine, contact in this position is on the transverse processes rather than the articular pillars.

Extension can also be checked by lifting the thoracic segments of the supine patient anteriorly. *Assess resiliency by springing your fingers towards the ceiling. Check for axial compression by approximating the segments.*

Treatment

The principles of engagement and treatment for the thoracic spine are similar to those described for the neck. The activation of the ligaments through use of the forearm fulcra and of postural and respiratory cooperation are equally useful here. Respiratory and postural cooperation are adapted to the kyphotic thoracic curve in contrast to those used for the cervical lordosis. This means that a flexed thoracic segment can be augmented by the patient holding exhalation, and an extended one by holding inhalation. An extended area or segment can also be augmented by lowering the shoulders, and a flexed one by raising the shoulders.

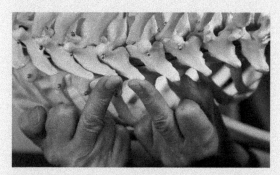

Figure 2.8 Supine thoracic finger hold on skeleton (two hands).

Supine balancing of thoracic group

Sensing the spine as whole organ, sit beside the supine patient with your forearms as fulcra on the table. Take the two ends of the thoracic spine, supporting the spinous processes on your fingertips, and suspend it from the ALSL as if holding a clothes line. Add a little axial compression until a sense of flow returns.

If there is a sense of discontinuity or strain between the upper and lower thoracic groups, support the areas immediately above and below the point of break in the curve. Approximate the two areas with a little axial compression to alter the strained fulcrum between them. This provides an opportunity for the ligaments to reorganise the segmental strain and regain continuity to integrate the thoracic curve.

Paraspinal muscle inhibition

Paraspinal inhibition was used frequently by A.T. Still (Hildreth 1942) and by the early osteopaths such as J.M. Littlejohn (Wernham 1975, 1999). The aim, through relaxing the spinal muscles, is to calm the facilitated segmental reflexes. This can have the effect of freeing intervertebral movement and calming sympathetic activity (see Chapter 16).

Lumbar spine (supine)

1. HANDHOLD AND EXAMINATION

The lumbar spine may be examined as described for the cervical and thoracic areas.

Sitting to the side of the supine patient, hold the tips of the sturdy lumbar spinous processes of adjacent vertebrae between the third and fourth fingertips of each hand. Single fingertips may also be used.

In a flexed segmental relationship, the spinous process of the superior of the two vertebrae will easily move cephalad. In an extended one, the inferior of the two will move cephalad.

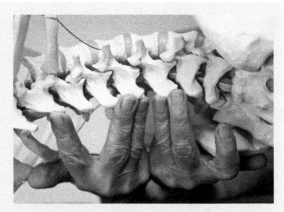

Figure 2.10 Lumbar spine supine contact.

If there is barely any movement in any direction, try approximating them by pushing the vertebrae together to match and relax any element of axial compression. Even if there is only a hair's breadth of movement in any direction, this is often sufficient to 'open the door' to the expression of other components of the strain, revealing the directional forces locked in the joint. Think of the ligaments as the 'power agents' with the vertebrae as secondary, suspended in the spinal stocking.

2. MATCHING THE BALANCE POINT

Support the segment in its position of balanced tension for all components of the strain, observing the respiratory action of the crura on the ALSL, until the joint fulcrum shifts and the strain resolves.

This is palpable, not only through spontaneous realignment of the segment but also a renewed rhythmic expression and lengthening, often with improvement of the natural lumbar curve.

3. POSTURAL AND RESPIRATORY COOPERATION

To empower the balance point, a lumbar segmental flexion strain may be augmented by asking the patient to dorsiflex the feet and inhale; vice versa for extension. Reversal of the strain often coincides with the moment that the patient can hold the breath no longer.

To empower the balance point for a sidebending strain, the patient can lift one hip to the point that matches the strain. For rotation, the patient can turn the head in the direction of the rotated segment. All elements of postural cooperation are returned to normal at the end of the procedure.

Balanced tension in direct action

If 'the gentle exaggeration of the lesion' is not yielding any response, direct action for derotation of a lumbar vertebra may prove effective. *Sit beside the patient, hooking your fingers round the relevant lumbar spinous process. Initially, take the segment or group to the position of ease to take the strain out of the ligaments. Then, keeping the original notochordal midline 'blueprint' in mind, steadily hold it towards you in the direction of derotation, precisely matching its resistance and wait for easing.* This quiet insistence could be called the 'I am not going away until you budge' technique. Maintain your hold until the tissues yield and reposition.

In juvenile functional scoliosis, direct action may be applied on one or more spinal groups. *Sit at the side of the supine patient's spinal concavity. Hook the fingertips of both hands around the spinous processes, to encompass as much of the sidebent and rotated group as possible. Gently but steadily hold the spinous processes towards you, matching the resistance at the motion barrier. Wait, as each thoracic respiration works on the ALSL to gradually allow the curve to yield a little.* This may be repeated weekly and parents can also be taught how to continue between sessions.

Lap technique for lumbar spine

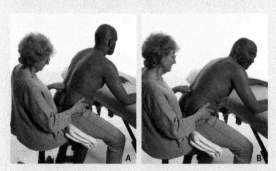

Figure 2.11A & B Lumbar lap technique.

If it is either too painful or difficult to lie down, this approach to the lumbar spine is especially useful, following the lap technique for reseating the sacrum (see Chapter 3). This is also useful to encompass the often complex components of a scoliosis, as it is equally applicable to the thoracic spine.

The main drive here comes from the patient's postural cooperation where his or her active postural flexion, extension, sidebending or rotation matches the ligamentous balance for the state of strain in the lumbar segment addressed. The operator's hands play a secondary role to monitor and also guide the vertebra by contact on the spinous process.

Keep in mind that in the lumbar spine, the superior articular processes of the lower of two vertebrae cup the inferior articular processes of the vertebra above, laterally and anteriorly. This allows the articular facets to glide up and down in relation to each other.

1. POSITION AND CONTACT

Following a preliminary examination, the patient sits on a lap pad on your knees, facing the treatment table. You can localise the field of operation, stabilising the patient's pelvis, either by wrapping a forearm around the anterior superior iliac spine (ASIS) on both sides or holding one ASIS only, on the restricted side. The other hand holds the spinous process of the vertebra being addressed between index finger and thumb.

2. POSTURAL COOPERATION

Flexion strain: *Ask the patient to 'walk' his or her hands forward on the table to the point where this matches the position of ligamentous balance for the strained segment. Hold the spinous process cephalad to match the position of the flexion strain.*

Extension strain: *The patient moves his or her hands forward on the table as above and then 'walks' them back again towards the position of balance for the extended segment. You can further augment the extension pattern by holding the spinous process of the lower of the two vertebrae towards the head.*

Sidebending pattern: *Lift your knee on the side of concavity. Hold the spinous process of the involved segment, to monitor the point when the strain is matched in BLT. The other hand holds the ASIS back on the side of the convexity.*

Rotational component: *Ask the patient to turn his or her head and shoulder towards the side the involved segment has rotated. Sliding one forearm forward relative to the other is also useful.*

3. ACTIVE RESPIRATORY COOPERATION
If respiratory cooperation is needed, to match a flexion segment the patient may inhale and hold until the final exhalation assists resolution of the strain. For an extension strain, the patient exhales and holds.

4. BALANCE AND RESOLUTION
When all these components are gathered in a composite state of ligamentous balance, *support and monitor through your contact on the spinous process.* Pay attention to the front of the ALSL ligamentous stocking, as rhythmic respiratory action on the crura shifts the segmental fulcrum, enabling the ligaments to correct the strain. When you perceive a sense of softening and the beginning of new movement under your hands, the correction has happened at a reflexive level. *The patient completes the reversal of the positional strain by then actively returning to an upright position. Your contact on the spinous process assists this by actively guiding the vertebral realignment in this final stage.*

PART 2: TRANSITIONAL AREAS

'The position of balanced ligamentous tension is the position of health (function) for that segment.'

Anne Wales

The transitional areas of the spine considered here are the cranio-cervical (occiput–C1–C2–C3), cervico-thoracic (C3–T3), thoraco-lumbar (T10–L3), lumbo-sacral (L5–S1) and sacro-coccygeal junctions. The spheno-basilar junction is also an important interface between the sphenoidal and occipital spheres of influence within the cranium, but here Dr Sutherland's approach outside the cranium is explored.

These areas are vulnerable to strain, not only because they coincide with the meeting of mobile and less mobile regions, but also because they are crucial to arteriovenous and lymphatic flow and suspension of the anterior fascial column and visceral organs from the ALSL. (See also Chapter 5 and Chapter 15).

THE CRANIO-CERVICAL JUNCTION

In Sutherland's model, the cranio-cervical junction consisting of occiput, atlas, axis and the articulation between C2 and C3 constitute a 'universal joint' and belong to the cranial sphere, while the neck proper begins at C3.

The occipito-atlantal (OA) joint is structurally adapted for flexion/extension (nodding as in saying 'yes'), the atlanto-axial joint, mainly for rotation (as in saying 'no') with C2/C3 allowing for sidebending (Vigo *et al.* 2020).

The occipital condyles are convex, converging anteriorly and inferiorly to match the concavity of the anterior and inferior convergence of the articular facets of the atlas. The relationship of the occipital condyles to the atlas facets resembles the anterior half of an ellipsoid cone with its long axis transverse. This matches the 'half cup' of the atlas articular facets, functionally forming a single ovoid joint. Another way of visualising this is as pigeon-toed feet in matching slippers.

This arrangement of a 'cone within a cup' predisposes the occipital condyles to becoming compressed in the anterior convergence of the atlas facets with resulting limitation of articular movement. This, in turn, imposes far-reaching limitations through the whole neurospinal axis and potential inhibition of the vertebrobasilar circulation.

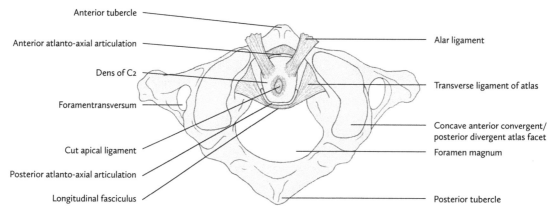

Figure 2.12 Superior articular facets of the atlas, showing anterior convergence/posterior divergence and median atlanto-axial joint.

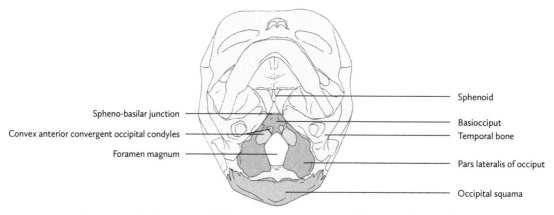

Figure 2.13 Inferior surface of infant cranium showing condylar parts of the occiput.

OA compression can come about through various situations, including the axially compressive and rotational forces of intrauterine moulding and birth, or traumatic impact to the head and sacrum. Collapsing postural habits can also cause the suboccipital muscles to compensate for increased thoracic kyphosis/cervical lordosis or scoliosis.

Falls on the sacrum involve an upward vectorial force that is often absorbed by the OA joint. It has frequently been found that lumbosacral and OA compression occur together and influence each other reciprocally (Sutherland 1998, COT p. 225). For this reason, to ensure the durability of articular freedom of the one, it is wise to check that the other is also free.

Post-partum sacral sag (see Chapter 3, anterior sacral approach) appears to predispose OA compression, dragging on the occiput and intracranial structures via the dural tube and longitudinal spinal ligaments (Sutherland 1990, COT p. 278–283). This tends to draw the cranio-cervical junction together and strains both the PVF and anterior fascial column (see Chapter 5). In the author's experience, meningeal scarring from lumbar puncture, spinal anaesthetic or failed epidural also appear to be occasionally associated with this effect.

Sutherland observed that if the condylar parts have significantly moved anteriorly into the anterior convergence of the atlas facets, this can strain the transverse ligament of the atlas and potentially narrow the antero-posterior (A/P) diameter of the spinal canal. He was concerned by this phenomenon as a consequence of difficult birth (Sutherland 1945).

OA compression is especially common in an infant following difficult delivery because it is at this joint that the compressive and rotational forces of labour tend to converge, from vault, pelvis and laterally. Where there are retained intraosseous strains in the condylar parts of the occiput, the body's inherent forces are sometimes unsuccessful in resolving them until they can move freely within the atlas facets. On palpation there is a sense of narrowing the A/P and transverse diameters of the spinal canal in OA compression. The inherent fluid drive stimulated by crying, suckling and thoracic respiration are Nature's way of resolving these strains to the degree possible.

LIGAMENTOUS ANATOMY

OA joint

The atlas attaches to the cranium via:

- its articular capsules connecting the occipital condyles and atlas facets
- the posterior and anterior atlanto-occipital membranes
- the lateral ligament between its transverse processes and the jugular processes of the temporal bones on the cranial base.

The cranio-cervical junction as a whole

The atlas and axis are the only vertebrae to have their articular processes anterior to the neural arch. In the case of the atlas, this applies to both its superior and inferior articular facets. However, although the axis has a unique morphology when viewed from above, it appears typical when viewed from below in its relationship with C3.

The atlas is the widest vertebra in the spine apart from its equal in the 3rd lumbar. Its vertebral body is largely replaced by the odontoid peg ('dens') of C2, which is suspended from the anterior border of the foramen magnum by the *apical ligament*. This ligament is the only place where the residual cells of the embryological notochord are not surrounded by an intervertebral disc.

The axis has further ligamentous connections with the cranium that bypass the atlas (Dove 1982):

- The *transverse ligament of the atlas* binds the odontoid peg to the anterior arch of the atlas. The *superior cruciate ligament* which is a vertical extension of the transverse ligament connects the axis to the foramen magnum. The *inferior cruciate ligament* connects it with the body of C2.
- The bilateral *alar ligaments* connect the odontoid peg of C2 with the medial borders of the foramen magnum. These allow flexion and extension, e.g., nodding, but limit sidebending and rotation (Offlah and Day 2017).

- The *tectorial membrane*, an upper extension of the PLSL, originates on the intracranial surface of the basiocciput, blending with the dura. It attaches to the posterior surface of the body of the axis, covering the cruciate ligament and bypassing the atlas.
- The cranial dura mater lines the skull and its infoldings between the lobes of the brain that form the falx cerebri, falx cerebelli, tentorium cerebelli and (in infancy) the anterior dural girdle. The spinal dura attaches to the rim of the foramen magnum, bypassing the atlas to attach firmly to the vertebral bodies of C2 and C3. The dural tube continues through the spinal canal to the sacrum, encompassing the spinal cord within its inner leptomeningeal layers of arachnoid and pia mater.
- The rectus capitis posterior minor muscle attaches to the dura at the OA joint, forming a 'myodural bridge'. There are also myodural bridges from the fascia of rectus capitis posterior major and inferior oblique muscles to the cervical dura between C1 and C2. Through this connection, dural irritation can result from force vectors induced by whiplash injury from rear impact (Enix *et al.* 2014).

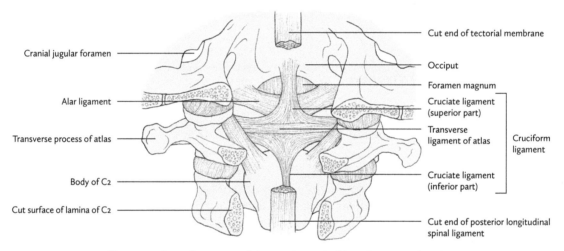

Figure 2.14 Deep ligaments of the cranio-cervical junction, posterior view.

(See Figure 2.2 for the ligamentous relationships of the cranio-cervical junction.)

The axis has a large sphere of muscular attachments connecting it functionally to the skull, the atlas, the rest of the cervical spine, the scapula, the 1st ribs and T1–T5 (Dove 1982).

THERAPEUTIC ENGAGEMENT

OA joint
The operator holds the bolt while the patient turns the nut.

Dr Wales called this manoeuvre for releasing the OA joint 'one of the neatest techniques that Dr Sutherland ever devised because you don't have to take the transverse processes of the atlas into consideration' (Wales 1987). She emphasised that there are no contraindications to it and that it is often advisable to free the OA joint before diagnosing and treating the cranium. She also noted that the postural reflexes in the upper neck are so proprioceptively responsive to any changes in the body or cranium during an osteopathic treatment that the OA joint often needs rebalancing at the end of the session also. In her words, 'Under many circumstances you get a change in the cranial base and the O/A locks up.'

Aim: For normal movement to be restored, the tendency of the OA joint to become locked in the anterior/inferior convergence of the atlas facets requires it to release towards the freedom of the posterior divergence. The flexing of the occiput, while fixing the atlas, draws the condyles towards the posterior divergence.

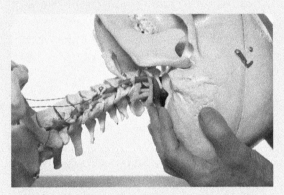

Figure 2.15 Occipito-atlantal joint supine hold on skeleton.

1. HANDHOLD
Sitting behind the head of the supine patient, support the head with the middle ray of one hand, in line with the patient's sagittal line. The tip of your middle finger is as close as possible to the posterior tubercle of the atlas. As this is deep to the suboccipital muscles, it is possible initially only to sense its presence beneath them. It is important to avoid the larger spinous process of C2. The other hand may lightly support the vault or the supraocciput.

2. POSTURAL COOPERATION
For an adult or child old enough to take instructions, *ask the patient to slightly tuck in the chin or 'nod the nose towards the chest'.* This should be just enough to bring the atlas posterior tubercle into more direct contact with your middle finger, but without flexing the rest of the neck.

This action rotates the occiput posteriorly while your middle finger stabilises the atlas, as if 'mentally directing it towards the toes' to prevent it from moving back with the occiput. This posterior rotation of the occiput, relative to the atlas, brings the occipital condyles towards the posterior divergence of the atlas facets. The patient maintains this position until the end of the procedure.

3. HOLDING THE ATLAS AND WAITING FOR RESOLUTION
Wait until after about 30 seconds, when the ligaments will usually yield and rebalance. This allows the occipital condyles to move from their fixity in the anterior convergence to greater freedom in the posterior divergence of the pits of the atlas facets, without carrying the atlas with them.

When this happens, the atlas appears to 'move away' from your stabilising finger.

Other signs that the manoeuvre has been effective are that the suboccipital muscles relax.

4. RESPIRATORY AND POSTURAL COOPERATION
To make this manoeuvre more potent, the patient may inhale and hold the breath and/or dorsiflex the feet.

5. UNILATERAL OA RELEASE
If one side is found to be resistant on completion of the manoeuvre, *it is repeated by asking the patient to dorsiflex only the opposite foot.* This creates a contralateral fluid drive towards the restricted side of the OA joint.

6. RESPONSE

The effects can be surprising. When the condyles regain articular freedom with the atlas, it is as if there is greater intraosseous expression within the occiput. This gives an impression of a change in the spatial environment of the posterior cranial fossa, as if the cerebrospinal fluid cisternae are better able to float the brainstem and cerebellum. There may be an impression of the tentorium cerebelli lifting and the occipitomastoid sutures releasing enough to facilitate cranial venous drainage, with freer passage for the vagus, glossopharyngeal and accessory nerves. Simple OA release has been shown to immediately improve cranial arterial flow (Roberts et al. 2021). (Intraosseous strains of the atlas are described in Chapter 17.)

Atlanto-axial joint (occiput, C1, C2 and C3)

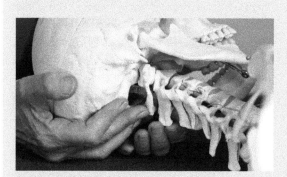

Figure 2.16 C1–C2 supine hold on skeleton.

The axis almost always compensates to OA compression, unilaterally or bilaterally. Because the atlanto-axial joint is an intrinsic part of this functional unit, integration is often needed following release of the OA joint. The axis also has to compensate to prevent scoliotic influences from below from disturbing the horizontal position of the eyes (Dove 1982).

1. OPERATOR POSITION

With the patient supine, sit at the corner of the table 45 degrees to the left side of the patient's head.

2. HANDHOLD

Cup your right hand under the occiput so that the tip of the middle finger supports the arch of the atlas. The left hand cradles the cervical spine with the 5th finger under C2.

3. POSITION OF COMPOSITE BALANCED TENSION

Find the most comfortable and 'easy neutral' position for the patient's head and note the motion pattern at the junction. Also note the position of the occipital condyles within the elliptical half cup of the atlas and any compression on either side. Note any rotational strain between atlas/axis and any sidebending strain between axis/C3.

4. ENGAGEMENT AND LIGAMENTOUS ACTIVATION

If you *add a little tone to your forearm muscles* it becomes easier to feel how the pattern intensifies and begins to seek a resolution for the junction as a whole.

5. RESOLUTION

Honour the stillness of the balance point, followed by the individual path that the tissues take through to resolution of the strain.

This can also be adapted for the seated patient.

(For suboccipital muscle inhibition see Chapter 16.)

Cervico-thoracic junction (C3–T3)

Because so many neck problems originate from the 'baseline' of T3–T4, this transitional area is extremely important for the whole unit of function from T4 upwards, involving upper ribs, thoracic inlet, shoulders and arms.

Considerations to keep in mind

- The ALSL is, as ever, a helpful reference when addressing the integration of this group. The LC muscle, which is prone to becoming hypertonic after whiplash, covers the ALSL anteriorly between C2 and T2.

- In front of that is the *prevertebral fascial sleeve* running unattached to the vertebral bodies between the basiocciput and T3. Anterior to this is the sleeve of the *pretracheal fascia* (PTF) which only connects with the PVF via the carotid sheaths bilaterally.

- Suspended from the pretracheal 'tube' are the aortic arch and the pericardium which are continuous with the central tendon of the diaphragm. When we consider the relationship of these anterior structures to the mechanical balance of this area, it is easy to see why Dr Sutherland recommended taking these into the picture when addressing spinal problems. This is particularly relevant to the short flexion fixation at the CT junction known as the 'dowager's hump', referred to by Sutherland as the 'old age centre' (Sutherland 1998, COT p. 279) (see Chapter 5).

- The sympathetic chain and the stellate ganglion in particular provide much of the sympathetic innervation to the head, neck, arms and part of the upper thorax. This area is also important for drainage of the lymphatics into the venous system (see Chapter 7 and Chapter 15).

The following manoeuvre is useful, either for integration of the whole group or to clear the field to reveal an individual segment needing specific attention.

Engaging C3–T3 as a group

1. HANDHOLD
Sit behind the head of the supine patient, broadly cradling the occiput with the middle ray of one hand, aligned with the sagittal midline of the patient's head. The tip of your middle finger stabilises the occiput/C1/C2. The aim here is to 'localise the field of operation' between C3 and T3 to avoid distraction

from the powerful proprioceptive responses of the cranio-cervical junction (Wales 1995).

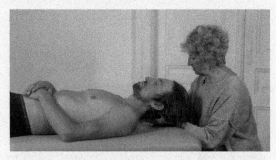

Figure 2.17 C3–T3 live model.

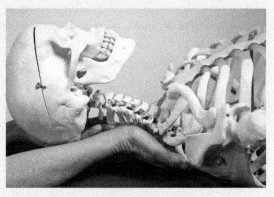

Figure 2.18 C3–T3 supine hold on skeleton.

Your other hand supports C3 to T3 with the middle ray of the palm and third finger under the spinous processes. C3 and C4 rest between the thenar and hypothenar eminences. The shape of your hand moulds to the individual morphology of the patient's cervico-thoracic junction. This enables you to support and encompass every segment between C3 and T3, in the positional state in which you find it, within its spinal stocking.

2. ENGAGEMENT
To match the tone, pattern and force that is holding the strain as one unit, put a little weight through your forearms by moving your lumbar spine forward slightly. This will produce some leverage to slightly lift your wrists and alert your finger proprioceptors, enabling the soft receptivity of the hands to 'meet' the tone of the ALSL through this area.

A precise amount of leverage is met by an enlivened tissue response. *When the internal forces maintaining the strain pattern in the ALSL are exactly matched by your support, it is as if the whole ligamentous stocking in this area starts to actively move, expressing and even exaggerating its pattern and shape.* The vertebral bodies within the stocking reveal their idiosyncratic individual arrangement in a composite state of balanced tension for the spinal group.

It may be surprising how much weight it is necessary to put through the forearm fulcra to match the pattern of this frequently heavily burdened area. For this reason, Rollin Becker advised increasing your leverage very slowly to a point where, between too much and too little support, an enlivening tissue response is perceived (Becker 1989).

3. BALANCE POINT AND RESOLUTION
Maintain unwavering support as the whole vertebral group, under your hand, rests in the stillness of its state of composite balanced tension, until it begins to spontaneously reorganise. This is sometimes accompanied by a sense of upward flow as the area lengthens, untwists and begins to 'breathe' longitudinally. Only then do you withdraw your hands and rest the patient's head on the pillow.

N.B. If either a contracted LC muscle or the PVF are involved, then in addition to matching the tone of the ALSL, it may be necessary to engage more anteriorly to include them. When they are involved in holding the pattern, *your hands may feel as if the tissues 'invite' them to add some axial compression, relieving the strain by drawing them together* (see Figure 2.4, longus colli muscle).

Thoraco-lumbar junction (T10–L3) and crura

The thoraco-lumbar junction is often found to be buckled, both by forces absorbed from the external impact of falls on the pelvis and from diaphragmatic pull of the crura on the ALSL at L1–L3. This is also an area that is subject to torsional strains between the upper and lower body (see Chapter 4, 12th rib, Chapter 5, fascia and Chapter 15, lymphatics.)

This area is potent physiologically, involving vascular, lymphatic, organic, neural and endocrine elements, so be receptive to what peripherally calls your attention as you engage the tissues. This area is strongly affected by fascial drag from the viscera. It can also impose drag on the whole spine from occiput to sacrum when the diaphragmatic crura exert too much tension on the ALSL (Wales 1995).

If this area is compromised by static strain on the arcuate ligaments (lumbocostal arches) attached to the 12th ribs and their association with the quadratus lumborum, TLF and psoas muscles, the 11th and 12th ribs may also need attention.

1. HANDHOLD
Sit beside the supine patient, supporting the spinous processes of T10–L3 with three fingertips of each hand. Note and support any strain pattern in this area, e.g., flexion, rotation, axial compression.

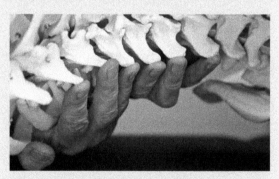

Figure 2.19 T10–L3 supine hold on skeleton.

2. ENGAGEMENT
From your lumbar spine, lean into your forearm fulcra until the force applied through your forearms matches the internal force and pattern, maintaining the strain in this group. Keep the ALSL in mind, as a 'stocking' wrapping the vertebral bodies. Also note

and match any anterior force exerted on the spine by the crura that may be contributing to axial compression, buckling, hyperflexion etc. Retained shock held in the diaphragm can chronically mould this area, sometimes disturbing the development of the spinal curves.

When the ALSL and crura register your *precise matching and consistent support*, there is sometimes a sense of the vertebral group exaggerating its strain pattern. *It is as if an active exploration in the tissues 'invites' your hands to move together to match and mirror a hidden element of axial compression, torsion, sheer or other elements of a pattern that had been previously concealed.*

3. BALANCE POINT AND RESOLUTION
Stay present as the whole T/L group rests at a position of balance within its strain pattern, awake to the reorganisation and realignment that follows. Note any change in the tissues, signifying the return of fluid interchange, axial breathing or lengthening.

Lumbo-sacral (LS) junction
This area is vulnerable to force impact from below through falls and also to downward compressive forces absorbed from lifting injuries. It is subject to static strain from a sedentary lifestyle. Childbirth, whiplash injury, disequilibrium of the spinal curves, loss of resiliency in the arches of the feet, loss of postural tone and many other factors can negatively affect it. It is therefore not surprising that the lower lumbar segments are the most common site of intervertebral disc injuries (see also Chapter 3).

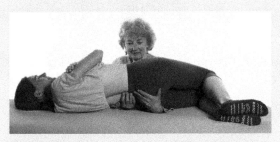

Figure 2.20 Lumbo-sacral junction hold.

1. HANDHOLD
Sitting to the side of the supine patient and facing towards the head, support the sacrum with fingertips on the sacral base and the heel of the hand towards the sacral apex and coccyx. The other hand supports the spinous processes of L3, L4 and L5.

Keep the connection in mind between cranium/ cranio-cervical junction and sacrum via the longitudinal ligaments and ligamentous chains, dural tube and spinal cord wisth its filum terminale as a 'pial tail'. The sacrum also has a reciprocal relationship with the intracranial dura and Sutherland fulcrum (see Key Terms).

2. TESTING FOR EASE OF MOTION
The sacrum is suspended between the ilia by its ligaments. *Motion test for its position of ease, comparing left and right sidebending (A/P axis), rotation left and right (around vertical axis), flexion and extension (transverse axis) etc. Support it in the composite neutral position for all these components.* Note whether it feels dense, hard and dry, denoting intraosseous compression, or whether it is resilient and 'breathing'.

With the fingers of the other hand, test the relationship of the sacrum with L5 and lower lumbars. Move the spinous processes of each segment to check for ease in rotation and sidebending. Move them cephalad and caudad to check for flexion or extension. Approximate L5 and the sacrum to check for axial compression. Support L5, and also L4 and L3, if necessary, in the neutral position for their pattern.

3. ENGAGEMENT
Lean forward slightly from your lumbar spine into your forearm fulcra to provide some leverage through which your two hands are able to engage with the pattern and force that is holding the strain pattern. Aim to match the tone of the ALSL where it merges with the sacral periosteum, acknowledging the shape of the disc spaces between the vertebral bodies. When matched precisely the ligaments are relieved of the strain and can spontaneously refine balanced tension.

In this process, force vectors that have been absorbed, often many years before, may reveal themselves. You may feel your upper hand on the lower lumbars being pulled downwards towards the sacrum, signifying the vectorial resultant of an old lifting injury or head trauma. Conversely you may feel the sacrum tending to move cephalad towards the lower lumbars into a lumbosacral compression pattern that reveals the upward force vector of a past fall on the sacrum.

Acknowledging the intraosseous potential fluid spaces within the five segments of the sacrum, you may become aware of a process of fluid reorganisation within the sacrum, discs and vertebrae as well as their ligamentous-articular relationships.

As always, when treating the spine, observe the shape of the space *between* the vertebrae as the point of orientation of the segment, i.e., of the intervertebral disc and notochordal remnant in the nucleus pulposus.

4. BALANCED TENSION AND RESOLUTION
Continue to support the expression of balanced tension as it finds rest in the resolution point for the opposing forces of the strain pattern. The tissues can then find their own path to resolution of the strain pattern, self-organising and rehydrating.

The sacro-coccygeal junction (sidelying)
This sidelying external approach to the coccyx and sacro-coccygeal junction was shown to this author in 1997 by Brookes Walker DO whose mother was trained by A.T. Still (and whom he met as a very small child). Besides being effective as a balanced tension approach to coccygeal strain patterns, it can have a calming effect on the whole nervous system, central and autonomic, with which it is strategically interrelated.

The tail of the pia mater, i.e., the filum terminale, below the distal end of the spinal cord, attaches to the coccyx, where it blends with the dorsal sacrococcygeal ligament. This makes it a place of remote contact with the central nervous system. Within the second sacral segment is the membranous attachment of the dural tube and the lowest fluid compartment of the spinal canal.

The sacrospinous ligament attaches to the lower two sacral segments, blending with the anterior sacrococcygeal ligaments and appears, in some cases, to contribute to postpartum coccygeal pain. The sacrotuberous and sacrospinous ligaments play a protective role in childbirth in restraining extremes of sacral nutation (see Chapter 3). It is not hard to see how strain and unequal tension between the sacrospinous ligaments could irritate the sacro-coccygeal junction.

The ganglion impar ('coccygeal ganglion') is situated immediately anterior to the sacrococcygeal joint and coccyx and is the meeting place between the two sides of the sympathetic trunk. The sacrum itself carries outflow for the parasympathetic nervous system.

1. HANDHOLD
The patient is sidelying with flexed hips and knees with a pillow between them. *Sitting behind the patient, wrap the palm of your hand around the sacrum, with the third finger around the sacro-coccygeal junction to the tip of the coccyx. Let your fingers mould to whatever positional shape you find it in, e.g., hyperflexion, sidebending, torsion. The other hand can make contact on the spine or occiput.*

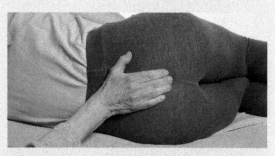

Figure 2.21 Sacro-coccygeal junction sidelying hold.

2. ENGAGEMENT

Just as the ALSL is useful for orientation when treating the spine, so are the anterior coccygeal ligaments when treating the sacro-coccygeal junction.

Acknowledge that the sacrum consists originally of five individual vertebral segments. Engage with these osseous elements of the sacrum and coccyx as fluid systems suspended within their membranous, periosteal and ligamentous web. This approach is also an intraosseous release of the sacrum.

Allow your hands to become receptive to the way the sacrum and coccyx require to be matched, in position and tissue quality, supporting and mirroring the expression of the strain in its various components. This frees the fluid forces within the tissues to seek a resolving point of balance in stillness, from which spontaneous reorganisation emerges.

Prone approach to the sacro-coccygeal junction

The same approach may be applied with the patient lying prone. *The hand cradles the sacrum while the pad of the middle finger contacts the first coccygeal segment and motion tests for the point of balance.*

Sacral intraosseous strains are described more fully in Chapter 17.

VIDEOS FOR CHAPTER 2

Scan the QR code or visit https://www.youtube.com/playlist?list=PL3j_YuMBqigE4AJ22fa7K-M16sja_RaTa to find a playlist of the videos that accompany this chapter.

REFERENCES

Becker, R. (1989) Postgraduate lecture at British School of Osteopathy, London.

Bogduk, N. (1994) Cervical causes of headache and dizziness. *Grieve's Modern Manual Therapy. The Vertebral Column,* 2nd edition. Edinburgh: Churchill Livingstone; pp. 317–331.

Christ, B. & Wilting, J. (1992) From somites to vertebral column. *Ann Anat 174* (1), 23–32. https://doi.org/10.1016/s0940-9602(11)80337-7.

Chu, G., Shi, C., Wang, H., *et al.* (2018) Strategies for annulus fibrosus regeneration: from biological therapies to tissue engineering. *Frontiers in Bioengineering and Regenerative Medicine 6* (90). https://doi.org/10.3389/fbioe.2018.00090.

Cox, J.M., Gorbis, S., Dick, L.M, Rogers, J.C., Rogers, F.J. (1983) Palpable musculoskeletal findings in coronary artery disease: : results of a double-blind study. *J Am Osteopath Assoc. 82* (11) 832-836.

Cunningham, D.J. (1984) *Cunningham's Manual of Practical Anatomy.* Oxford Medical Publications.

de Bree, K., de Bakker, B.S., Oostra, R-J. (2018) The development of the human notochord. *PLoS One 13* (10), e0205752. https://doi.org/10.1371/journal.pone.0205752.

Denslow, J.S., Korr, I.M., Krems, A.D. (1947) Quantitive studies of chronic facilitation in the human motoneuron pool. *Am J Physiol 105,* 229–238.

Dove, C.I. (1982) The occipito-atlanto-axial complex. *Manuelle Medizin 20,* 11–15.

Enix, D., Scali, F., Pontell, M.E. (2014) The cervical myodural bridge, a review of the literature and clinical implications. *The Journal of the Canadian Chiropractic Association 58* (2), 184–192.

Ettlinger, H. (2003) *Foundations for Osteopathic Medicine,* 2nd edition. Philadelphia, PA: American Osteopathic Association/Lippincott Williams and Wilkins; pp. 1118–1119, 1135.

Ettlinger, H. (2017) Personal communication.

Filler, A.G. (2007) *The Upright Ape: A New Origin of the Species.* Hitchin: New Page Books.

Fryer, G. (2016) Somatic dysfunction: an osteopathic conundrum. *International Journal of Osteopathic Medicine 22,* 52–63.

Hildreth, A.G. (1942) *The Lengthening Shadow of Dr. Andrew Taylor Still,* 2nd edition. Paw Paw, MI: A.G. Hildreth & A.E. Van Vleck; pp. 186, 194, 195.

Korr, I.M. (1947) The neural basis of the osteopathic lesion. *The Journal of the American Osteopathic Association 47*, 191–198.

Korr, I.M. (1986) Somatic dysfunction, osteopathic manipulative treatment, and the nervous system: a few facts, some theories, many questions. *The Journal of the American Osteopathic Association 86* (2), 97–102.

Martinez Santos, J.L. & Kalhorn, S.P. (2021) Anatomy of the posterolateral spine epidural ligaments. *Surg Neurol Int 12*, 33.

Offlah, C.E. & Day, E. (2017) The craniocervical junction: embryology, anatomy, biomechanics and imaging in blunt trauma. *Insights Into Imaging 8*, 29–47.

Roberts, B., Makar, A.E., Canaan, R., Pazdernik, V., Kondrashova, T. (2021) Effect of occipitoatlantal decompression on cerebral blood flow dynamics as evaluated by Doppler ultrasonography. *J Osteopath Med 121* (2), 171–179. https://doi.org/10.1515/jom-2020-0100.

Scarr, G. (2018) *Biotensegrity. The Structural Basis of Life,* 2nd edition. Edinburgh: Handspring Publishing Ltd; pp. 76, 85–86.

Slijper, E.J. (1946) Comparative biologic-anatomical investigations of the vertebral column and spinal musculature of mammals. Amsterdam: North-Holland Publishing Co.

Snelson, K. (1968) *Needle Tower.* Hirschhorn Museum, Washington, D.C.

Sutherland, W.G. (1945) *The Hole in the Tree. Condylar Parts of the Occiput.* Mankato, MN: Free Press Company.

Sutherland, W.G. (1971) *Contributions of Thought.* A.L. Wales and A.S. Sutherland (eds). Fort Worth, TX: Sutherland Cranial Teaching Foundation, Inc.; p. 94.

Sutherland, W.G. (1990) *Teachings in the Science of Osteopathy.* A.L. Wales (ed.). Fort Worth, TX: Sutherland Cranial Teaching Foundation, Inc./Rudra Press; pp. 179, 213, 250.

Sutherland, W.G. (1998) *Contributions of Thought,* 2nd edition. A.L. Wales and A.S. Sutherland (eds). Fort Worth, TX: Sutherland Cranial Teaching Foundation, Inc.; pp. 32–33, 225, 278–283, 279.

Switters, J.M. (2021) A splenic cyst causing a viscerosomatic reflex in the thoracic spine. A case report. *Int J of Osteopathic Medicine 20*, 21–25. https://doi.org/10.1016/j.ijosm.2020.10.005.

Tardieu, G.G., Fisahn, C., Loukas, M., *et al.* (2016) The epidural ligaments (of Hofmann): a comprehensive review of the literature. *Cureus 8* (9), e779. https://doi.org/10.7759/cureus.779.

Te Poorten, B.A. (1979) Spinal palpatory diagnosis of visceral disease. *Osteo Ann,* August, 52–53.

Unal, M. & Sezgin, A.B. (2021) Dura mater: anatomy and clinical implication. *J of Behavioural and Brain Science 11* (10), 239–247.

Van Buskirk, R.L. (1990) Nociceptive reflexes and the somatic dysfunction: a model. *The Journal of the American Osteopathic Association 90* (9), 792–809.

Vigo, V., Hirpara, A., Yassin, M., *et al.* (2020) Immersive surgical anatomy of the craniocervical junction. *Cureus 12*, 9. http://dx.doi.org/10.7759/cureus.10364.

Von Lanz, T. (1929) Uber die Rückenmarkshäute. *W. Roux' Archiv f. Entwicklungmechanik 118*, 252–307.

Wales, A.L. (1987) Unpublished paper.

Wales, A.L. (1995) Personal communication.

Weaver, C. (1938) The cranial vertebrae. *The Journal of the American Osteopathic Association,* March.

Wernham, J. (1975) Personal communication.

Wernham, J. (1981) *Yearbook of the Osteopathic Institute of Applied Technique* (later the Institute of Classical Osteopathy). First published by J.M. Littlejohn (ed.). *The Journal of the Science of Osteopathy 1*, 6, 254–255.

Wernham, J. (1999) *The Life and Times of Littlejohn.* Maidstone: John Wernham College of Osteopathy Publishing Company.

Whyte, F.L. (2017) Adolescent idiopathic scoliosis: the tethered spine III. Is fascial spiral the key? *Journal of Bodywork and Movement Therapies 21* (4), 948–971.

Willard, F. (1995) Personal communication.

Willard, F. H, Vleeming, A., Schuenke, M.D., Danneels, L., Schleip, R. (2012) The thoracolumbar fascia: anatomy, function and clinical considerations. *Journal of Anatomy 221* (6), 507–536. https://doi.org/10.1111/j.1469-7580.2012.01511.x.

Woolf, C.J. (2011) Central sensitisation: implications for the diagnosis and treatment of pain. *Pain 152* (3), S2–S15.

Wright, H.M. (1955) Sympathetic activity in facilitated segments: vasomotor studies. *The Journal of the American Osteopathic Association 54* (5), 273–276.

CHAPTER 3

The Pelvis

LYNN HALLER AND ZENNA ZWIERZCHOWSKA

PART 1: ANATOMICAL OVERVIEW

In Sutherland's model there is an 'intimate correlation' between the 'pelvic bowl' and 'cranial bowl' as analogous mechanisms that exert a strong mutual influence (Sutherland 1998, COT pp. 224–225). Osteopathic diagnosis and treatment of the pelvis requires the flexibility to shift between the modes of 'watchmaker' and 'mechanic' (Sutherland 1998, COT p. 160) according to whether the forces of weight bearing or more subtle membranous-articular and intraosseous dimensions are being engaged.

The sacrum takes its name from the Latin *os sacrum* inspired by the Greek *heiron osteon*, meaning 'sacred bone'. In the ancient world it was seen as holy, both because of its role in protecting the genital organs whose sacred function is to house the seeds of new life, and also because of its relative indestructibility in the skeleton after death. This linked it with the idea of resurrection or immortality. This association was also reflected throughout the early Christian, Jewish, Islamic and ancient Egyptian traditions (Ojumah and Loukas 2018).

THE INNOMINATE COMPONENTS

The specialised ligaments of the pelvis unite the two innominate bones with the weight-bearing sacrum behind and the 'tie beam' of the pubic symphysis in front, to form the pelvis into a bony ring. This is transformed into a bowl or basket by the support of the pelvic floor and coccyx ('pelvis' is Latin for 'basin'). It needs to be resilient enough to accommodate to body movements such as walking and running, while being stable enough to support the weight of the spine and body above and protect the foetus in gestation.

This would not be possible without the tensile support of the soft tissues, especially the ligaments. These act in dynamic counterbalance to the compressive forces borne by the bones, and ligamentous proprioceptive responsiveness allows moment-to-moment retuning and adaptation. The pelvis demonstrates the principle of biotensegrity, where the soft tissues provide tensile support and proprioception through continuous tension, while the bones act as discontinuous spacers absorbing compressive forces (Pardeshenas 2014).

The relationship of the pelvis to the lumbar spine, hip joints and lower limbs needs to be approached as one unit of function. The pelvis is adapted to absorb the forces transmitted upwards from the feet via the talocalcaneal joints to hips, sacroiliac (SI) joints, sacrum and lumbar spine. Conversely the upper three sacral segments transmit weight from the vertebral column above through the SI joints, ilia and acetabula to the femora and feet. This transmission of forces, from both above and below, is illustrated in the arrangement of the intraosseous trabeculae which are aligned, not only through the bones, but straight through the hip and SI joints, almost as if ignoring the existence of these joints. The first sacral segment is the largest and has the densest trabecular arrangement, indicating its major weight-bearing function for the sacrum (Diel *et al.* 2001).

Developmentally, the sacrum is formed of five vertebral segments which are initially separated by intervertebral discs. The sacral segments begin fusion from the age of 18 upwards and may complete between 25 and 33 years of age, and sometimes a decade later (Cheng and Song 2003). The ischial, iliac and pubic parts of the innominate bones which meet in a 'Y' shape at the acetabulum fuse between 11 and 18 years, although full replacement of the triradiate cartilage completes between 20 and 25 years of age. The possibility of intraosseous strains in the five-part sacrum and three-part acetabulum should be considered in osteopathic diagnosis and treatment for patients of any age.

In terms of habitual posture, patients may need to be reminded to think of their own sacrum and coccyx as a 'tail' and sit with their weight transmitted through the ischial tuberosities so that the coccyx is suspended between the ischia. This allows balanced weight transmission and, paradoxically, makes use of gravity to strengthen the tensile support of the spinal connective tissue network to give a sense of being uplifted rather than collapsed. There is an increasing tendency, however, to act as if the sacrum and coccyx were weight-bearing structures by sitting slumped backwards. This not only creates interarticular and intraosseous compression of the sacrum, SI joints and coccyx but weakens the tone of the lumbar spine long term.

THE PELVIC LIGAMENTS IN WEIGHT TRANSMISSION

Sutherland perceived the sacrum to be suspended between the ilia, in a similar way to the suspension of the sphenoid from the triangular articulations beneath the frontal bones (Sutherland 1990, TSO p. 23). In a sense, the sacrum hangs its load off the ilia by a flexible tension link. It is suspended from the transverse processes of L5 by the *lateral lumbosacral ligaments* and the lumbosacral extension of the iliolumbar ligaments. L5 itself is suspended from the iliac crests by the ilio-lumbar ligaments in a way that is reminiscent of a suspension bridge.

The *ilio-lumbar ligaments* are crucial to both the bilateral stabilisation of the SI joints and the support of the vertebral relationship to the pelvic ring, to resist forward glide of the sacrum on L5. These ligaments are a strongly thickened part of the thoracolumbar fascia (TLF; paraspinal reticular sheath) covering the quadratus lumborum muscle (Willard *et al.* 2012). They originate on the apex of the transverse processes of L5 and sometimes L4, to attach on the anterior margin of the iliac crest and extend down to the superior surface of the SI synovial capsule (Vleeming *et al.* 2012).

It would be natural to expect that the SI joint, through which all of the load is transferred from the spine on its way to the lower extremity, would be subject to great downward force and therefore need a strong, rigid connection. Yet the sacrum is not wedged between the ilia but held in a ligamentous sling which permits constant play as ligamentous, fascial and muscular tension balances and shifts in response to ever-changing loads being taken up, distributed and released (Armitage 1990; Levin 2007a).

The weight of the spine, transmitted from L5 to the sacral base, is also countered on each side by the strong *SI interosseous ligaments* which stabilise the interlocking surfaces of the SI joints. This action is reinforced by the powerful *short and long dorsal SI ligaments* overlying them posteriorly, together with the *sacrospinous and sacrotuberous ligaments* below.

On standing upright, the lumbosacral angle may become subject to shearing forces. In this position, the lordosis of the lumbar spine, together with the weight of the vertebral column, tends to tip the sacral base forward and rotate the sacral apex and coccyx posteriorly. This tendency is countered by the strong *posterior pelvic ligaments* which suspend the sacrum from above, while the weaker *anterior ligaments* support the sacrum from below like a sling. When standing, the *interosseous SI ligaments* and whole posterior ligamentous sheet become taut, drawing the ilia closer together to lock the auricular surfaces of the SI joints (Grant 1966; Vleeming *et al.* 2012).

The tone of the pelvic floor is also important in restraining the sacral apex from rotating anteriorly beyond physiological limits. This assists the *sacrotuberous and sacrospinous ligaments* and together these indirectly support the lumbar spine in restraining a tendency to hyperlordosis.

Weight bearing through the posterior structures, and also force transmission from the legs and feet, is partially dispersed anteriorly to the pubic arch and the strong ligaments uniting the symphysis. When a person is standing, the symphysis resists the forcing together of the acetabula and pelvic sidewalls. When sitting or falling on the buttocks, it resists being pulled apart as weight is transmitted through the ischial tuberosities. Thus it counterbalances the forces of both distraction and compression (Basmajian 1982; Grant 1966).

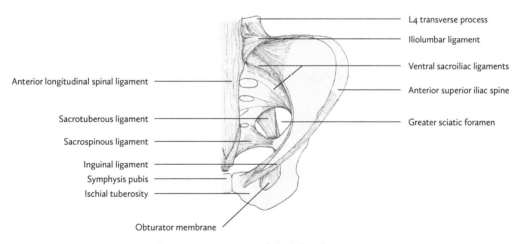

Figure 3.1 Ligaments of the left pelvis, anterior view.

INTERWEAVING OF THE PELVIC LIGAMENTS

Overlying the SI interosseous ligaments, the reinforcing fibres of the *long dorsal SI ligaments* descend vertically from the posterior superior iliac spine (PSIS) to the third and fourth transverse tubercles of the sacrum. Including the wider field we see these ligaments blending above, with the tendinous aponeurosis of erector spinae and TLF, and below, with the biceps femoris tendon and the sacrotuberous and sacrospinous ligaments (Vleeming *et al.* 1996).

The *sacrotuberous ligament*, in turn, blends with the fascia of the obturator internus muscle and provides partial attachment for the pelvic fascia, gluteus maximus, biceps femoris and piriformis muscles.

The *sacrospinous ligament* blends with the *dorsal sacrococcygeal ligament* and coccygeus muscle, transforming the greater sciatic notch into a foramen. Its cephalad end blends with the ventral surface of the SI synovial capsule (Vleeming *et al.* 2012).

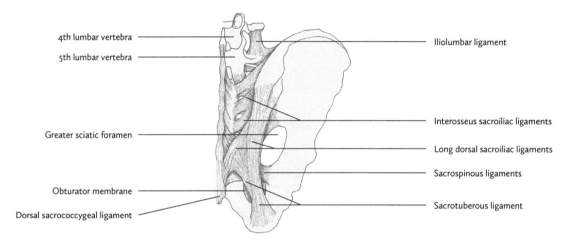

4th lumbar vertebra
5th lumbar vertebra
Greater sciatic foramen
Obturator membrane
Dorsal sacrococcygeal ligament

Iliolumbar ligament
Interosseus sacroiliac ligaments
Long dorsal sacroiliac ligaments
Sacrospinous ligaments
Sacrotuberous ligament

Figure 3.2 Posterior view of pelvic ligaments.

If we consider that it is the proprioceptive response of the ligaments that activates the muscles to react, it is perhaps significant that these important muscles are in direct contact with these powerful ligaments (see Chapter 1).

On the anterior sacral surface are the *iliolumbar, lumbosacral and ventral SI ligaments*. The latter is a smooth sheet of dense connective tissue spanning the ventral surface of the sacral alae and ilium and contributing to the anterior border of the synovial capsule (Vleeming *et al.* 2012).

Although the SI ligaments are named individually, they are functionally continuous sheets posteriorly and anteriorly. This blending and interweaving of the soft tissues can be seen to continue in either and all directions through the body, revealing the mechanism by which loads can be distributed instantly through the body's tensional network (Armitage 1990; Ashby *et al.* 2021).

Symphysis pubis

Anteriorly the pelvic bowl is completed by the union of the two pubic bones at the symphysis pubis. Its ligaments are strong and tightly bind the two sides together. The pubic symphysis is a cartilaginous joint which consists of a fibrocartilaginous interpubic disc (Aslan and Fynes 2007) connected by four ligaments. The superior pubic ligaments span from the superior pubis to the pubic tubercles. The strong arcuate ligaments form the lower border of the symphysis and blend with the fibrocartilaginous disc, maintaining joint stability. The four ligaments together neutralise shear and tensile stresses (Jain *et al.* 2006), but accommodate for limited rotational motion between the pubic bones in walking.

The superior border of the pubic bone provides attachment for the rectus abdominis, pectineus and conjoint tendon (union of aponeuroses of internal oblique and transversus abdominis). The external surface of the pubic bone supports gracilis, adductor brevis, obturator externus and adductor longus muscles.

The obturator membrane

This almost covers the obturator foramen and may be considered an interosseous membrane (IoM) between the ischial and pubic bones. The membrane may be put under stress by intra-osseous strains between the pelvic bones or by tension in the obturator internus muscle, causing discomfort in sitting (see Chapter 16, obturator internus release).

The SI joint

When treating the pelvis, it is useful to keep in mind the different ligamentous layers in addition to the auricular surfaces of the synovial part of the joint.

The SI joint fulfils the need for both movement and stability through the combined action of its anterior and posterior parts. Its anterior synovial part consists of an *'L' shaped 'auricular' articulation*, between the levels of S1 and S3. Its rough interlocking surfaces assist in resisting the downward and forward tendency described above (Bowen and Cassidy 1981; Vleeming *et al.* 1996). The convex iliac surface is covered with fibrocartilage and the concave sacral surface with hyaline cartilage.

The posterior part of the SI joint is a syndesmosis (Kapandji 1974; Williams 1995) whose rough surfaces provide attachment for the many short fibres of the strong *interosseous ligament* between the two bones. The joint is further strengthened posteriorly by the long and short dorsal SI ligaments.

MOVEMENT OF THE SACRUM BETWEEN THE ILIA

Sutherland drew attention to a small but significant anteriorly convergent area at the level of S2, where a curved ridge on the auricular surface of the ilium corresponds to a groove on the sacrum. In the words of Howard Lippincott, 'This arrangement of the ligaments is such that the sacrum can swing between the ilia along the line of those ridges without materially changing the tension', as it rotates around a horizontal transverse axis of motion through the lamina of S2 (Sutherland 1990, TSO p. 251).

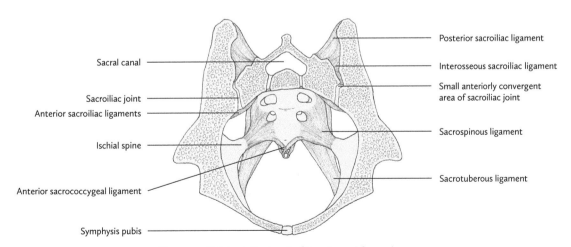

Figure 3.3 Pelvis at the level of S2, viewed from above.

In Sutherland's model of the craniosacral mechanism (see Key Terms), the sacrum is seen as expressing a rhythmic and very fine biphasic rotatory motion synchronously with the rotation of the sphenoid within the cranium. He saw the 'core link' of the intracranial and intraspinal dura connecting the two as an expression of what he referred to as the 'primary respiratory mechanism' (PRM) (Sutherland 1990, TSO p. 251). This involuntary motion is not limited to the inter-articular framework but expresses itself through the extracellular matrix (ECM) of the whole body.

W.G. Sutherland made a clear distinction between the postural movement of the ilia on the sacrum and the involuntary or 'respiratory' motion of the sacrum between the ilia. In his words, 'The involuntary operates through the accommodation of the intraspinal membranes during respiratory periods, and the postural, through the accommodation of the SI and sacrosciatic (sacrotuberous and sacrospinous) ligaments brought about by gravity and indirect leverage' (Sutherland 1998, COT p. 131).

On the so-called 'flexion' or 'primary inhalation' phase of the PRM, the sacral base theoretically rotates posteriorly and its apex anteriorly around its horizontal transverse axis of motion through the lamina/spinous process of S2. On the 'extension' or 'primary exhalation' phase its base rotates anteriorly and its apex posteriorly. On the flexion phase, the sacrum should also rise cephalad as the ilia externally rotate slightly; on the extension phase it descends as the ilia internally rotate (Mitchell and Pruzzo 1971).

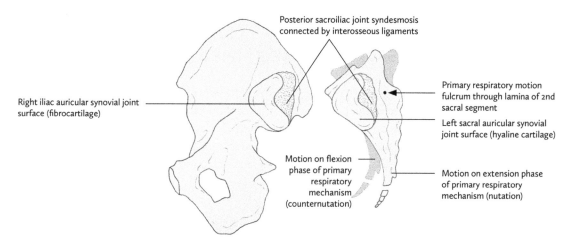

Posterior sacroiliac joint syndesmosis connected by interosseous ligaments

Right iliac auricular synovial joint surface (fibrocartilage)

Primary respiratory motion fulcrum through lamina of 2nd sacral segment

Left sacral auricular synovial joint surface (hyaline cartilage)

Motion on flexion phase of primary respiratory mechanism (counternutation)

Motion on extension phase of primary respiratory mechanism (nutation)

Figure 3.4 Side view of sacral involuntary movement on ilium.

The biphasic primary motion is not explicable in terms of any muscular forces acting on the sacrum or SI joints. This suggests that this is an involuntary ligamentous-articular mechanism rather than a voluntary neuromusculoskeletal one. The sacrum is also 'membranous-articular' through its relationship to the intraspinal and intracranial dural membrane.

The sacrum and ilia make a similar biphasic movement in response to thoracic respiration, though at a different frequency and not necessarily around the same axis of motion.

The anterior rotation of the sacral base was first referred to as 'nutation' ('nodding') by Kapandji (1974) and its posterior rotation as 'counternutation'. These movements, once again, do not necessarily orientate around the same axis of motion as in primary respiratory motion. Nutation and counternutation theoretically occur around the main accessory SI joint (with its interosseous ligament) at the level of S2 (Bakland and Hansen 2012; Vleeming et al. 2012). This is slightly anterior to the theoretical primary respiratory axis of sacral motion in Sutherland's model.

Since the whole living human body is one functional unit, any disturbed sacral pattern of function, be it compression between the ilia, sidebending/rotation, torsion etc., will be reflected in the whole neurospinal axis, including the cranium, nervous system, anterior fascial column (see Chapter 5), legs and feet. The hip joints are also influenced by the orientation of the acetabula, so any positional distortion of the innominate bones needs to be taken into the picture when addressing any problems of the lower limb.

Where the membranous-articular or ligamentous-articular movements of the pelvis are distorted, the 'geometry of the space', encompassed by the osseous container, inevitably affects the physiology of the contents. This includes visceral position, fascial arrangement and neurotrophic, vascular and lymphatic flow affecting the pelvic organs. Ligamentous-articular strains will also create tensions in the pelvic floor by altering the relationship between the origin and insertion of the pelvic floor muscles and fascia. The drainage function of the venous and lymphatic plexi close to the pelvic floor, which permeate the pelvic organs, is dependent on the rhythmic response of the pelvic floor and sacral plexus to both thoracic and primary respiratory movement of the sacrum and innominate bones.

PART 2: ANTERIOR APPROACH TO THE SACRAL ALAE

'Remember that any cranial strain will affect a sacral strain, and any sacral strain will affect a cranial strain. Therefore, when there is a sacral strain you should think of the effect on the cranium.'

(Sutherland 1990, TSO p. 205)

An 'anterior sacral alae contact technique' described in this chapter is used to resolve what Dr Sutherland referred to as a 'bilateral antero-inferior displacement of the sacrum between the ilia' or 'depressed sacrum' (Lippincott 1965). Sutherland was one of the first osteopaths to acknowledge the mechanical effect and full significance of this problem (Lippincott 1958) which he descriptively referred to as 'Sacral Sag' (Sutherland 1998, COT p. 286).

In this approach the osteopath stabilises the ilia via the legs of the seated patient, setting up the conditions for the ilia to glide free of the sacrum. With the operator's assistance, the patient's active postural and respiratory action is then able to lift and reseat the sacrum. This is a powerful and specific procedure which, where indicated, has sometimes proved helpful for lifting the spirits in addition to the sacrum, especially postpartum. Dr Sutherland's saying that 'Fascial drags and sacral sags make chronic rags' describes his observation of the potential somatico-psychic effect of sags of the sacrum which he viewed as 'a disturbing factor leading to mental complications' (Sutherland 1998, COT p. 285).

He devised this procedure after an 'obstetric mission' when he was called out to a rural patient who was giving birth at home. He was delayed by a broken axle on his buggy on a muddy track, so he mounted one of the horses and led the other. About a mile from the farm he met the woman he had come to see walking along the road, having already given birth. In his own words he 'noticed immediately the disturbed or irrational state of mind that occasionally follows birth delivery'. He persuaded her to sit on the horse he was leading and accompanied her back home. By the time they arrived the woman's 'state of mind had changed from irrational to normal during that eventful ride' (Sutherland 1998, COT p. 286).

Many would have simply been relieved and left it at that but, being a true student of A.T. Still, he needed to understand the cause. On consideration of this mysterious event, he surmised that her sacrum had sagged during labour, creating fascial and dural drag through her body, resulting in a membranous articular strain in the cranium. He concluded that this must have caused the tentorium cerebelli to lock the cerebellum down on the brainstem, 4th ventricle and cisterna magna (Sutherland 1998, TSO p. 205).

If all these factors were indeed involved, it is not difficult to see how this contributed to her distraught state. Recent studies suggest a connection between 'brain sag' and cognitive dysfunction (Robeson et al. 2012; Sugiyama et al. 2022) and also the role of the cerebrospinal fluid (CSF) in clearing the brain of toxic metabolic byproducts (Iliff et al. 2012; Mollgard et al. 2023; Wicklund et al. 2011).

But how had she recovered? He concluded that, seated on the horse, the fixation of her ischia had freed the ilia in relation to the sacrum, while the rhythmic movement of the walking horse also fluctuated the CSF, enabling the sacrum to reposition (Sutherland 1998, COT p. 286). In analysing this surprising event he considered how the forces involved in his patient's recovery might be applied therapeutically. He saw that 'sacral sag' could be corrected from the front: 'Therefore an anterior approach to the alae of the sacrum, in an operation that would hold the ilia or turn them laterally while the operator pushed, was devised' (Sutherland 1998, COT p. 286).

APPLIED ANATOMY

The dynamic stability of the sacrum and lumbar vertebrae is dependent on the tone of the ligaments and fascia which guide and support the bony articulations of the pelvis, while also playing an important role in evoking appropriate muscle response. The precise position of the sacrum between the ilia plays a key role in sacral mobility, as well as the overall integrity of the pelvis (Kiapour et al. 2020).

Sutherland perceived the sacrum to be suspended between the ilia from above by the L-shaped articulations and strong SI and iliolumbar ligaments. The posterior SI ligaments limit the downward and forward tilt of the sacral base in response to the weight transmitted from the lumbar spine when standing. The sacrum is supported from below by the 'sling' of the anterior SI ligaments. The sacrospinous and sacrotuberous ligaments also play an important role in drawing the sacral apex forward and countering the tendency for the weight of the spine from above to tip the sacral apex posteriorly to an unphysiological degree. This balanced tension is key, both in weight bearing through the hips and in providing a platform for support and tensegrity of the spinal column above (Levin 2007b) (see Part 1: Anatomical overview).

Because the sacrum's ligamentous support is weaker anteriorly than posteriorly, when strained, it has a tendency for its base to rotate more antero-inferiorly than posteriorly. Hyperlordosis of the lumbar spine or lack of abdominal tone can augment this tendency, as can the posture of late pregnancy with its large anterior load and ligamentous laxity. The process of giving birth especially involves a strong degree of anteroinferior sacral rotation (nutation), as described below, but ideally only for the duration of labour and delivery itself.

INVOLUNTARY ROTATION OF THE SACRUM

In Sutherland's model of the craniosacral mechanism, PRM of the sacrum between the ilia expresses biphasic anterior and posterior rotation about a transverse axis through the laminae or spinous process of S2. As a membranous-articular mechanism, in the primary inhalation ('flexion') phase the sacrum should lift slightly cephalad, while the base rotates posteriorly and the apex anteriorly as in counternutation. The reverse motion happens on primary exhalation ('extension' or 'nutation'). A similar motion, on a larger scale, is expressed during thoracic inhalation and exhalation. On a different scale again, this pivoting action also happens in postural movements such as sitting, standing or bending and especially in labour and delivery.

To allow for this minute physiological rotation the 'fit' of the 'L' shaped auricular surfaces of the sacrum with the ilia is necessarily precise and firmly supported by the ligaments. The sacrum's 'L' shaped auricular surfaces flare anteriorly to match the corresponding surfaces of the ilia. Sutherland, however, drew attention to the significance of 'a small anteriorly convergent area at the level of S2. Here a groove on the sacrum corresponds to a curved ridge on the auricular surface of the ilium.' This tiny interlocking arrangement allows the sacrum to 'swing within limits between the ilia along the line of those ridges without materially changing the tension' (Sutherland 1990, TSO p. 251).

DISTURBANCE OF NORMAL MOTION

In most injuries affecting the pelvis and sacrum that involve a ligamentous articular strain, the articulation remains within or only slightly beyond its normal range of motion. What is different about the depressed sacrum or 'sacral sag' is that the sacrum has become displaced anteriorly and inferiorly beyond its physiological limits. This puts undue strain on the SI ligaments. The horizontal axis of rotatory motion of the sacrum between the ilia becomes displaced from the laminae of S2 to the sacrotuberous and sacrospinous ligaments (Sutherland 1990, TSO p. 251). The axis of motion may also be simply shifted forward to the vertebral body of S2. In either case, when this happens the sacrum actually *descends on* primary or thoracic inhalation instead of rising. Deprived of normal rhythmic cephalad rising of the sacrum between the ilia, a downward drag is exerted on the body above, through the anterior fascial column, the long ligamentous stocking of the spine

and the whole dural tube to the cranium (Sutherland 1998, COT pp. 278–283) (see Chapter 5).

> 'This, then, becomes the axis in which the sacrum rotates anteriorly and downward in relation to the ilia and the whole sacrum except the apex is depressed, violating the normal transverse axis. Consequently, in addition to anterior rotation to the extreme limit of its range, the sacrum will be in an unphysiological relationship to the innominates. The little prominence will be removed from its niche, the groove will not fit the ridge, and none of the irregularities of the articular surfaces will mesh properly with their counterparts on the surfaces of the ilium. Also, the ligaments of the joint will be under severe strain. This constitutes a downward dislocation of the sacrum between the ilia, even though it may be slight in amount in many cases.' (Lippincott 1965)

PHYSIOLOGICAL IMPLICATIONS

Destabilisation of the pelvis, especially post-partum, will affect the ability of the pelvic floor to support the sacrum from below, with both mechanical and physiological implications. The extensive lymphatic and venous plexi that rest on the pelvic floor depend, for efficient drainage, on the support of physiological motion of the sacrum and pelvic floor. Circulatory and lymphatic stasis predispose the local tissues to passive congestion, while loss of tone and organisation of the endopelvic fascia diminishes support for the pelvic viscera (Roch *et al.* 2021). These factors may contribute to the functional problems in bladder, uterus and bowel that sometimes follow difficult obstetric delivery. If tensegrity is not restored, the altered pelvic shape may lead to progressive loss of tone in the pelvic fascia and ligaments and a predisposition to pelvic organ prolapse.

The sacral plexus is formed by the spinal nerves exiting the foramina of L4–S4 and sits on the anterior surface of the sacrum. Increased angulation of the lumbosacral junction or anterior displacement of the sacrum (sacral sag) may compromise the sensory and motor innervation to the pelvis, genitals and lower limbs by mechanically stressing the vasa nervorum and nervi nervorum of the plexus. Effects may extend to the tibial and fibular branches of the sciatic nerve. The pudendal nerve (S2, S3, S4) may be compromised in its passage through the pudendal (Alcock's) canal, formed within the fascia of obturator internus. When damaged, this may be implicated in urinary incontinence, pudendal neuralgia or sexual dysfunction (Beco *et al.* 2004; Vancaillie *et al.* 2012). In practice the motion pattern of the sacrum should be checked in anyone suffering from depleted vitality, lower back pain, brain fog or problems with prostate, bladder, rectum or erectile dysfunction. Sacral sag has also been found, on occasion, to be a key factor impeding resolution of otherwise inexplicable foot pain.

CAUSES OF SACRAL SAG

The most common cause of 'sacral sag' appears to be either a long and difficult labour or sometimes a very fast one. However, this is not limited to the effects of pregnancy and labour as it can affect men, women or children. The sacrum can be displaced antero-inferiorly by lifting heavy objects while bending forward with the legs spread wide apart. Sit-down falls where the impact goes equally through both legs or ischial tuberosities can create a similar downward displacement, wedging the sacrum between the ilia. Occasionally, sacral sag can be the result of a force vector from a fall on the vertex.

Sacral sag can be found in both men and women experiencing depression. Sometimes it is difficult to discern whether the cause is somatico-psychic or psycho-somatic, as it also appears that sacral sag can occasionally happen purely as an expression of depression where both the body and psyche have lost their sense of 'lift'.

Factors associated with labour and delivery

In a normal second stage of labour, the innominates change from flaring superiorly to flaring inferiorly, widening the space between the ischia. Meanwhile the sacrum rotates towards a nutation position with the base tilting forward and the apex and coccyx posteriorly. Together, these adaptations spatially increase the pelvic outlet for emergence of the baby's head. A problem arises only when the sacrum is unable to spring back into its normal apposition to the ilia when delivery is complete.

Higher levels of relaxin, oestrogen and progesterone in pregnancy permit a necessary increase in ligamentous laxity (Kumar andMagon 2012). In a prolonged second stage of labour, exhaustion also can result in diminished ligamentous resilience. If intervention is needed from ventouse or forceps, excessive downward traction may transmit its force to the uterus and through the sacro-uterine ligaments to the sacrum. These appear to be contributory factors in anteroinferior sacral displacement and associated ligamentous strain. If, however, labour is overly quick and the delivery 'explosive', the ilia may spring back quickly around the sacrum on delivery. If this happens before the sacrum has spontaneously returned to its normal position, it may become caught in 'sacral sag'.

Although potentially effective at any stage, osteopathic examination and treatment should ideally be available as soon as possible after birth, when experience has shown that there is a special window of opportunity to easily reverse pelvic strain patterns. This may minimise any possible long-term effects of fascial drag affecting the psyche and body as a whole.

Where postpartum depression is involved, there may also be other contributory factors including past or present mental or physical stresses, social circumstances, financial worries, etc. As osteopaths our particular role is to assist the resolution of any physical component, while other professional support may also be necessary alongside.

DIAGNOSIS OF THE 'ANTERIOR SACRUM' OR SACRAL SAG

A visual impression of postural collapse often accompanies sacral sag because of the weight imposed by an anchored sacrum on the whole fascial and dural continuum. There are several other especially useful indicators for an anterior sacrum or sacral sag:

- On physical examination the posterior SI ligaments may feel loose and boggy while the sacrotuberous and sacrospinous ligaments are under greater strain and may be tender on palpation. The PSIS may be prominent with deep sulci, and the sacral base angled anteriorly. The sacrum may feel hard and dry, lacking the fluid sense of intraosseous 'breathing' that healthy bone expresses. These signs are variable.
- On either primary respiratory inhalation (flexion) or thoracic inhalation, check to see whether or not the sacrum rises cephalad, because in true sacral sag there is no independent rising cephalad of the sacrum between the ilia. This may give an impression of the sacrum as an inert anchor against which the rest of the body has to exert effort to attain any sense of uplift or defiance of gravity. On occasion it may even give the impression of actually descending on the flexion phase as a result of the axis of motion having shifted anteriorly from the lamina to the body of S2.
- As the patient bends forward as if to touch the toes, the sacrum does not demonstrate an easy cephalad lift between PSIS points which also fail to widen.

THERAPEUTIC ENGAGEMENT

Anterior approach to the sacral alae

Sutherland discovered in 1919, when he handled Virgil Halladay's seated ligamentous-articular dissection of the pelvis and spine, that femoral *adduction caused the ilia to rotate anteriorly while causing the sacral base to rotate posteriorly, widening the pelvic diameter* (Sutherland 1998, COT p. 287). In the following procedure, adduction of the patient's thighs, through the action of the operator's knees, will apply this principle to increase the space between the ilia superiorly and posteriorly and posteriorise the sacral base. 'The ischia can function as fulcra to allow a lateral gliding away by the ilia from the sacral alae' (Sutherland 1998, COT p. 286). Thus the patient is then able to lift the freed sacrum and reseat it between the ilia, restoring stability.

This helps to restore its normal mobility and motility, with benefit to the stability of the pelvis and its contents. Since 'sacral sags' usually occur together with 'fascial drags' through the whole body, it is beneficial to check the free movement of the anterior fascial compartments and cranium. These often benefit from being addressed following the procedure (see Chapter 5).

Clarity of explanation and permission

An explanation as to why this approach is appropriate is helpful in gaining the patient's permission. Clear instructions are also important so the patient knows what to expect and what to do. It is advisable to demonstrate or rehearse the required actions in advance.

1. PATIENT AND PRACTITIONER POSITIONING

Sit well-grounded facing the patient, who sits on a plinth slightly above you. The patient should allow the weight to be borne through the ischial tuberosities which will act as fulcra for the positioning of the ilia. Place your knees laterally to the patient's knees.

2. HANDHOLD

Ask the patient to place both hands or forearms on your shoulders.

With your thumbs in line with your straight arms to avoid straining them, reach forward and place your palms over the patient's iliac crests, advancing them so that your thumbs rest just anterior to the insertion of quadratus lumborum.

Then roll your thumbs over the medial surface of the iliac crests as deep as comfortably possible onto the fascia, internal to the iliac crests. If the patient lifts one side of the pelvis and then the other, this will help your thumbs to enter this space more easily.

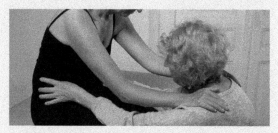

Figure 3.5 Anterior approach to sacral alae.

3. 'PLACING THE GLOVE OVER THE HAND RATHER THAN THE HAND INTO THE GLOVE'

Avoid pushing your thumbs into position as this will meet resistance from your patient's abdominal muscles. Further postural cooperation is helpful:

- *Ask the patient to drop the head, slump forward and lean into your thumbs, thus folding the tissues over them.*

    This allows you to drop your thumbs downwards to advance closer to the sacral alae without patient discomfort.

- *You lean forward also, with your arms straight, matching your weight to that of the patient, so that you are each mutually and effortlessly supported. Continue to lean some of your weight towards the posterior ilia, so as to prepare them to be able to glide slightly laterally away from the sacral alae.*

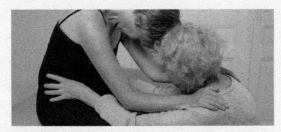

Figure 3.6 Anterior approach to sacral alae.

4. GAINING DEEPER CONTACT

The patient may be asked to sit back while keeping the head dropped. Meanwhile, you move forward towards him or her, advancing your thumbs to keep the contact you have already made, close to the alae.

Maintain your thumb position as the patient again leans forward into your thumbs, slumping towards you as you match each other's weight as before.

This may be repeated several times, so that a progressively deeper but comfortable contact closer to the sacral alae can be achieved each time.

5. A PAUSE WHILE THE TISSUES BALANCE

Continuing to lean against each other, read the tissues and wait for a sense of relaxation and balancing through the fascia and ligaments of the posterior pelvis and sacral alae. The patient's natural breathing assists this. There often comes a moment of stillness indicating that the system is ready for the final positional correction.

6. CORRECTIVE ACTION OF THE OPERATOR

To flare the ilia, allowing them to rotate anteriorly while the sacral base rotates posteriorly, adduct the patient's femurs by bringing your knees together around his or her knees. Maintain this position until after the end of the manoeuvre.

7. THE PATIENT'S ACTIVE LIFTING AND POSTERIORISING OF THE SACRAL BASE

As you continue to hold the ilia, the patient is asked to exhale fully and then to breathe in, sit back and sit tall, this time straightening the head and neck. The lumbar spine should roll back from the base rather than being extended.

The patient's in-breath assists the lifting and posteriorising of the sacral base as he or she pivots on the ischial tuberosities. You may feel the turning of the sacrum.

As the patient moves away from you, it is important that you try to maintain the same matching contact with the posterior ilia/sacral alae that you had before the patient began to sit up straight. At the same time your thumbs gently, but firmly, maintain the lateral flaring of the posterior ilia.

8. RESEATING OF THE SACRUM

On exhalation the patient reseats the sacrum between the ilia by sinking back down with the weight falling vertically through the ischial tuberosities.

You maintain adduction of the patient's femurs by your continuing to hold their knees together with your knees until the sacrum has fully settled between the ilia.

Dr Sutherland said, 'This is where you are backing the car into the garage', the 'car' being the sacrum and the 'garage' being the space between the ilia.

The aim of restoring the integrity of ligamentous and fascial relationships within the pelvis is to give lift to the lumbar vertebrae and a balanced platform for the hips, resetting proprioceptive feedback in the pelvis, hips and internal organs. This will hopefully improve local circulation, pelvic floor function and organ suspension. Although the drag on both posterior and anterior fascial columns is removed, it may be indicated to follow through by lifting of the anterior fascias (see Chapter 5). This is especially important with a patient suffering from postpartum depression.

PART 3: THE 'DIFFERENTIAL' TECHNIQUE

The 'differential technique' refers to a safe, gentle and precise long lever approach devised by Dr Sutherland for correcting ligamentous articular strains of the sacrum between the ilia and also the lumbar spine. The osteopath sets up a field of BLT for the pelvis from below, while the seated patient turns the sacrum to its position of balance from above. It is then the patient who provides the final corrective action as the operator stabilises the legs. This illustrates the concept of the sacrum as balanced on a tripod with the third leg turned upward as the spinal column (Wales 1995).

HISTORY

Dr Sutherland recommended the 'differential' approach to his student, Alvira Millar, for her patient who had undergone several lower lumbar surgical operations which had been only partially successful. Dr Millar was extremely cautious about what approach to choose but knew how much this patient needed help. This procedure was so-called because of the analogy between the ability of the ilia to turn independently of each other and the slip differential of a car which allows it to turn corners by having one wheel turning faster than the other (Wales 1996).

The analogy of the human pelvic-hip unit to the differential of a car is illustrated by the way we accommodate in walking round corners. When walking, the weight-bearing side increases tension and stabilises as the ilium rotates slightly anteriorly. This allows the non-weight-bearing side to swing the leg through with an accommodative movement at the SI joint, rotating the ilium on that side posteriorly in its release (Cibulka *et al.* 2019; Dontigny 2011).

In referring to this approach, Dr Wales recalled Alvira Miller saying that, in her experience of patients with clinical problems in the lumbar discs, the patient's own ligamentous articular mechanism was much the safest agency to use for correction (Wales 1996). She also mentioned that Sutherland had emphasised this.

Osteopathic diagnosis and treatment are inseparable. Dr Wales often used this procedure as part of her initial general assessment and diagnostic routine as well as treatment. After listening to her patients, she would assess them, testing for movement while all the time observing and palpating. She would then sit her patient on the table, seating herself on a stool at a lower level and facing the patient. In her words, 'sitting below at your patient's feet puts you (the osteopath) in the proper relationship to your patient' (Wales 1992).

Dr James Jealous described the first time he visited Dr Ruby Day, a student of Dr Sutherland, who was to become his mentor and a transformational influence on his osteopathic journey. Sitting in her kitchen he mentioned to her that he had been suffering for some time with lower back pain. She sat him up on the kitchen dresser, held his feet and then said 'that should be alright now'. This was the 'differential'. He privately thought she must be a crazy old lady until, driving home, he realised that, for the first time in many months, he was free of pain. Fascinated and mystified by this experience, he knew he needed to learn from her, and so began a long and formative relationship (Jealous 1988).

HOW DID THIS PROCEDURE EVOLVE?

Sutherland's realisation as a student, that 'it is the ligaments, not the muscles, that are the natural agencies for this purpose of correcting the relations and positions of joints' (Sutherland 1998, COT p. 160), regained momentum in 1919 when he first saw Virgil Halladay's dissection at the AOA Convention in Chicago. The dissection left only the skeleton and ligaments in situ with the ligaments treated so as to preserve their pliability. This lumbar-pelvic specimen enabled Sutherland to manually explore the relationship between ligamentous-articular movement of the pelvis, hip joints and lumbar spine. As the specimen was placed in a sitting position the ischial tuberosities were fixed on the table, enabling them to act as fulcra for the anterior and posterior rotation of the ilia. By pulling one femur and pushing the other he discovered that the anterior rotation of the ilium was associated with the pulled or 'longer' leg and the posterior iliac rotation with the pushed or 'shorter' leg (Sutherland 1998, COT pp. 287–288). He then understood how the legs of a seated patient could be used therapeutically to match ligamentous articular strains of the pelvis, bringing the whole unit of function to a position of BLT.

WHEN IS THIS USEFUL?

The differential technique can address a variety of ligamentous articular strain patterns involving the hips, sacrum, lumbar spine or the whole unity of the pelvis. An advantage is that it requires minimal effort on the part of the practitioner.

It can be safely adapted for all ages. An infant or young child can sit on the carer's lap while you hold the feet, using the legs as long levers to find the position of ease of the innominates around the sacrum. Meanwhile, toys can engage the child's attention to encourage turning of the trunk to one side or the other and then back to centre.

The differential is especially helpful in addressing the many common injuries that can occur through a combination of twisting and lifting. An example is when a patient in acute pain says, 'I don't know what happened. I only leant over slightly and turned to pick up a toothbrush and my back went!' In this approach, the position taken up by the patient often recreates the position that created the strain, from which a natural resolution is made possible.

In Sutherland's view, pain in the lower lumbar and sacral iliac joint region, very often, 'are secondary indications of a primary femoroacetabular lesion, or twist of the hip capsule produced by the psoas and iliacus muscles' (Sutherland 1998, COT p. 125; see also Sutherland 1990, TSO p. 199). Iliopsoas contractions cause pelvic changes to the acetabulum, the SI joints and lumbar spine. This manoeuvre allows the operator to bring the SI and hip joints and iliopsoas muscles into a composite field of BLT.

Patients with acute psoas spasm have difficulty lying down and possibly even more difficulty sitting back up again. In the sitting position the hip joints can be brought into BLT via the legs while the patient leans forward slightly to approximate the psoas origins to their insertion on the lesser trochanter to allow the possibility of relaxation (Lippincott 1958, 1965; Wales 1988).

Diagnostically, locking the seated patient's ankles steadily against the lateral surface of the operator's thighs is an ideal position from which to simultaneously assess the feet, tibiofibular IoM, knees and hip joints. It can also provide insight into more specific patterns in the pelvis and lumbar spine and their integration with the rest of the body.

This procedure is very forgiving of the operator's ability to diagnose. An initial recognition of even just one component of a SI strain evolves into a more nuanced and detailed diagnosis of the region throughout the BLT process and resolution phase. In this way, the diagnostic process continues as we treat. The direction of the pattern of ease taken up from below and above often mimics the direction of the original position of injury, giving insight into the complex aetiological forces involved. This exaggeration of the 'lesion' helps release the original trauma and allows the innate self-correcting forces to resolve the injury, restoring dynamic balance by retracing the steps that produced it.

ANALYSIS

The movement of forward bending and twisting is best viewed in the context of the tensegrity of the whole pelvic ligamentous and fascial 'basket'. When lifting in this awkward position there is a risk of the sacrum becoming unilaterally strained inferiorly on the ilium. In turn this may cause the whole pelvic-sacral-lumbar-hip complex to become unstable and prone to further injury.

The action of lifting a heavy object while forward bending and twisting also involves the hip internally rotating on the side toward which the pelvis has twisted. This involves contraction of psoas and antero-inferior rotation of the sacrum on the ilium on that side. The opposite hip will tend to turn towards external rotation, with tightening of the sacrospinous, sacrotuberous and SI ligaments on that side. Although the TLF and quadratus lumborum assist stability, this creates an unstable situation for the sacrum and lumbar spine with compensatory rotation of the ilia (Vleeming *et al.* 2012). In this torsional position the annulus fibrosus of the intervertebral discs is also at its weakest. This illustrates how much the lumbar spine, hip joints and pelvis operate as a unit of function, challenging the whole body's capacity to accommodate when the ligaments have been challenged beyond their physiological limits.

It may be helpful to keep in mind that the motion of the sacrum, suspended between the ilia, may take place in combination with up to three axes, i.e., transverse, anteroposterior or vertical. Respectively, these will permit sacral flexion/extension (nutation/counternutation), sidebending and rotation (Goode *et al.* 2008; Walker 1992).

SUMMARY

With the patient seated on the ischial tuberosities, the seated operator holds the ankles, using the legs to rotate the ilia towards the direction of ease or injury. This establishes a stabilised field of ligamentous balance for the ilia from below. The patient then actively rotates the sacrum towards the direction of ease to create a field of balanced tension for the SI joints from above. Once a release is felt the patient is instructed to sit up tall to reverse the sacral rotation by facing forwards. The osteopath continues to stabilise the innominate bones from below until the patient's sacrum is reseated through his or her own agency. Thus, the patient has control over the whole procedure by providing the corrective forces. Dr Sutherland asked: 'Why is it safe? Because patients won't hurt themselves.'

THERAPEUTIC ENGAGEMENT

Differential technique

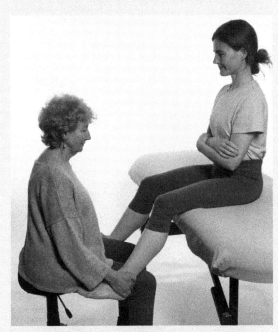

Figure 3.7 Differential technique.

1. POSITIONING

The patient sits on the treatment table on his or her 'sitting bones' (ischial tuberosities) with legs hanging off the side. You sit facing the patient, also keeping your weight through your sitting bones and your feet flat on the floor.

Many patients (and especially teenagers) have no concept of how to sit up straight without slumping onto the sacrum and collapsing the lumbar curve. If a patient is asked to 'walk' forward on the sitting bones, then 'walk' back to the original spot, it becomes easier to understand what it means to be planted on them.

2. HANDHOLD

Pick up the patient's feet with your fingers wrapped around the heels and your thenar eminences over the lateral malleoli.

This cupped handhold can also be used to engage the IoM between the tibia and fibula for comparative diagnosis and to sense the pattern and quality of the whole lower limb.

3. ENGAGING THE PELVIS THROUGH (VIA) THE LEGS

Lift up the patient's relaxed legs to as nearly horizontal as the hamstrings will allow, without tipping the patient backwards. Look for the place where you 'connect' with the pelvis via the legs.

The patient's weight needs to be transmitted vertically through the fulcra of the ischial tuberosities throughout. The point here is to stabilise the legs enough to use them as long levers to engage the whole pelvis through to the hips and SI joints. To avoid dissipating the continuity between your contact and SI joints it can be helpful to lock the patient's hips by holding them slightly towards internal rotation via the ankles.

4. FORMING A PARALLELOGRAM WITH THE PATIENT

Staying well-grounded through your own ischial tuberosities, lock the patient's malleoli firmly against the lateral surface of your thighs. This will enable you to form a parallelogram between your pelvis and that of the patient.

5. MOTION TESTING

Rotate your own pelvis and thigh forward on one side, back to neutral and then forward on the other. This reveals which direction the patient's innominates rotate most easily and enables you to match the pattern of ease of the ilia in relation to the sacrum.

This position of balance for the innominates via the feet is steadily held until after the end of the procedure.

As the patient's leg is pushed proximally on one side, this will engage with the acetabulum to rotate that iliac wheel posteriorly on the fulcrum of the ischial tuberosities. On the side that you cannot easily push proximally (as if it feels longer) the patient's ilium will be rotated anteriorly (Sutherland 1998, COT p. 288). *In this way, as your thighs and pelvis are moved forward on one side and back on the other, you will be 'turning the wheels' of the patient's ilia on the ischial tuberosities to match their natural position.* This is made possible by the patient's medial malleoli being locked against your lateral thighs.

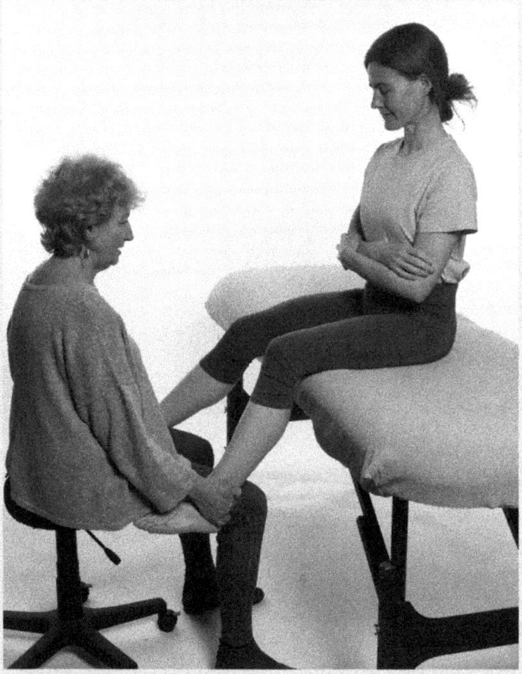

It is often easier for the patient to be asked to turn in the direction of a landmark such as a window or door, rather than left or right.

Be sure that the patient is turning from the waist to engage the lumbar spine and sacrum, rather than just the upper trunk.

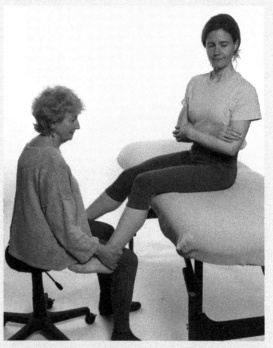

Figure 3.9 Differential technique: holding pelvic rotation as patient turns sacrum.

Figure 3.8 Differential technique: holding pelvic rotation via patient's feet.

The patient should not turn the sacrum so far that the ilia and hips also begin to be moved.

6. PATIENT POSTURAL COOPERATION

While stabilising the ilia via the ankles, ask the patient to either fold the arms or place a hand over the opposite thigh and turn the waist (sacrum) towards the direction of ease, left or right. The sacrum and lumbar spine will often turn towards the side of anterior iliac rotation, i.e., the side of the 'longer' leg (Sutherland 1998, COT p. 288). This will bring the sacrum into a state of balance at the SI joints from above, the operator having established a state of balance for the ilia from below.

7. READING SI RELEASE

A release of the SI joints often coincides with a sense of softening and 'fluid breathing' through the interosseous membranes at the ankles. This will usually happen on one side before the other, so wait until change is felt on both sides.

8. PATIENT'S ACTIVE POSITIONAL DE-ROTATION

Continue to hold the patient's innominates firmly via the ankles and ask the patient to breathe in, sit tall, de-rotate the trunk and turn back to face the front.

This final stage is a *direct action* correction by the patient, of the sacrum in relation to the ilia. This is made possible by the fact that, after local ligamentous articular release, there is no resistance to easy reversal of the strain pattern, allowing mechanical repositioning of the sacrum between the ilia.

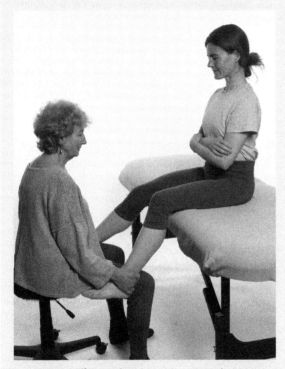

Figure 3.10 Differential technique: patient de-rotates trunk to realign sacrum.

Wait a few moments for the reseating of the sacrum to settle before you lighten your support, replacing the patient's legs at the side of the table and removing your contact.

9. RETESTING

Once this is completed, retest for symmetry and freedom of movement. Retesting at the end of a procedure helps in 'giving the body back to itself' as it re-establishes its proprioceptive sense of a renewed ease and freedom of movement.

Further refinements to the 'differential'

Inclusion of the hip joints: *While holding the innominate bones steady via the legs, subtle refinements can be included in this manoeuvre, e.g., the legs can be held, either in external or internal rotation by the operator, to match the position of BLT for the hip joints.*

In this way, a state of balance is built up in the entire tensile pelvic bowl, hips, SI joints and lumbar spine.

Inclusion of psoas: In addition, *the patient may be asked to lean forward or slump slightly from the hips to give slack to a unilateral or bilateral hypertonic psoas muscle.*

Respiratory cooperation

While you maintain balance from below, the patient's natural breathing will gradually work to shift the fulcra of balance in the SI joints. Active respiratory cooperation can also be added by *asking the patient to exhale and hold the breath out to further exaggerate a unilateral depression of the sacrum* (Lippincott 1958, 1965).

PART 4: LAP TECHNIQUE TO 'RESEAT' THE SACRUM

'BACKING THE CAR INTO THE GARAGE'

'One way to view the architecture of the human skeleton is to see it as a tripod with the sacrum at the centre of the tripod. In this view, the 3rd leg is raised up over the other two and functions as a tension spring and shock absorber.'

(Wales 1996)

(For the lap technique for the lumbar spine and above, see Chapter 2.)

Early osteopaths often treated their patients either on a treatment stool or standing, rather than supine. Dr Sutherland frequently used 'lap techniques' which he referred to as 'bedside techniques'. These can be especially helpful on home visits where treatment tables are not available, but they are also invaluable in a clinic setting.

The lap technique for the sacrum involves the patient sitting on the knees of the seated operator and facing the treatment table. Through BLT of the SI joints and whole pelvic bowl, the operator creates the conditions for the patient to be able to actively lift and then reseat the sacrum in a more balanced position between the ilia. This approach was humorously referred to by Sutherland as 'backing the car into the garage'.

There are times when it is difficult for the patient to lie down, as in later stages of pregnancy, acute pain or conditions such as congestive heart failure or pulmonary distress. When sitting, the upright position of the patient's torso makes effective use of gravity, helping the operator to therapeutically engage and precisely match the tone in the tissues. This may enable profound reorganisation with less physical effort for the operator. Another advantage is that for a patient in acute pain, the seated position allows relaxation of any iliopsoas hypertonicity. It is also easy to treat toddlers on parents' or the operator's knees while occupying them with toys or books.

The inclusion of lap techniques in this book is not just for their historical value or because the patient cannot lie down. One of the advantages of this procedure is that the thighs and hands of the operator together provide a four-point contact, freeing the hands to be used as required. This three-dimensional support makes the composite position of ligamentous balance of the pelvis easier to find since it is possible to encompass the various components of the strain pattern simultaneously. The thighs of the operator can match the sidebending and rotational components of the pelvic pattern in a way that the flat surface of a table cannot.

The four-point contact is especially useful for understanding complex patterns of the pelvis where various force vectors have been absorbed by the tissues over time. These may include torsional and sheering strains but also compressive vectors, making the total situation difficult to analyse. Picture, for instance, a patient who has recently had a difficult vaginal delivery, who has a history of falls and who may have further strains as a result of lifting and carrying a heavy baby.

The most common ligamentous articular strains in the SI joints include some degree of bilateral or unilateral strain of the sacrum between the ilia. By guiding the patient's pelvis to move towards the direction of ease, a field of balance can be obtained which mimics the position in which the injury occurred, often revealing factors that the operator may not have originally considered.

The additional use of the patient's active postural and respiratory cooperation adds speed and effectiveness, bringing focus and precision to the field of operation.

THERAPEUTIC ENGAGEMENT

Lap technique to reseat the sacrum
Consent and explanation

The near disappearance of lap techniques from the osteopathic tool kit may stem from hesitancy at the prospect of having a patient on the operator's lap. Care is needed to avoid misunderstanding so that gaining the patient's permission, confidence and cooperation at the outset requires clarity as to what to expect and why this is the most appropriate approach in that case.

Assure the patient to let you know if there is discomfort at any stage. It is suggested that a lap pad or cushion is used over the operator's legs.

This is to create a physical boundary, to reinforce the patient's sense of safety and also to protect the operator's thighs from sharp sitting bones!

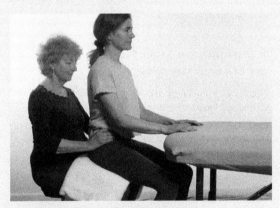

Figure 3.11 Lap technique for sacrum (1).

1. POSITIONING THE PATIENT

Sit behind the patient who stands facing the treatment table.

Guide him or her, with your hands on the iliac crests, into a seated position on your covered lap so that the sitting bones are positioned on your thighs just behind your knees.

The weight of the patient is thus transmitted directly into the ground via your legs for more comfort and less effort on your part.

If the patient and practitioner are of similar height it should be possible for the operator to have the knees at a right angle. If the patient is shorter the knees may be more flexed.

2. TESTING FOR PELVIC TILT AND ROTATION ETC.

With the patient seated upright on your lap, test for the position of ease of the pelvic bowl by moving your thigh contact on the ischial tuberosities as follows:

- *To test for a sidebending component, raise one leg and drop the other, comparing the position of ease on each side. Allow a pause before comparing one side with the other.*
- *To test for a tendency for outflare or inflare of the ischia, abduct and adduct your thighs.*
- *To test for pelvic rotation, move your thighs forward on one side and back on the other; the side where the ischial tuberosity most easily moves posteriorly indicates an anterior rotation of that innominate and vice versa.*

3. POSITION OF BALANCED TENSION OF THE ILIA IN RELATION TO THE SACRUM

With your thighs and guiding hands, support the patient's pelvis in the composite position of ease for all the components found.

This will place the SI ligaments in an approximate position of BLT, maximum ease and minimum resistance to the inherent self-corrective forces. Your hands are free to contact the iliac crests, anterior spines and/or sacrum to further support the pattern of ease.

4. PATIENT POSTURAL COOPERATION

Ask the patient to place his/her hands on the treatment table and 'walk' them slowly forward, as you hold the innominates steady in the balanced tension position through your thighs and hands.

The forward bending of the patient's trunk slightly disengages the sacrum from its wedged position between the ilia. It also takes up the tension from above and will engage the whole body down to the sacrum and pelvis, including the TLF and lumbosacral ligaments.

Use your hands to monitor the moment that the innominates start to move forward together with the sacrum and ask the patient to pause. When resistance is felt this is a sign that the ligaments you are focusing on are engaged.

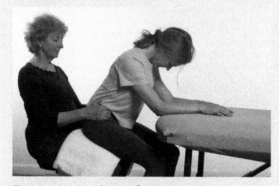

Figure 3.12 Lap technique for sacrum (2).

5. READJUSTING THE INNOMINATE POSITION TO BLT OF THE SI JOINTS IN STAGES

Retest for the neutral position of the innominates relative to the sacrum for this new level, using your knees as before. The aim here is to find a new position of balanced tension for the SI joints for the more forward position of the sacrum and patient's trunk. This is because we are progressively engaging the posterior to anterior ligamentous layers and also the different levels of the SI joints.

Wait for a release at the SI joints before asking the patient to now place his/her elbows on the table and walk them forward a little further as before. The patient is also asked to drop the head and neck forward so that the longitudinal spinal ligaments and dura can assist the lifting of the sacrum between the ilia.

6. A PAUSE BEFORE THE FINAL ACTION

As before, with your hands around the innominates, restrain any tendency for the ilia to begin moving forward with the sacrum. When you feel this tendency, ask the patient to pause as you once more readjust the innominates to the new position of balanced tension.

Lean back slightly, holding the iliac crests or anterior superior iliac spine (ASIS) to create a stable field, against which the weight of the patient's dropped head further acts on the long ligaments to lift the sacrum.

Meanwhile a deepening of the patient's thoracic respiration is working to assist ligamentous-articular and also membranous-articular release.

7. 'OPENING THE GARAGE DOORS'

To open the upper pelvis and flare the ilia, adduct the patient's ischial tuberosities by bringing your knees together beneath them. Hold that position until the end of the manoeuvre.

8. RESEATING THE SACRUM OR 'BACKING THE CAR INTO THE GARAGE'

Maintain the flaring on the upper pelvis with your adducted knees as you ask the patient to breathe in deeply and sit tall, slowly uncurling the spine by rolling upwards from the lumbar spine. The patient's thoracic inhalation and posture further act to lift the sacrum.

To reseat the sacrum, the patient then slowly breathes out and sits back down to sink into the pelvis. Only when fully settled do you let your knees part into their normal position.

This action also helps 'turn' the sacrum by moving the sacral base posteriorly.

9. RETESTING

Reassess the patient as before, to examine for improved symmetry and mobility of the pelvis and body as a whole, first sitting and then standing, to give back voluntary postural control.

Modification for specific sacral patterns

This approach can be adapted for specific liga-mentous articular strains of the sacrum between the ilia, e.g., in fixed respiratory (PRM) 'flexion', 'extension' or unilateral restrictions of the SI joint as below (Lippincott 1949).

Extension (nutation) fixation of the sacrum between the ilia

1. POSITIONING

The patient sits on your knees, over a lap pad as above, and faces the plinth.

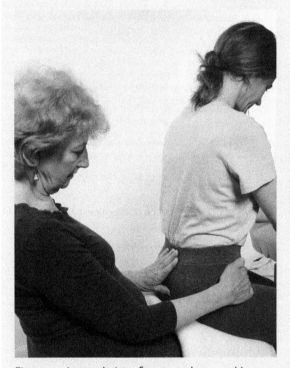

Figure 3.13 Lap technique for nutated sacrum (1).

You stabilise the ASIS on the side of the restricted SI joint with one hand or forearm, restraining it from moving anteriorly.

The fingers of your other hand are on the sacral base and your thumb on the apex.

Slightly exaggerate the sacral extension strain pattern by holding the base forward and down and the apex posteriorly.

2. POSTURAL AND RESPIRATORY COOPERATION BY THE PATIENT

The patient is asked to 'walk' the forearms slowly forward on the table just to the point where you feel the first point of lifting or balanced tension in the ligaments. The patient holds still at that point.

Meanwhile you move your knees to match and support the position of balance for the innominates as described above, taking in sidebending, torsion and in-flare/out-flare etc.

Ask the patient to exhale deeply for as long as possible to exaggerate the extension position of the sacrum.

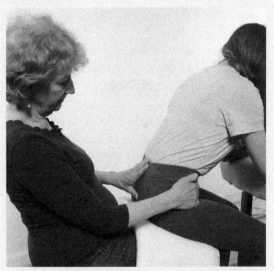

Figure 3.14 Lap technique for nutated sacrum (2).

3. BALANCE POINT

This is achieved between:

- the precise degree of pull on the sacrum from the forward position of the patient's trunk
- the precise degree of exaggeration of the sacral extension position held by your hand
- matching of the innominate position through the ischial contact of your knees
- the power of the patient's held thoracic exhalation.

4. RESOLUTION

The softening and sense of ligamentous reorganisation often happens just as the patient can hold the breath out no longer. *The final integration happens as the patient breathes in deeply and sits up.*

Flexion (counternutation) fixation of the sacrum

This is where the sacral base is found to be drawn cephalad and posterior with the apex anterior.

1. POSITIONING

With the patient seated on your knees as above, simply steady the pelvis with one hand on the side of the SI restriction.

With the other hand, exaggerate the sacral flexion strain position with your thumb on the sacral apex and your fingers on the base.

2. POSTURAL AND RESPIRATORY COOPERATION

The patient walks hands or elbows forward on the plinth, just enough to allow the sacral base to begin to move posteriorly to exaggerate the flexion strain position.

By moving your knees, find the position of ease for the innominates, via the fulcra of the ischial tuberosities, to bring the whole pelvic bowl into a position of BLT with the sacrum.

The patient is asked to inhale fully for as long as possible, further exaggerating the position of sacral strain, to enable a refinement of the point of BLT.

3. RESOLUTION

After a change is perceived in the ligamentous quality, the positional correction completes as the patient breathes out and slowly sits up.

Sidebending or rotational sacral strains

The sacral flexion or extension engagement above may include other elements of a pattern.

The operator's hands can match sidebending or rotational components of the sacrum between the ilia by emphasising them with the hands, as described above. *The patient assists with postural cooperation by sliding one forearm forward on the table to exaggerate the sacral position and fine-tune BLT of the SI joints.*

Balancing the pregnant uterus within the pelvis

A further very simple adaptation is helpful in later pregnancy to balance the uterosacral ligaments to create the best conditions for delivery.

1. POSITIONING

The patient sits on your knees, facing the plinth, as above.

2. CONTACT

Place your hands around the patient's lower belly to test for the position of ease of the uterus in sidebending, torsion etc., keeping in mind its relationship to the sacrum via the uterosacral ligaments.

With your thighs under the ischial tuberosities, test for the position of ease of the pelvis in relation to the uterus.

Once an easy sense of balance between the uterus and pelvic bowl is found, the patient's natural breathing will be working to shift the fulcrum towards resolution of the strain. This may be perceived by a spontaneous realignment and harmonisation, felt within both the position of the uterus and the pelvic bowl (Molinari 2010).

Supine pelvic spread

The principle of freeing the sacrum of restriction between the ilia is applicable to infants and young children and is often key in postpartum recovery. The pelvis sometimes remains compressed or slightly displaced after long or difficult delivery, with implications for the whole body.

1. HANDHOLD

With the child supine, hold the posterior ilia very gently apart, just up to the first point of resistance.

Wait, as the balanced tension between your

sensitive lateral distraction and the patient's tissues enables the SI ligaments to seek balanced tension.

This process may give an impression of the ligaments guiding the ilia to reveal any asymmetry and finding balanced tension within that pattern. *Simply hold, as the inherent fluid and respiratory forces shift the articular fulcra to free the sacrum.*

Recheck the pelvis, inherent sacral motion and textural quality, noting the response in the rest of the body and cranium.

PART 5: STANDING ILIOSACRAL CORRECTION

This approach involves the patient standing with the weight primarily borne through the contralateral foot to the side being treated. The osteopath supports the innominate on the non-weight-bearing side, holding it between ischial tuberosity and iliac crest or ASIS. This makes it possible to float it to a point of ligamentous balance with the sacrum as the patient 'sits down' slightly on the osteopath's hand. This is followed by direct action towards the direction of correction. The final correction takes place when the patient stands up and takes weight equally on both feet again, while the osteopath stabilises the innominate. This manoeuvre is designed for 'postural lesions', i.e., where the innominate has gone into a positional strain on the sacrum, rather than a sacral positional strain between the ilia.

Dr Sutherland often treated the pelvis and hips in the standing position as did Dr Still. We remember stories of the Old Doctor stopping and treating people in the street with no couch or even a stool at hand. A lot of problems arise while the patient is on his or her feet, whether bending and twisting or coming down heavily on one side or the other. The advantage of not having the patient reclining passively is that it is easier to take into the picture all possible components of a strain pattern, by recreating the exact position in which the injury occurred. Because the correction is performed with the innominate bone in a suspended field, with the help of the patient's postural cooperation, it can be relatively easy to enhance a point of balanced tension.

Many different pelvic and SI strain patterns can be treated with the patient standing. In this instance we will take a very specific strain of the ileum on the sacrum, i.e., when the ileum has been shunted upwards on the auricular surface of the sacrum on one side, such as may happen with a heavy landing on one leg or possibly onto one buttock or ischial tuberosity. This type of injury is typical of displacement of the ilium in relation to the sacrum (iliosacral strain) rather than the sacrum being turned in relation to the ilium (sacroiliac).

AN IMAGE OF THE PELVIS

For the operator it can be helpful to think of the pelvis as a basket where the innominates are the struts held in place by a tensile ligamentous web, like the weave in a basket. As the osteopath supports the whole innominate, holding the iliac crest with one hand and supporting the ischial tuberosity with the other, this replaces the patient's leg as a support for that side of the pelvis. In this way, the whole ligamentous 'basket' will be suspended, balanced between the two hands.

THERAPEUTIC ENGAGEMENT

Standing approach to postural sacroiliac or iliosacral ligamentous-articular strains
Demonstration and explanation

This procedure requires a lot of cooperation from the patient, so it is very important to explain in advance exactly what will be done and what the patient is required to do. It is best to demonstrate how to follow the instructions you will be giving by getting the patient to copy the movements before starting to treat. As being treated standing may be a new experience, you will need to explain why this is the best way to approach the problem. Normally, patients can easily understand that correcting a problem in the position it was originally created is very effective and that, when upright, the pelvis is 'free floating' rather than fixed at one point as in sitting or lying down.

Diagnosis

The diagnosis of postural SI or iliosacral lesions can be done in several ways. A history of the injury will often give a clue. The operator is looking for lack of free motion of the ilium pivoting on the sacrum with the release of weight bearing especially, where the ilium has been shunted upwards in relation to the sacrum.

1. EXPLANATION, DEMONSTRATION AND CONSENT

Explain the exact hold you will be taking and, as it is close to an intimate area, always ask for the patient's consent. If possible, *demonstrate your hold on a skeleton model,* showing the radial surface of the distal phalanges of your index finger under the ischial tuberosity and the other hand spanning the iliac crest and ASIS.

It is also helpful to *demonstrate the movements you will be asking the patient to perform* as, although keen to cooperate, patients often have difficulties following verbal instructions without a rehearsal.

2. PATIENT AND PRACTITIONER POSITION AND HANDHOLD

Ask the patient to stand with hands lightly resting, but not leaning, on the table or back of a chair for stability, as weight will be shifted onto one leg.

Sit facing the side of the patient, well-grounded with feet flat on the floor if possible, for stable support. It is usual to start on the side of the upward shunt.

As your lower hand will be under the ischial tuberosity, taking up some of the weight of the pelvis, it will be more comfortable for you to *have one elbow resting on a pillow positioned on your thigh.* This will allow any weight to pass through your forearm, elbow, knee, leg and into the ground, reducing the muscular effort of supporting the weight of the patient's pelvis.

3. OPERATOR HAND POSITION

First take up your hold with one hand from behind, under the ischial tuberosity, and the other around the front on the ASIS, and find an approximate position of balanced tension within the SI joint. Check that this is comfortable for the patient.

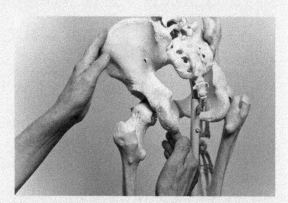

Figure 3.15 Standing iliosacral hold on skeleton.

4. PATIENT'S WEIGHT TRANSFER

Then ask the patient to transfer weight onto the opposite leg while relaxing and bending the knee on the supported side while you adjust your hold.

Patients often find this hard to understand but it is no more than the way we all stand at times, with the weight mainly on one side rather than equally distributed between two feet.

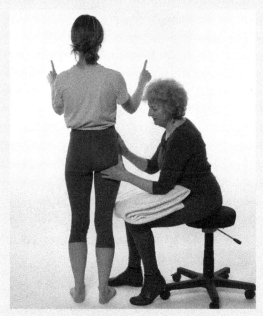

Figure 3.16 Standing iliosacral hold on live model.

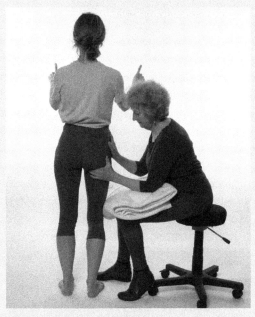

Figure 3.17 Dropping one hip.

5. PATIENT'S FOOT CROSSES OVER

The patient then turns the non-weight-bearing knee outwards and crosses the foot over to the other side of the weight-bearing foot. This allows the suspended hip, leg and foot to hang freely as the foot rests on its side.

You may observe a tendency for the innominate to rotate posteriorly or anteriorly or into in-flare or out-flare etc.

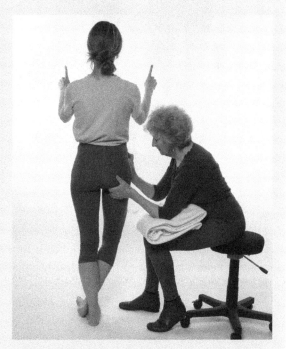

Figure 3.18 Foot crosses over.

6. PATIENT 'SITS' ON YOUR SUPPORTING HAND

Ask the patient to bend the weight-bearing knee as if starting to sit on your supporting hand under the ischial tuberosity. It is important that the non-weight-bearing hip is allowed to dangle.

This allows the 'wheel' of the innominate to be suspended on the supporting hand and the sacral base to drop forward.

With each change of the patient's position, your hold adapts to fully support the suspended field of operation that has been created. This allows you to work in three dimensions taking into account the whole ligamentous field of the pelvic bowl.

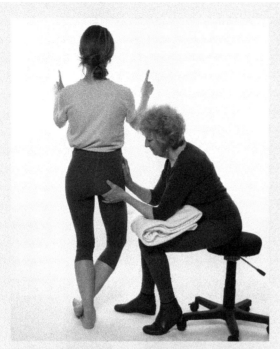

Figure 3.19 Patient 'sitting' slightly on operator's hand.

7. FLOATING FREE
Hold and support the innominate as the ligaments explore. In this position the innominate is in a floating field, enabling it to spontaneously move towards the direction of the strain for further adjustment and refinement of the point of BLT.

The innominate should begin to 'float' free of the sacrum.

8. HOLDING STEADY AS THE PATIENT STANDS UP
Ask the patient to straighten the weight-bearing leg while you hold the innominate 'wheel' still and steady. This action of the patient lifts and turns the sacrum back into correct apposition to the ileum which you hold firmly to allow this to occur.

9. RESOLUTION
Finally, ask the patient to uncross the leg and return to normal standing posture while you maintain a hold of the 'wheel' in a 'direct action' until the very end. Do not let go until the patient is standing with the weight settled firmly on both feet.

'Direct action' refers to guiding the innominate

directly towards the position of correction. As the essential proprioceptive change in the ligamentous relationship will have already happened, there is normally no resistance to this guidance.

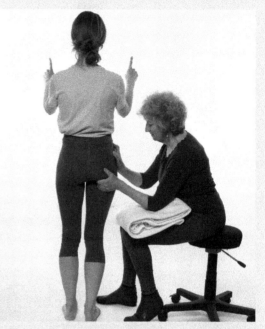

Figure 3.20 Patient replaces both feet equally on the ground.

As the pelvic bowl operates as a unit, the procedure should normally be repeated on the other side to integrate the whole. Sometimes, however, this procedure also resolves a problem on the opposite side, since the whole pelvis is engaged.

Importance of comfort for both
It is important that at every stage of the procedure the practitioner feels comfortable and not strained and that the patient feels supported in such a way that postural control can be handed over to the operator. *The operator must be firmly grounded to maintain this stable supportive hold.*

Application to other strain patterns
In this instance we have been looking at a specific injury of the ilium shunted cephalad on the sacrum.

Anterior rotation

If the ilium is rotated anteriorly the ischium will rotate posteriorly and vice versa. Following the point of balance, *the operator holds the innominate towards the direction of reversal of the strain and maintains this hold as the patient slowly straightens the knee and replaces the contralateral foot, equalising the weight.*

Downslip

If there is a *downslip of the innominate* this will often be felt as a strong inferior dropping of the ischial tuberosity into the hand as the patient bends the knee (Carreiro 2003). *Resist this downward movement as the patient bends the knee until you feel the ilium engage with the resistance of the sacrum. Hold the innominate steady as the patient slowly straightens the knee.*

Working in this suspended field, this same handhold and standing approach can be applied to a variety of pelvic, SI and even hip problems by bringing attention to different parts of the pelvic basket. It is possible to address strains within the whole network of pelvic ligaments, whether in the different ligamentous and fascial layers of the SI joint or as these extend into the hip joint.

PART 6: PUBIC SYMPHYSIS AND PELVIC FLOOR

The procedure described below is a comfortable and effective way to assess and balance the pelvic floor of the seated patient, preparing the tissues for a modified muscle energy approach to engage the pubic symphysis. This can be helpful for treating pubic symphysis dysfunction (PSD) both in the later months of pregnancy and postpartum. It is also useful for addressing congestive conditions in the urogenital triangle in both women and men.

FUNCTIONAL ANATOMY OF THE PUBIC SYMPHYSIS AND PELVIC FLOOR

The pubic symphysis draws attention mainly when PSD causes pain in pregnancy. It is otherwise not often given the credit it deserves as an essential element of the tensegrity of the pelvis in anteriorly uniting the two sides of the bony ring.

Whereas the function of the posterior pelvis is mainly weight bearing, the pubic arch is often likened to a 'tie beam' to resist tension when sitting or compression when standing. It also has a role in resisting the forces of weight bearing as they are distributed throughout the pelvis from the spine and sacrum.

The symphysis pubis is a cartilaginous joint consisting of an interpubic disc of fibrocartilage with hyaline cartilage lining the bones at each end. Strong ligaments tightly bind the two sides, working together to neutralise tensile and shearing forces, while accommodating limited torsional motion in walking (Volinski *et al.* 2018). The superior pubic ligament spans the superior part of the pubis between the tubercles. The inferior 'arcuate' pubic ligament forms the lower border of the pubic symphysis and blends with the disc. This is the strongest of the pubic ligaments, providing the greatest degree of stability (Mathieu *et al.* 2020).

The two medial surfaces of the pubic arch form the border of the thin sheet of muscle forming the urogenital diaphragm. The deep transverse perineal muscle runs transversely, blending with the urogenital diaphragm to surround the urethral sphincter. The superior and inferior layers of the perineal membrane are formed by the fascia of this diaphragm. The sponge-like superficial perineal fascia of Colles is attached to the base of the perineal membrane and pubic arch. This arrangement perhaps offers a clue as to why A.T. Still treated misalignment of the pubic symphysis in children with enuresis, since efficient sphincter function requires equally balanced tension of its fibres. Poor apposition of the pubic symphysis may distort this (Cooperstein *et al.* 2014; He *et al.* 2022).

The fibrous perineal body is an important point of attachment for the bulbospongiosus, levator ani and superficial transverse peronei muscles as well as the right and left sides of the external anal sphincter. The deep part of the external anal sphincter surrounds the anal canal and blends with the superficial transverse peronei and levator ani. The whole pelvic floor should be considered as a unit of function.

PUBIC SYMPHYSIS DYSFUNCTION

The interpubic disc is very small in children, with a greater proportion of hyaline cartilage. It is higher and narrower in men (Aslan and Fynes 2007; Jain *et al.* 2006). In women it widens by 2–3 mm during the last trimester of pregnancy to facilitate delivery. When the gap is equal to or more than 10 mm, there's a diastasis of the pubic symphysis.

There is limited agreement as to the diagnosis and causes of PSD, also referred to as pelvic pain syndrome (PPS). The discomfort may be local or referred (Kanakaris *et al.* 2011), and may be aching or sharp at the symphysis, in the perineum or the lumbosacral area. Pain is normally made worse by movements such as walking, standing on one leg or even turning over in bed. Increased levels of relaxin and progesterone in pregnancy allow softening of the pelvic ligaments to accommodate labour, also making the symphysis more vulnerable to malalignment (Wang *et al.* 2021). Because of this, PSD in pregnancy and postpartum can leave the pelvis unstable if untreated.

A history of previous pelvic injuries appears to predispose some women to PSD in pregnancy, when hitherto symptom-free pelvic and lower spinal strains become challenged by postural changes and increased ligamentous laxity. The pubic symphysis has to accommodate any ligamentous imbalance of the hip, SI joint or lumbosacral region, and also childhood injuries to an as-yet unfused acetabulum.

In most pregnancies, the pubic symphysis is easily corrected, especially when any predisposing primary cause is also addressed (Showalter 2017). When a patient is hypermobile or involved in work activities that retrigger instability, it may need to be addressed several times.

Venous congestion within the anterior pubic triangle appears to benefit from the approach described below. Too often, a sedentary lifestyle and tense pelvic floor inhibit local venous and lymphatic drainage and the resulting passive congestion may be one of the precursors to prostate and bladder problems in older men. In women who have lack of tone in the pelvic floor or a degree of prolapse, this approach may be used to increase tone and circulation prior to any work that is indicated for the bladder or uterus.

Assessment of the pelvic floor and pubic symphysis should be routine for all pregnant and postpartum patients, especially after a difficult vaginal delivery. One of the benefits of addressing the pelvic floor and pubis indirectly, engaging the ischial tuberosities as 'handles', rather than by direct contact, is that it is comfortable for the patient even when the postpartum pelvic floor is injured and still tender.

THERAPEUTIC ENGAGEMENT

Pubic symphysis and pelvic floor
Balancing the pelvic floor

1. POSITIONING
Sit facing the patient who sits upright on the treatment table with weight transmitted through the ischial tuberosities which act as fulcra.

2. HANDHOLD
Scoop your hands under the patient's hips so that your fingers can contact the ischial tuberosities.

The patient may have to lift the pelvis on each side in turn to allow you to wrap your fingers around or under the tuberosities. *These become the bony handles* to allow for balancing of the complex fasciae and musculature of the pelvic floor.

The hand contact under the ischial tuberosities is useful for diagnosis as the operator's thenar eminences also cup the patient's greater trochanters. Using the ischial tuberosities as 'handles' makes it possible to feel any asymmetry of the hips and assess whether or not they contribute to the malalignment of the symphysis.

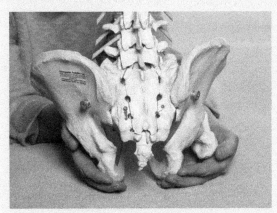

Figure 3.21 Ischial tuberosities hold for pubic symphysis on skeleton.

3. MOTION TESTING
Motion test for the position of ease of the pelvic floor through your ischial contact, e.g., forward, back, medial, lateral.

Tight areas, e.g., where there is perineal scarring, may invite your hands to engage more firmly by approximating the tissues via the tuberosities, to match their tone in the space between your hands.

4. FOREARM FULCRA
Lean your weight through your forearm or elbow fulcra to the degree needed to match and engage the tissue tone.

Thus you are supporting the entire pelvic bowl, with all its complex forces, to a composite point of balanced tension, being especially aware of the pelvic floor between your hands.

5. RESPIRATORY COOPERATION
The patient can help by mentally directing the breath into the pelvic floor.

6. SIMPLY MATCHING AND HOLDING
Maintain your support steadily as you observe the self-corrective forces engaging towards a composite position of balanced myofascial tension, followed by more harmonious balance in the tissues of the pelvic floor.

Realignment of the pubic symphysis
A modified 'muscle energy' approach (Wales 1995).

1. POSITIONING
Your hands remain under the patient's ischial tuberosities. From the 'eyes' in your fingers, visualise the superior and inferior pubic rami converging towards the pubic symphysis as you lean into your forearms to match the forces held there.

Place your knees lateral to the patient's knees.

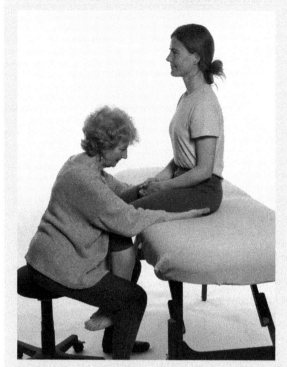

Figure 3.22 Ischial tuberosity hold to engage pubic symphysis.

2. ACTIVE PATIENT COOPERATION

Ask the patient to push her knees laterally against the resistance exerted by your knees and thighs. Adjust your adduction pressure to the individual tone of the patient and ask her to let you know when tension is felt at the pubic symphysis.

Men and non-pregnant women may need slightly stronger engagement.

The action of resisting the operator's femoral adduction will cause the pubic symphysis to resist the compressive forces exerted on it by the acetabula. This has the effect of slightly laterally distracting the symphysis. This activates the self-corrective action of the pubic ligaments, giving space for the symphysis to spontaneously align. The feedback from the ligaments holding the pubic symphysis is usually clear when alignment is again correct.

3. RESOLUTION

Once realignment is perceived, ask the patient to relax her knees before you relax yours. This will avoid injury to the patient.

VIDEOS FOR CHAPTER 3

Scan the QR code or visit https://www.youtube.com/playlist?list=PL3j_YuMBqigFwPiXPiUCm6ZWCH8woWSyW to find a playlist of the videos that accompany this chapter.

REFERENCES

Armitage, P.J. (1990) Tensegrity (unpublished article).

Ashby, K., Yilmaz, E., Mathkour, M., *et al.* (2021) Ligaments stabilizing the sacrum and sacroiliac joint: a comprehensive review. *Neurosurg Rev 45* (1), 357-364.

Aslan, A. & Fynes, M. (2007) Symphyseal pelvic dysfunction. *Current Opinion Obstetrics and Gynaecology 19,* 133-139.

Bakland, O. & Hansen, J.H. (2012) The 'axial sacroiliac joint'. *Anat Clin 1984* (6), 29-36.

Basmajian, J.V. (1982) *Primary Anatomy,* 8th edition. Baltimore, MD: Williams and Wilkins.

Beco, J., Climov, D., Box, M., *et al.* (2004) Pudendal nerve decompression in perineology: a case series. *BMC Surgery 4,* 15.

Bowen, V. & Cassidy, J.D. (1981) Macroscopic and microscopic anatomy of the sacroiliac joint from embryonic life to the eighth decade. *Spine (Phila Pa 1976) 6,* 620-628.

Carreiro, J.E. (2003) *Foundations for Osteopathic Medicine,* 2nd edition. Baltimore, MD: Williams and Wilkins/American Osteopathic Association; pp. 920-921.

Cheng, J.S. & Song, J.K. (2003) Anatomy of the sacrum. *Neurosurg Focus 15,* 2.

Cibulka, M.T., Morr, B., Wedel, J., *et al.* (2019) Changes in pelvic tilt during three different reciprocal stance positions in patients with sacroiliac joint regional pain. *Int J Sports Phys Therapy 14* (6), 967–977.

Cooperstein, R., Lisi, A., Burd, A., *et al.* (2014) Chiropractic management of pubic symphysis shear dysfunction in a patient with overactive bladder. *Journal of Chiropractic Medicine 13,* 81–89.

Diel, J., Ortiz, O., Losada, R.A., Price, D.B., Hayt, M.W. & Katz, D. (2001) The sacrum: pathologic spectrum, multimodality imaging, and subspecialty approach. *Radiographics 21* (1), 83–104.

Dontigny, R.L. (2011) Sacroiliac 101: form and function – a biomechanical study. *Journal of Prolotherapy 3* (1), 561–567.

Goode, A., Hegedus, E.J., Sizer, P., *et al.* (2008) Three-dimensional movements of the sacroiliac joint: a systematic review of the literature and assessment of clinical utility. *J Man Manip Therapy 16* (1), 25–38.

Grant, J.C.B. (1966) *Grant's Method of Anatomy.* Baltimore, MD: Waverly Press; p. 320.

He, K., Wang, J., Zhao, H., *et al.* (2022) Lower urinary tract symptoms in an elderly woman caused by degeneration of the pubic symphysis. *BMC Urology 22,* 98. https://doi.org/10.1186/s12894-022-01052-1.

Iliff, J., Wang, M., Liao, Y., *et al.* (2012) A paravascular pathway facilitates CSF flow through the brain parenchyma and the clearance of interstitial solutes, including amyloid β. *Sci Transl Med 15* (4), 147ra111. https://doi.org/10.1126/scitranslmed.3003748.

Jain, S., Eedarapalli, P., Jamjute, P. & Sawdy, R. (2006) Symphysis pubis dysfunction: a practical approach to management. *The Obstetrician & Gynaecologist 8,* 153–158.

Jealous, J S. (1988) Personal communication.

Kanakaris, N.K., Roberts, C.S., Giannoudis, P.V., *et al.* (2011) Pregnancy-related pelvic girdle pain: an update. *BMC Med 9,* 15. https://doi.org/10.1186/1741-7015-9-15.

Kapandji, I.A. (1974) *The Physiology of the Joints. Vol. 3: The Trunk and Vertebral Column,* 2nd edition. Edinburgh: Churchill Livingstone.

Kiapour, A., Joukar, A., Elgafy, H., *et al.* (2020) Biomechanics of the sacroiliac joint: anatomy, function, biomechanics, sexual dimorphism, and causes of pain. *Int J of Spine Surg 14* (1), S3–S13.

Kumar, P. & Magon, N. (2012) Hormones in pregnancy. *Niger Med J 53* (4), 179–183. https://doi.org/10.4103/0300-1652.107549.

Levin, S.M. (2007a) A suspensory system for the sacrum in pelvic mechanics: biotensegrity. In: A. Vleeming, V. Mooney, R. Stoeckart (eds) *Movement, Stability and Lumbopelvic Pain,* 2nd edition. Edinburgh: Churchill Livingstone; pp. 229–237.

Levin, S.M. (2007b) Hang in there! The statics and dynamics of pelvic mechanics. In: A. Vleeming, V. Mooney, R. Stoeckart (eds) *Movement, Stability and Lumbopelvic Pain,* 2nd edition. Edinburgh: Churchill Livingstone.

Lippincott, H.A. (1949) The Osteopathic Technique of Wm. G. Sutherland, D.O. In: W.G. Sutherland (1990) *Teachings in the Science of Osteopathy*. A.L. Wales (ed.). Fort Worth, TX: Sutherland Cranial Teaching Foundation, Inc./Rudra Press.

Lippincott, H.A. (1958) Corrective technique for the sacrum. *AAO Year Book Vol II;* pp. 57–58.

Lippincott, H.A. (1965) AAO Year Book Vol. II, The Depressed Sacrum, 206–209.

Mathieu, T., Gielen, J., Vyncke, G., *et al.* (2020) Arcuate pubic ligament injury: an unknown cause of athletic pubalgia. *Clinical Journal of Sport Medicine 30* (5), e175–e177.

Mitchell, F.L. Jr & Pruzzo, N.L. (1971) Investigation of voluntary and primary respiratory mechanisms. *J Am Osteopath Assoc 70,* 149–153.

Molinari, R. (2010) Personal communication.

Mollgard, K., Beinlich, F.R., Kusk, P., *et al.* (2023) A mesothelium divides the subarachnoid space into functional compartments. *Science 379* (6627), 84–88. https://doi.org/10.1126/science.adc8810.

Ojumah, N. & Loukas, M. (2018) Intriguing history of the term sacrum. *Spine Scholar 2* (1), 17–18.

Pardeshenas, H., Maroufi, N., Sanjari, M., *et al.* (2014) Lumbopelvic muscle activation patterns in three stances under graded loading conditions: proposing a tensegrity model for load transfer through the sacroiliac joints. *J Bodywork Mov Ther 18* (4), 633–642.

Robeson, K., Blondin, N. & Szekely, A. (2012) Frontotemporal brain sagging syndrome due to minor head trauma. *Neurology 78* (1), 03.212.

Roch, M., Gaudreault, N., Cyr, M.P. *et al.* (2021) The female pelvic floor fascia anatomy: a systematic search and review. *Life 11* (9), 900.

Showalter, A. (2017) Osteopathic manipulation for pubic symphysis dysfunction during spontaneous labour: a case study. *MOJ Women's Health 5* (2), 213–215.

Sugiyama, A., Tamiya, A., Yokota, H., *et al.* (2022) Frontotemporal brain sagging syndrome as a treatable cause mimicking frontotemporal dementia: a case report. *Case Rep Neurol 14* (1), 82–87.

Sutherland, W.G. (1990) *Teachings in the Science of Osteopathy*. A.L. Wales (ed.). Fort Worth, TX: Sutherland Cranial Teaching Foundation, Inc./Rudra Press; pp. 23, 88, 199, 205, 251.

Sutherland, W.G. (1998) *Contributions of Thought,* 2nd edition. A.L. Wales and A.S. Sutherland (eds). Fort Worth, TX: Sutherland Cranial Teaching Foundation, Inc.; pp. 125, 131, 160, 224–225, 278–283, 285, 286, 287, 288.

Vancaillie, T., Eggermont, J., Armstrong, G., *et al.* (2012) Response to pudendal nerve block in women with pudendal neuralgia. *Pain Medicine 13* (4), 596–603.

Vleeming, A., Pool-Goudzwaard, A.L., Hammudoghlu, D., *et al.* (1996) The function of the long dorsal sacroiliac ligament: its implication for understanding low back pain. *Spine (Phila Pa 1976) 21* (5), 556–562.

Vleeming, A., Schuenke, M.D., Masi, A.T., *et al.* (2012) The sacroiliac joint: an overview of its anatomy, function and potential clinical implications. *Journal of Anatomy 221* (6), 537–567.

Volinski, B., Kalra, A. & Yang, K. (2018) Evaluation of full pelvic ring stresses using a bilateral static gait-phase finite element modelling method. *Journal of Mechanical Behavior of Biomedical Materials 78,* 175–187.

Wales, A.L. (1988) Andrew Still Sutherland Study Group (ASSSG). Rhode Island, USA.

Wales, A.L. (1992) Personal communication.

Wales, A.L. (1995) Personal communication.

Wales, A.L. (1996) Personal communication.

Walker, J.M. (1992) The sacroiliac joint: a critical review. *Physical Therapy 71,* 903–916.

Wang, Y., Li, M.R., Wang, N., *et al.* (2021) Role of relaxin in diastasis of the pubic symphysis peripartum. *World J Clin Cases 9* (1), 91–101.

Wicklund, M.R., Mokri, B., Drubach, D., *et al.* (2011) Frontotemporal brain-sagging syndrome. *Neurology 76* (16), 1377–1382. https://doi.org/10.1212/WNL.0b013e3182166e42.

Willard, F., Vleeming, A., Schuenke, M.D., Danneels, L. & Schleip, R. (2012) The thoracolumbar fascia: anatomy, function and clinical considerations. *J Anat 221* (6), 507–536.

Williams, P.L. (1995) *Gray's Anatomy,* 38th edition. Edinburgh: Churchill Livingstone.

CHAPTER 4

The Ribcage

SUSAN TURNER

PART 1: RIBS 1–10

'All you have to do is hold the bolt, that is the rib, in a position...and ask the patient to turn the nut, that is the facet or related facets of the related vertebrae. The patient does this by turning the opposite shoulder, or perhaps just his head, away. With respiratory cooperation, added to this postural cooperation, the ligaments related to the joints involved that have held the head of the rib in the facet will bring it back into normal relationship.'

(Sutherland 1990, TSO p. 143)

The three-dimensional shape of the ribcage, bounded by the diaphragm below and Sibson's fascia and cupola of the lung above, is beautifully adapted for integrated movement. Good mobility is essential for supporting oxygenation, cardiovascular function and lymphatic flow. The balance of the shoulder girdle, head and neck is only ever as good as the platform provided by the scaffolding of the ribcage.

The ribs are often referred to as the 'Cinderella' of osteopathy in generally lacking the attention they deserve. Strained ribs can cause extreme pain and adversely affect physiology. They may also limit respiratory excursion and spinal mobility. Drs Sutherland and Wales recommended resolving rib strains before addressing the thoracic spine. They also treated the ribs for beneficial effects on the autonomic nervous system, lymphatic flow and the whole lung field, especially during infection.

This approach to the ribs is effective, quick, precise and comfortable for the patient.

ANATOMY OF THE RIBS

When approaching the treatment of the ribs, we take the particular morphology of the different levels into the picture. Anteriorly, ribs 1–10 articulate with the costal cartilages at the costochondral junctions.

- The 'true' ribs (1–7) articulate directly with the sternum via the costal cartilages.

- The 'false' ribs (8, 9 and 10) adjoin the costal cartilages but not the sternum.
- The 'floating' ribs (11 and 12) are free of an anterior cartilaginous attachment. These have large heads but no tubercles so the necks are not defined.

Costovertebral joints

All ribs except the 1st, 10th, 11th and 12th articulate with two vertebral bodies and the transverse process of the inferior of the two segments. Each rib head has two articular facets with a crest between them. These form a double synovial 'socket' joint with the vertebral body above and below with the disc and interarticular ligament between them. The rib is named after the *inferior* of the two vertebral segments. Each rib, with its tuberosity and articular facets, points towards the nucleus pulposus at the centre of the intervertebral disc.

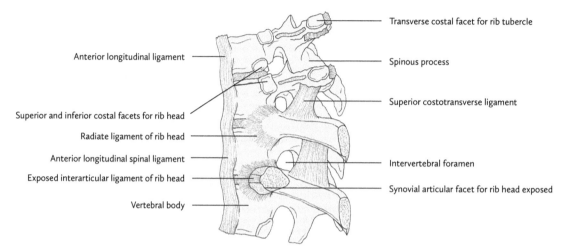

Figure 4.1 Lateral view of thoracic spine and rib relationship.

Costovertebral ligaments

Three main costovertebral ligaments guide and limit joint motion with the vertebral body. From superficial to deep, these are:

- The radiate ligament which fans out from the rib head to the disc and vertebral bodies above and below, merging with the sides of the anterior longitudinal ligament.
- The capsular ligament, surrounding the double synovial joint.
- The intra-articular ligament from the crest of the rib to the disc.

Costotransverse joints

The posterior aspect of the neck and tubercle of a typical rib articulates with the anterior aspect of the transverse process (TP) of its corresponding (inferior) vertebra. The ligaments involved are:

- The costotransverse ligament between the neck of the rib and the shaft of the transverse process.
- The articular fibrous capsule.
- The lateral costotransverse ligament which wraps the lateral TP and the non-articular part of the costal tubercle.

The intertransverse ligaments connect the costotransverse joint on the rib neck to the TP of the vertebra above.

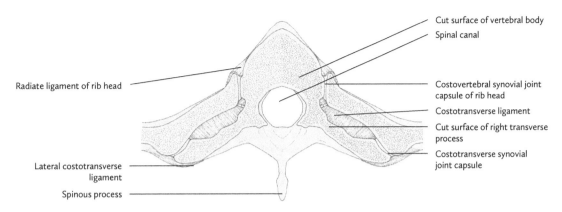

Figure 4.2 Transverse section through costovertebral junction, superior view.

Dr Sutherland likened the shape of a typical rib to a horseshoe. The long arm extends from the rib angle to the anterior end. The short arm extends from the angle to the rib head and costovertebral-costotransverse articulations (Lippincott 1949).

The endothoracic fascia is a layer of loose connective tissue uniting the thoracic cavity. It provides an interface between the ribs and intercostal muscles externally and the parietal pleural layer internal to it. In terms of treatment, we can think of this as acting analogously to the internal periosteal and meningeal dural layers lining the cranium. Just as the endosteal dura binds and unites the cranial bones and sutures, the endothoracic fascia assists the thorax in acting as one unit of function. This can be engaged in diagnosis and treatment of these regions as a whole.

RELEVANT MUSCULATURE

The 'double spiral' arrangement of the intercostal muscles of the thoracic wall is triple-layered with nerves and blood vessels passing between the layers. The intercostal nerve, artery and vein run along the inferior surface of each rib.

Transversus thoracis muscle

Anteriorly the fan-shaped transversus thoracis muscle arises from the internal surface of the xiphoid and lower two segments of the sternum. It spreads out to insert into the 3rd to 6th costochondral junctions. As it is very active in the action of coughing, it may remain palpably hypertonic after respiratory infection. Such retained tensions tend to anchor the anterior thorax and hold the ribcage in an exhalation position. This inhibits full respiratory excursion and therefore oxygenation and lymphatic flow. It may also exaggerate thoracic kyphosis. In the author's experience, this can be a factor in repeated respiratory infections if the tethering effect of this muscle on the sternum is not resolved. Efficient lymphatic flow, oxygenation and cardiovascular circulation, essential for optimum health, all depend on free thoracic and diaphragmatic respiratory movement.

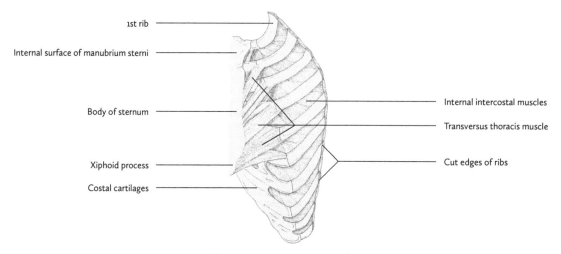

1st rib

Internal surface of manubrium sterni

Body of sternum

Xiphoid process

Costal cartilages

Internal intercostal muscles

Transversus thoracis muscle

Cut edges of ribs

Figure 4.3 Transversus thoracis muscle, internal surface of anterior ribcage.

Sternohyoid and sternothyroid muscles

The sternohyoid and sternothyroid muscles act on the manubrium sterni from above, enabling the sternum to contribute to the stabilisation of the hyoid bone and floor of the tongue in the actions of infant suckling and of speech (Konow *et al.* 2010; Mayeri *et al.* 2020).

COSTOVERTEBRAL 'WEDGING'

In normal respiratory inhalation, the rib heads rotate slightly posteriorly and into external rotation in relation to the socket formed by the vertebral demifacets and disc (Sutherland 1998, COT p. 270). Contrary to the general view of the time, Dr Sutherland perceived the sternal ends of the ribs to move posteriorly on respiratory inhalation and anteriorly on exhalation. He related this to a 'sickle motion' of the rib, together with a 'spinning motion' at the costovertebral end.

When in a state of strain, the dual articulation of the costovertebral junctions risks wedging of the rib heads into the socket, formed by the vertebral body above and below (Wales 1996). This braces the intersegmental relationship, causing restricted movement in the thoracic spine. This can also result in hyperextension or flattening of the thoracic spine (Sutherland 1990, TSO p. 250). Dr Sutherland likened the loss of normal thoracic curve to a flat foot, in that both have reduced resilience to impact.

CLINICAL CONSIDERATIONS

The lateral chain (sympathetic) ganglia are situated on the front of the rib heads, and when the heads of the ribs are released laterally, the tissues around the ganglia appear to relax, improving their blood flow. Experience suggests that this helps to 'set the stage' for the patient's respiratory movement to continue the normalisation of sympathetic activity, following the treatment session.

The author had an experience of the power of this when visiting Dr Anne Wales in a state of shock and high anxiety. After a brief chat she said, 'I'm going to beat you up.' She was 95 years old at the time and, knowing her sense of humour, I understood that she intended to give me a very comfortable osteopathic treatment. I lay down on the plinth as she sat beside me with her hands under the rib angles, creating a little anterior and lateral leverage to draw the rib heads laterally with each thoracic exhalation. Within minutes my anxiety calmed and I was relaxed. I was aware, not only of her hands seemingly melting with my tissues, but of her state of grounded and calm presence, as if aligned between Heaven and Earth.

She described using this same manoeuvre 70 years previously as a young intern in an osteopathic hospital, where she was required to treat patients with pneumonia. She graduated in 1926, before the discovery of antibiotics or even vitamin C, and was given the task of treating the supine patients for 5 minutes once an hour round the clock. Down on her knees with her hands contacting the rib angles under the bedclothes, her aim was to balance the sympathetic chain by laterally releasing the rib heads at the costovertebral junctions. Referring to the effect of this on the vasomotor system, she quoted Dr Still's advice to 'Turn on the blood supply' and declared 'It works! I've done it!'

Dr Wales once recounted how, in 1983, she had suffered from tachycardia until two colleagues, who were teaching on the same course, had simultaneously released her 4th rib on each side. She felt the benefit from this moment for many years (Wales 1995).

It is easy to see a parallel here between this approach and that of J.M. Littlejohn who would engage the function of the thoracic sympathetic segmental reflex pathways via stimulation or inhibition of the paraspinal muscles. This uses a different method but with similar intent (Wernham 1975). Dr Still himself frequently used paraspinal inhibition (Hildreth 1942) (see Chapter 16).

Where the 1st rib is raised and the clavicle depressed, compression of the neurovascular bundle supplying the upper limb can produce brachial symptoms, mimicking spinal nerve root entrapment. Strain of the costovertebral junction may cause facilitation of the stellate ganglia close to the heads of the 1st ribs. These exert strong sympathetic vasomotor and neural influence to the head as well as brachial plexus and upper chest, including the heart.

THERAPEUTIC ENGAGEMENT

Global assessment of the ribcage

1. A preliminary observation of natural breathing is helpful. The pattern of rib movement may reveal, for example, scoliosis, accessory muscle use or a visible sense of emotional holding. Intercostal retractions may show respiratory distress. In asthma and COPD there is difficulty with exhalation but in pneumonia and congestive heart failure there is resistance to inhalation. Internal organic factors can affect the resiliency of the thoracic cage, such as pleural adhesions and scarring from radiotherapy. A history of pneumothorax, pneumonia or an emotional weight on the heart feels 'heavy' on palpation. The strong impression of implosion or 'sucking in' of the ribs in a current pneumothorax is unmistakeable. (For anterior thoracic fascial influences see Chapter 5.)

2. A simple way to assess rib movement is to stand behind the seated patient and place your hands around the posterior aspect of the ribs bilaterally, observing *how your hands are moved* in inhalation and exhalation at each level. Take note of any rib that is 'out of step' with the rest. It is surprising how precisely a restricted rib often corresponds with a patient's site of pain.

3. *Standing behind the seated patient, the 1st ribs can be palpated by placing the hands over the middle portion of the trapezius muscles with the fingertips just behind the clavicles in the supraclavicular fossa. Note whether they rise and fall with equal ease on each inhalation and exhalation to discern any restriction in either phase.* The first rib may be raised by a hypertonic scalene muscle. It may also be depressed because of intrathoracic factors or a restricted rib on any level below, including the 12th rib. Special attention should be paid to congestion in the supraclavicular fossa with regard to the 1st rib and lymphatic return.

4. *Standing to the side of the seated patient, place one hand on the sternum and the other on the spine and ribs posteriorly.* As you feel the movement of the sternum and anterior ribs, notice any mismatch of the respiratory movement between the front and the back. The anteroposterior relationship of the thorax may reveal fascial or muscular anterior tethering which inhibits costosternal movement (see Chapter 5).

5. *Place the hands around the 11th and 12th ribs and check their symmetry of movement as the patient breathes in and out.* Unlike the rest of the ribcage, the 12th ribs should descend on inhalation rather than lift. If one side is unable to move with breathing and is tethering the whole thorax on that side, check the tone of the diaphragm and of quadratus lumborum.

Supine global ribcage engagement
1. CONTACT
Sitting behind the head of the supine patient, place the palms and outstretched fingers under the rib angles, encompassing as many ribs as possible. Sensitively leaning your weight into your forearm fulcra will enable your hands to engage and match the tone of the endothoracic fascia and parietal pleura.

Because the endothoracic fascia lines and

unites the thorax in a similar way to the endosteal dural layer lining the skull, it is possible, with this hold, to gain an impression of the global balance of the thorax. Matching areas of greater density will require more forearm leverage on the treatment table than where the tissues are free.

This hold is useful, both for a preliminary assessment and for bringing the whole thorax through a cycle of balanced tension, leading to more specific work.

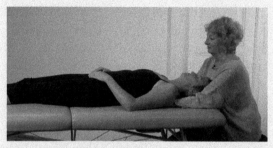

Figure 4.4 Supine global ribcage hold.

Supine simple lateral disengagement of a rib group
1. CONTACT
Sit beside the supine patient on the side to be addressed and place the palmar surface of the middle fingers of both hands under the rib angles. The two hands together can engage a group of up to six ribs at a time.

The aim is to exert enough leverage under the rib angles to *minimally lift the rib heads anteriorly and laterally, slightly disengaging them from impaction in the dual socket of the demifacets and disc*. This combined anterolateral movement, to engage and activate the ligaments, is enabled by leaning into your forearm fulcra to precisely match the forces holding the rib strain.

2. ENGAGEMENT AND USE OF FULCRA
To find this point of 'meeting' with the ligamentous-articular mechanism, find out what is too much or too little force and the 'sweet point' between them. *Slowly increase your leaning force*

through your forearm or elbow fulcra until you go beyond that point. Then lighten the weight on your fulcra so that, once again, you lose that meeting point. *Then slowly increase the force through them until, between too much and too little, you recognise the point of matching of forces by a sense of ligamentous enlivening* (Becker 1990). This sometimes feels like a wriggling or searching movement at the costovertebral end.

3. HOLDING STEADY
Maintain support of the ribs, matching the resistance, until the rhythmic movement of thoracic respiration shifts the costovertebral ligamentous-articular relationship towards free movement. This is often accompanied by a sense of easier lateral glide and improved tissue perfusion, warmth and pliability in the spinal and paraspinal tissues.

The same approach can be used on a single rib with one (active) hand supporting the other (sensory, afferent, monitoring) hand in contact with the rib angle.

Combining rib disengagement and intervertebral resolution
Intervertebral strain and costovertebral strain often occur together. In children especially, *gentle lateral release of a single rib with one hand can be combined with finding BLT for the two associated vertebrae segments. The index and third fingers of the other hand move the two adjacent spinous processes to their position of ease to match the strain.*

These positions are held and the tension matched until the patient's breathing shifts the articular fulcra via the anterior longitudinal spinal ligament (ALSL) and the strain realigns.

Supine 'nut and bolt' BLT for a single rib
1. DIAGNOSIS
As always, consider all components of the rib strain, e.g., compacted, distracted or held in inhalation or exhalation.

2. HANDHOLD
Sit at the side of the supine patient with the middle fingers and palms of each hand comfortably but firmly embracing the rib, back and front, matching the tone and position, e.g., fixed exhalation, impaction.

With the anterior hand, slightly draw the sternal end of the rib posteriorly as if 'squeezing' the rib a little while stabilising it.

3. STABILISATION OF THE FASCIA ON THE OPPOSITE SIDE
Ask the patient to dorsiflex the contralateral foot, to focus the field of operation.

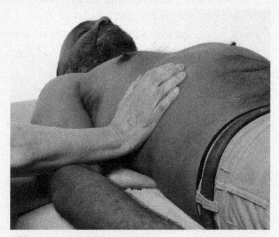

Figure 4.5 Supine single rib hold.

4. POSTURAL COOPERATION
To maximise effectiveness, *ask the patient to rotate the vertebral bodies away by 'slowly turning the head' to the opposite side.* This is only up to the first point of resistance or tension in the costovertebral ligaments. This rotation of the vertebral bodies will lift the rib head slightly anteriorly, disengaging it from its fixity in its costovertebral socket. Meanwhile the rib tubercle is brought to bear on the fulcrum of the costotransverse joint.

From your contact on the rib angle, you may 'read' the activation of the ligaments at the rib head as they seek their position of balanced tension.

Hold the rib steady throughout, to prevent it from moving with the rotation of the vertebral body, otherwise the leverage needed for the correction will be lost. You are 'holding the bolt' (the rib) while the patient 'turns the nut' (the vertebral end)!

5. RESPIRATORY COOPERATION
For a rib held in inspiration the patient augments this pattern by holding inhalation. The eventual spontaneous outbreath that follows local easing of the costovertebral joint will complete the correction by carrying the rib freely into exhalation, to regain its full range of movement.

Conversely, *for an exhalation rib strain, the patient holds the breath out to augment the position of strain.* Spontaneous inhalation completes reversal of the strain when he or she can no longer resist breathing in.

6. PATIENT RESUMES CONTROL
The patient is then asked to reverse all postural cooperation by relaxing the opposite foot and derotating the head and neck back to centre. This returns the socket to correct apposition with the rib head. Only then do you slowly withdraw your contact, leaning back slightly to gently float the rib away in its release.

Sitting unilateral 'nut and bolt' BLT for ribs 4–10
A more potent version of the supine rib correction described above can be used effectively with the patient sitting, as follows.

1. DIAGNOSIS
Consider all components of the rib strain as above.

2. CONTACT
The patient sits at the end of the treatment table with the involved side towards you. Take a broad-based stance for stability.

Wrap both hands around the side of the patient's thorax nearest to you. The middle fingers and middle

ray of your palms contact the involved rib, anteriorly, towards the sternal end and posteriorly, at the angle.

Your connected hands 'blend' with the rib with a firm and steady contact throughout the procedure.

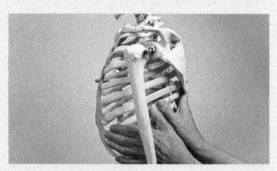

Figure 4.6 Middle rib hold on skeleton.

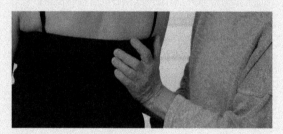

Figure 4.7 Handhold on sitting model.

3. MATCHING OF OPERATOR'S AND PATIENT'S WEIGHT
Initially, the costovertebral junction is approximated to relax the ligaments by *asking the patient, 'present your rib to me'.* You then lean towards the patient so that you each match the other's weight effortlessly like a 'card house'.

If the patient finds it difficult to give his or her weight to you, make sure you have not lost contact with the support of the ground as you may not be communicating steady support. We constantly need to check our own centre of gravity.

4. POSTURAL COOPERATION FOR LIGAMENTOUS ENGAGEMENT
As you stabilise the rib, ask the patient to draw the opposite shoulder back slightly as if turning away. This is just to the point where you feel the first

hint of tension at the costovertebral junction. The aim is to bring the rib to bear upon the fulcrum of the costotransverse joint and slightly disengage the rib head from the vertebral demifacets. This also activates the ligaments to explore for the point of balance.

5. RESPIRATORY COOPERATION
For a rib fixed in inhalation, the patient is asked to augment the pattern by inhaling and holding. When local ligamentous change is perceived at the costovertebral junction, the patient's full exhalation completes the correction. The converse is enlisted for a rib fixed in exhalation. A sense of ease and greater freedom of movement may then be perceived.

6. RESUMING POSTURAL CONTROL
Ask the patient to sit up slowly, reversing the rotation and taking back postural control. Only then do you slowly withdraw contact, having 'escorted them home' first.

Sitting release of ribs 2 and 3
The method for ribs 2 and 3 is similar to the sitting release for ribs 4–10 apart from a small adaptation to contact the ribs overlaid by the scapula.

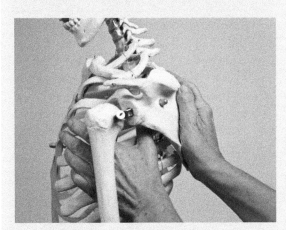

Figure 4.8 Upper rib contact on skeleton.

1. CONTACT: 'PUTTING THE GLOVE OVER THE HAND RATHER THAN THE HAND INTO THE GLOVE'
Stand beside the seated patient.

The index or middle finger of the posterior hand contacts the rib close to the transverse process while the thumb and palm hold the lower lateral border of the scapula upward and medially.

The index or middle finger of the anterior hand contacts the sternal end of the rib concerned, while the thumb makes a soft but stable fulcrum contact on the mid-axillary line of the involved rib.

To do this *ask the patient to lift the shoulder up towards the ear. As the shoulder lifts, advance your thumb from the lateral scapular border up along the mid-axillary line towards the rib to be addressed.* Maintain the advance as the patient then comfortably settles the shoulder back down over the thumb. This may be repeated several times, so that you advance further each time, until contact is made on the lateral surface of the rib you seek to engage. Be careful not to flex your thumb in this tender area.

Give clear instructions such as 'lift your shoulder up towards your ear', then 'slowly allow your shoulder to comfortably settle over my thumb'.

2. RECIPROCAL LEANING TO MATCH WEIGHT
The patient slowly leans the involved rib towards your secure and grounded contact so that your two weights effortlessly match.

3. POSTURAL COOPERATION
As before, ask the patient to slightly turn the opposite shoulder back to the first point of ligamentous resistance. As the vertebral body rotates away, the rib head disengages and the costal tubercle is brought to bear on the fulcrum of the transverse process, activating the ligaments.

The further cephalad the ribs are, the less the shoulder needs to turn to find the point of engagement. To avoid over-enthusiastic trunk rotation *a helpful instruction might be: 'As you lean against me, until I say stop, slowly turn your opposite shoulder back.'*

4. HOLDING STEADY

As with the middle ribs described above, *hold the rib steady and wait while the costovertebral ligaments reach a point of balanced tension, and a local proprioceptive change is perceived.* This may be aided by the patient's active respiratory cooperation where the return breath, after holding, restores the full range of rib excursion.

5. RESUMING POSTURAL CONTROL

Ask the patient to reverse the postural rotation and sit up as you escort him or her back to full postural control.

Sitting unilateral correction of rib 1

The principles described above for both the sitting and supine approach can be modified for the 1st rib, while taking into account its unique features.

The 1st and the 12th ribs both balance complex myofascial forces acting on the thorax from above, below and transversely. For this reason, Dr Anne Wales advised that intermediate ribs are often easier to engage therapeutically when we have first made sure that the 1st and the 12th are free.

Specific anatomy

The first rib is short, wide and flat and is the strongest and most curved of all the ribs. Strong muscular forces act upon it from scalenus anterior and medius, serratus anterior and levator costae. The suprapleural membrane (Sibson's fascia) attaches to the transverse process of C7 and suspends the lung from the inferior surface of the 1st rib, rendering the rib vulnerable to strain from intrathoracic fascial and organic forces. For this reason, take note of any history of pneumonia, asthma, pneumothorax, cardiovascular events or immune deficiency.

The 1st costal cartilage attaches to the inter-articular disc of the sternoclavicular joint, costo-clavicular joint and the origin of subclavius.

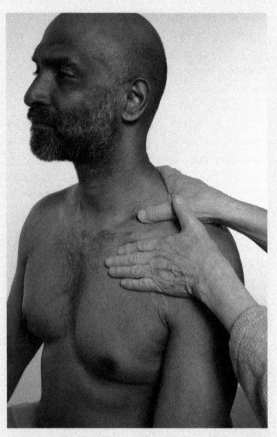

Figure 4.9 Handhold on 1st rib.

The complexity of the forces acting on the 1st rib render it prone to positional distortion and also to intraosseous strains, which can be painful and may sometimes refer to the shoulder. Both the 1st and the 2nd rib are essential to the function of the whole shoulder.

1. SUGGESTED HAND CONTACT

Standing beside the patient who is seated on the treatment table, make an anterior, lateral and posterior contact on the 1st rib. Fold your posterior hand over the trapezius muscles of the seated patient's shoulder, with the index finger immediately lateral to the transverse process of T1. Your thumb rests on the lateral superior surface of the first rib between trapezius and the clavicle.

The index finger of the anterior hand contacts the anterior surface of rib 1 below the clavicle. Link the thumb with the posterior hand, to enable the two hands to work as a unit.

2. POSTURAL COOPERATION

As for the other ribs, *hold the rib stable with both hands while the patient leans very slightly towards you for a minimal degree of approximation of the costovertebral junction. To engage the costovertebral ligaments at T1, ask the patient to 'just think about' turning the opposite shoulder posteriorly, but only minutely so as to avoid involving the neck.*

3. RESPIRATORY COOPERATION

For a raised 1st rib, ask the patient to inhale and hold; vice versa for a depressed position. 'Read' the changes at work in the costovertebral ligaments and also note any intraosseous reorganisation within the 1st rib itself. The patient lets the breath go when

it can no longer be held in or out to complete the correction.

4. 'ESCORTING THE PATIENT HOME'

Support the patient back to vertical postural control and then gently withdraw contact. Treat both sides if necessary.

Alternative hold for the 1st rib

The first rib may also be engaged with the thumb under the anterior border of trapezius, advancing with each respiratory cycle to contact the anterior edge of the posterior part of the rib shaft. With the other hand, hold the trapezius back and slightly disengage the costovertebral junction by hooking a finger around the spinous process of T1 and drawing it towards you. Hold steady as the patient's natural breathing shifts the fulcrum and the rib releases.

(See Part 2 for supine unilateral release of ribs 11 and 12.)

PART 2: RIBS 11 AND 12 AND THEIR INFLUENCE ON PHYSIOLOGY

'The crura of the diaphragm have more effect on physiology than almost any other structure.'

(W.G. Sutherland as quoted by Anne Wales 1988)

By virtue of their position and attachment to the lumbocostal arches or 'arcuate ligaments', the 12th ribs are well placed to exert a key influence on both the body's structural balance and its physiology. Together with the diaphragmatic crura, the lumbocostal arches form the posterior attachments of the diaphragm and contribute to the posterior abdominal wall.

The 12th ribs provide a useful contact for

positively influencing freedom of respiratory movement and benefitting the related organs and vessels. Pertinent to this, Dr Wales often spoke of the skeleton as a 'handle' through which our external contact enables us to perceive the shape, texture and motion quality of the physiological environment within. She described a handhold on the skeleton as being analogous to holding a door handle while being aware that it was also held by someone else on the other side of the door, i.e., on the inside of the body (Wales 1981). This piece of advice has proved invaluable for opening perception in palpation.

The shape and mobility of an anatomical 'container' defines the spatial environment of the encompassed organs, vessels and nerves. Tissues and organs need to be free from restraint imposed by the skeletal and fascial system in order to express their inherent motion. Stasis is one of the greatest enemies of healthy physiology. Three-dimensional rhythmic shape change anywhere in the body constitutes a physiological pump for the vital interchange of fluids. Nowhere is this more obvious than in the ribcage and diaphragm. If 'unwellness is an undesirable change of space' (Wales 1988) then one of our aims in restoring healthy function must be simply 'changing the geometry of the space'.

ANATOMY

The anatomy of the lower ribs reveals what a perfect handle the 12th ribs are for engaging the lumbocostal arches, crura, diaphragm and encompassed pertinent interior structures. The 12th ribs attach to the superficial layer of the thoracolumbar fascia (TLF) while the lateral arcuate ligaments suspend the TLF middle layer (see Chapter 5).

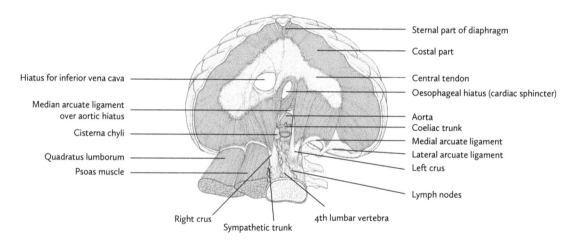

Figure 4.10 12th ribs, lumbocostal arches (arcuate ligaments) and crura.

Lumbocostal arches (arcuate ligaments)

- Each *lateral lumbocostal arch* spans from the middle of the 12th rib to the transverse process (TP) of L1 or 2. It is a thickened band covering the fascia of quadratus lumborum and provides the upper attachment of the middle layer of the TLF complex. Here it blends with the anterior fascial sheath of the TLF, covering quadratus lumborum (Willard *et al.* 2012). When the 12th ribs are displaced inferiorly this may strain the lateral arcuate ligaments, compressing the quadratus lumborum muscles and also the ilioinguinal and iliohypogastric nerves.
- The *medial arch* spans the TP of L1 to the side of the body of L1 and blends with the lateral margins of the ipsilateral diaphragmatic crus. It is a tendinous arch in the fascia covering psoas.
- The *median arch* is formed of a fibrous band linking the two crura. It covers the cisterna chyli and the aorta at the level of L1, just cephalad to the coeliac trunk.

- The *crura* lie over the vertebral bodies, and blend with the ALSL, the right one normally at L3 and the left at L2. The aorta passes under the crura, as does the cisterna chyli where it enters the lymphatic 'highway' of the thoracic duct.
- The *right crus* loops around the oesophagus, contributing to the cardiac sphincter of the stomach at the oesoph-ageal hiatus. The vagus nerve also passes through this sphincter. The ligament of Treitz, which is partly muscular and partly ligamentous, suspends the duodenal-jejunal (DJ) junction from the right crus (Nassar *et al.* 2021).

PHYSIOLOGICAL RELEVANCE

Free motion of the 12th ribs and their lumbocos-tal arches, with each breathing cycle, provides physiological support by transmitting rhythmic motion to the encompassed organs. The sub-phrenic organs of elimination and detoxification, e.g., liver, spleen, kidneys and colon, are strategi-cally positioned to benefit from this stimulus to their tissue motion.

If the lower ribs are held in a static strain pat-tern however, the arterial, venous and lymphatic flow in the encompassed vital organs may suffer. This carries a risk of stasis, resulting in poor fluid interchange in the cellular environment, and is potentially undermining to homoeostasis (see Chapter 15). The ability of the individual to 'breathe into the back', spontaneously moving the lower ribs with thoracic respiration, is fundamen-tal to the healthy environment of the vital organs.

The fascial envelopes of the kidneys and adrenal glands are closely connected and rest on the psoas fascia and crura. Dr Wales noted that chronic static strain in this area is often present in patients who tend to form renal calculi and gallstones. On rare occasions, the passing of gall-stones or kidney stones may follow release of the 12th rib. This is not advocated as a treatment for these conditions however, as general medi-cal procedures are safer and more comfortable.

The crura and median arcuate ligament
W.G. Sutherland referred to the crura of the dia-phragm as having 'more influence on physiology than almost any other structure', calling them a 'central physiological plug for the body' (Wales 1988). This is an extraordinary statement for someone who spent much of his adult life explor-ing the container of the brain.

Lymphatic flow
The thoracic respiratory movement of the crura is central to the flow of lymph through the thoracic duct, assisting the passage of lymph from the lower body, under the median arcuate ligamentous 'bridge'. The upward flow of lymph into the venous system is also supported by the biphasic motion of the diaphragm as a whole which functions as a 'lymphatic sponge', drawing excess intra-abdominal fluid through its lacunae into the retrosternal lymphatics (Abu-Hijleh *et al.* 1995) (see Chapter 5 and Chapter 15).

Arterial flow: 'Goat and boulder'
A.T. Still perceived chronic fixity of the dia-phragmatic crura to restrict the downward flow of aortic blood, 'predisposing the development of cardiac valvular pathology' (Sutherland 1998, COT p. 262). This is illustrated by Still's parable of 'the goat and the boulder' (Sutherland 1990, TSO p. 214). Here, a goat, determined to move a boulder in its mountain path, rushed at it repeatedly with no success. The first time 'his tail flopped up'. The second time 'his tail and hind legs flopped up'. The third time he rushed at it so hard that 'the whole damn works flopped up'. He

left his students to work out that the goat represented the valves of the heart, and the mountain path the arterial stream of the aorta. The boulder represented the crura with the median arcuate ligament between them, potentially compressing the aorta (Still 1902). His point was that resistance to the downward flow of aortic blood potentially created back pressure which, over time, would damage the mitral valve (see Chapter 5, diaphragm section).

This metaphor may be worth considering in cardio-compromised patients of any age. Even in neonates, the establishment of the new circulatory pathways involving closure of the atrial septum is sensitive to the balance of fluid pressures between the left and right heart. It is therefore important to release any retained tensions in the infant diaphragm to avoid any increased pressure on the left side of the heart (Severino and Severino 2017).

Cardiac venous return

'He cannot expect blood to quietly pass through the diaphragm if impeded by muscular constriction around the aorta, vena cava or thoracic duct. The diaphragm can be/is often pulled down on both the vena cava and thoracic duct, obstructing blood and chyle (lymph) from returning to the heart.'

(Still 1899, p. 36)

Where there is poor respiratory motion or asymmetrical forces are acting on the diaphragm, restraint on the inferior vena cava (IVC) may inhibit venous return to the heart (Kimura *et al.* 2011). This is, in part, because the IVC is valveless and its return flow of blood is dependent on the pumping action of free diaphragmatic movement.

Renal arterial flow and hypertension

Several studies suggest that compression of the left renal artery against the aorta, exerted by the left crus, can cause renal artery stenosis. The resulting diminished renal arterial flow has been shown, in some cases, to trigger the renin-angiotensin response resulting in hypertension (Bagnet and Thony 2003; Dove-Smith and Bloch 1998; Gaebel *et al.* 2009; Lazareth *et al.* 2009).

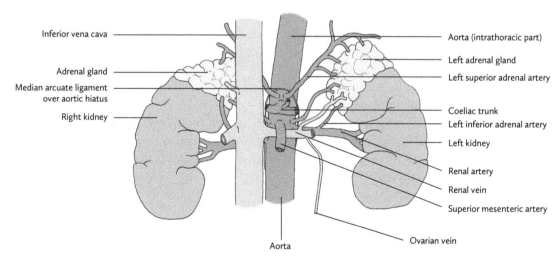

Figure 4.11 Adrenal and renal circulation.

Adrenal arterial supply

The anatomical position of the three suprarenal arteries would suggest that they could be even more vulnerable to compression than the renal and coeliac arteries. The suprarenal arteries branch from the inferior phrenic artery, the renal artery and the abdominal aorta. The superior and middle suprarenal arteries leave the aorta in a more cephalad position, relative to the median arcuate ligament, than the renal artery. This suggests that adrenal blood flow is at an even greater risk of impingement and compromise than that of the left kidney.

Ovarian venous drainage

In physiological disturbances of the *left ovary*, it is worth noting that the left ovarian vein drains into the left renal vein (Ghosh and Chaudhury 2019). This suggests the possibility that a contributory factor in ovarian circulatory stasis could sometimes be related to renal venous drainage, compromised by static strain in the diaphragm.

Coeliac artery compression

'Median arcuate ligament syndrome' has been known to occur where hypertrophy, tightness or low position of this ligament has caused compression of the coeliac artery. The resulting symptoms are epigastric pain and weight loss (Arazinska and Polgui 2016; Horton *et al.* 2005).

It is often possible to ease undue tension in the medial arcuate ligament by bringing it to a state of BLT through bilateral posterior contact on the supine 12th ribs. This can have pleasing results, although, with babies and young children, there are also many other positive developmental forces at work.

Experience in osteopathic practice has shown a calming effect on the sympathetic nervous system when the crura and arcuate ligaments are released via the 12th ribs. Among the many possible processes at work in the body, this may ease the pathways of renal and adrenal blood flow and improve the spatial environment of these organs.

Although the interactions within body physiology are too complex to involve just one phenomenon, a shift in just one component will sometimes 'begin to loosen the knot' enough to enable the body's innate self-correcting forces to restore homoeostasis.

Stomach and duodenum

Where the 12th ribs are not free to move with the diaphragm, the stomach, duodenum and pancreas are also deprived of the supportive effect of rhythmic shape change on their vascular perfusion. The resulting stasis may diminish their functional efficiency.

The *cardiac sphincter* of the stomach is largely formed by the loop of the right crus around the lower oesophagus. This anatomical arrangement is likely to make the sphincter responsive to alterations in crural tension which is a consideration in cases of reflux. The pathogenesis of gastro-oesophageal reflux (GERD) is thought to be related to factors such as lower oesophageal sphincter pressure or relaxation and crural diaphragmatic dysfunction (Ettlinger 2003; Zheng *et al.* 2021). A study by Eguaras *et al.* (2019) explored the application of osteopathic manual treatment in subjects with GERD with positive outcomes one week after treatment.

Dr Wales observed that, in her many decades of experience, static strain of the lumbocostal arches was often present in cases of hiatus hernia. She had also noticed an association with spasms of the sphincter of Oddi, the pancreatic duct and pyloric sphincter (Wales 1988; Zheng *et al.* 2021).

The *ligament of Treitz* passes across the anterior surface of the aorta where it suspends the duodenal-jejunal (DJ) junction from the right crus. Because of this arrangement, fascial drag on the ligament from visceroptosis is likely to compress the median arcuate ligament, the aorta and cisterna chyli (Sutherland 1990, TSO p. 214) (for the effects of visceroptosis, see Chapter 5).

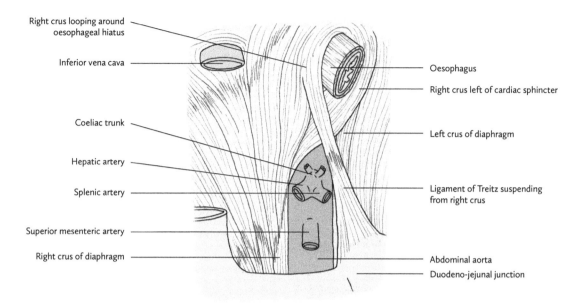

Figure 4.12 Ligament of Treitz suspending duodeno-jejunal junction from right crus.

Constipation

Sutherland wrote in 1915 of 'reaching the ascending colon without the use of high enemas'. He described treating a man with chronic constipation. With the patient sidelying, his approach was to wrap a well-padded, six-inch-wide belt around ribs 9–12. This was then attached to a suspension strap for 3–4 minutes. The results were dramatically successful (Sutherland 1998, COT pp. 7–8). Perhaps he had in mind the 'splanchnic' osteopathic spinal centres and also the effect of the rib heads on the lateral chain ganglia at that spinal level.

The spine and lower extremities

The influence exerted by the crura on the whole ALSL, spinal curves and intraspinal circulation is described in Chapter 2 and Chapter 5.

The psoas muscles, whose fascia blend with the medial arcuate ligaments, make a mechanical link between the posterior diaphragm and the femoral lesser trochanters, influencing hip function. Because of this, undue tension in the lumbocostal arches is capable of exerting upward fascial drag on the lower extremities, disturbing the fascial balance of the legs.

Nerve irritation

When the 12th ribs are displaced inferiorly this may strain the lateral arcuate ligaments, compressing the quadratus lumborum muscles and also the ilioinguinal and iliohypogastric nerves. This can result in pain in the thigh, scrotum, buttocks or groin (Carreiro 2003).

The sympathetic chain of paraspinal ganglia passes under the medial arcuate ligaments. It has been suggested that alterations in the tension of these ligaments around the sympathetic ganglia may alter their function (Patriquin 1992; Sutherland 1998, COT p. 260).

THERAPEUTIC ENGAGEMENT

Releasing static strain in the 11th and 12th ribs and lumbocostal arches

1. ASSESSMENT

Examine the lower ribs, noting their position and degree of respiratory excursion in both phases of thoracic respiration. Unlike the other ribs, the 12th rib normally descends on thoracic inhalation. The 12th rib on the right is often orientated more inferiorly than the left. Take time to feel the movement of each 12th rib with natural respiration, sensing the quality of the space above and below to gain an impression of the environment of the encompassed organs in the context of the body as a whole.

Aim: *The aim of the first stage is to free the costovertebral articulation* between the rib head and the body of T12 (or T11 if addressing the 11th rib). This is a direct approach using sensitively applied balanced tension through lateral disengagement, in cooperation with thoracic respiration.

2. SUGGESTED HAND CONTACT

Sit beside the supine patient on the side to be addressed. With one hand, make a plastic, sensory (afferent) contact along the 11th or the 12th rib with fingertips just lateral to the TP.

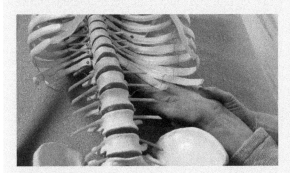

Figure 4.13 Hand position under 12th rib.

The other (active) hand supports and reinforces the sensory hand from beneath it. For leverage, the supporting hand may be best placed closer to the lateral tip of the rib, under the knuckles of the sensory hand.

3. ENGAGEMENT WITH THE COSTOVERTEBRAL JUNCTION

The body responds powerfully to where therapeutic attention is directed, especially where this is combined with the precise manual application of mechanical forces. *If you direct your intention towards the costovertebral junction, your hands will tend to spontaneously adapt as appropriate, to engage with the tissues.*

Each time the patient exhales, take advantage of the rib's natural movement towards you as the costovertebral junction relaxes. Take up the slack by leaning back a little, using your body weight to draw the rib towards you, just up to the first hint of resistance but no more. You are then in balanced tension with the patient's tissues.

On each inhalation resist the tendency of the rib to be pulled back into the trunk. With each exhalation a little more lateral release is gained. In this way, the costovertebral junction releases progressively with each respiratory cycle.

The effectiveness of this manoeuvre is because the forces applied are gentle enough to be below the level of tissue resistance.

4. BALANCED TENSION AND RESOLUTION

In the process, the rib may spontaneously move towards either a more horizontal or a more oblique position, as it seeks balanced tension within its position of strain. As the rib changes its orientation, it is helpful to align your own body to the direction it is pointing.

Maintain your steady and grounded contact as the inherent therapeutic agencies of the body take over and the strained position reverses. An obliquely orientated rib tends to become more horizontal as it releases. This new balance brings more space and amplitude of respiratory motion into the posterior abdominal wall and diaphragm.

5. LUMBOCOSTAL ARCHES

Aim: The aim of the second stage is to free the lumbocostal arches (arcuate ligaments) through contact on the 12th rib.

Maintaining your hand contact, now shift your attention to the lumbocostal arches on the anterior side of the 12th rib 'handle'. These ligaments attach one or two segments lower than the costovertebral junctions. Because of this, your engagement is now addressed more horizontally than in the first stage.

Now sitting at a right angle to the patient, lean back just enough to take up the slack in the lateral lumbocostal arch, putting it under a hint of tension. The degree of lateral traction should precisely match the degree of resistance, creating a state of balanced tension. *Hold it and observe as thoracic respiration slowly eases the tension and presents the medial arcuate ligament to your attention.* When you sense this also releasing, *direct your forces toward the median arcuate ligament between the crura.*

It will be remembered that both the medial and median arcuate ligaments blend with the crura.

An involuntary deep inhalation frequently accompanies the freeing of the lumbocostal arches. The response can often be felt through the whole diaphragm and its associated viscera and spinal segments. An amplification of both primary and secondary respiratory movement brings a sense of spaciousness, health and rhythm perfusing the tissues. It often feels as if the diaphragm rises cephalad as the thorax 'reclaims' it.

6. ADDRESS BOTH SIDES

Although sometimes the lumbocostal arches also release on the opposite side, *it is advisable to address the second side as well.*

7. POSSIBLE VISCEROSOMATIC INFLUENCE

If there is a viscerosomatic component to the tension held in the 11th or 12th ribs and ligaments, it may be necessary to include the compromised organ in the conceptual frame to complete the process successfully.

This is an effective way to ease the spatial environment of the subphrenic organs, especially the kidneys, adrenal glands, liver and spleen with benefit to their circulation and drainage. It also changes the spatial environment of the thoracic organs, with benefit to the heart, lungs, oesophagus and great vessels.

The 12th rib release forms part of Sutherland's treatment sequence for the lymphatics (see Chapter 15).

For releasing the crura, see Chapter 2 (transitional areas) and Chapter 5 (diaphragm lift).

Supine bilateral 12th rib spread in infants

In infants who have suffered stress during delivery or for whom the first breaths were difficult or failed to achieve full thoracic expansion, tensions may remain in the diaphragm and ribcage. For the reasons described above, this may have physiological effects, making it more difficult for the baby to settle.

A gentle bilateral release of the 12th ribs can enable the posterior attachments of the diaphragm to express normal respiratory movement, with potential benefit to cardiovascular and lymphatic function and more.

1. CONTACT

With the palmar surfaces of the fingers of each hand in empathetic contact around the 12th and lower ribs, *very gently hold the ribs laterally, but only to the degree that feels in balanced tension with the resistance of the tissues.* Keep the costovertebral junctions, posterior diaphragmatic attachments and totality of the body in mind.

Wait for a natural relaxation of the lower ribs

and diaphragm. If one side releases first, then simply wait for the other side.

This approach can be used for any rib, gently releasing the costovertebral junctions of both the lower and upper groups. Keep in mind the lateral chain of sympathetic ganglia, three-dimensional space and tissue quality of all that is contained between your hands.

VIDEOS FOR CHAPTER 4

Scan the QR code or visit https://www.youtube.com/playlist?list=PL3j_YuMBqigFQUuWVv9owhNgrLlko6HTZ to find a playlist of the videos that accompany this chapter.

REFERENCES

Abu-Hijleh, M.F., Habbal, O.A., Moqattash, S.T. (1995) The role of the diaphragm in lymphatic absorption from the peritoneal cavity. *J Anat 186* (Pt 3), 453–467.

Arazinska, A. & Polgui, M. (2016) An unusual case of left renal artery compression: a rare type of median arcuate ligament syndrome. *Surgical and Radiologic Anatomy 38,* 379–382.

Bagnet, J.P. & Thony, F. (2003) Stenting of a renal artery compressed by the diaphragm. *Journal of Human Hypertension 17,* 213–214.

Becker, R.F. (1990) British School of Osteopathy postgraduate seminar.

Carreiro, J.E. (2003) Osteopathic considerations in palpatory diagnosis and manipulative treatment. In: R.C. Ward (ed.) *Foundations for Osteopathic Medicine,* 2nd edition. Philadelphia, PA: Lippincott, Williams & Wilkins; p. 922.

Dove-Smith, P. & Bloch, R.D. (1998) Renal artery entrapment by the diaphragmatic crus revealed by helical CT angiography. *American Journal of Roentgenology 170,* 1291–1292.

Eguaras, N., Rodríguez-López, E.S., Lopez-Dicastillo, O., *et al.* (2019) Effects of osteopathic visceral treatment in patients with gastroesophageal reflux: a randomized controlled trial. *J Clin Med 8* (10), 1738.

Ettlinger, H. (2003) Treatment of the acutely ill hospitalized patient. In: R.C. Ward (ed.) *Foundations for Osteopathic Medicine,* 2nd edition. Philadelphia, PA: Lippincott, Williams & Wilkins; p. 1132.

Gaebel, G., Hinterseher, I., Saeger, H.D., Bergert, H. (2009) Compression of the left renal artery and celiac trunk by diaphragmatic crura. *Journal of Vascular Surgery 50,* 910–914.

Ghosh, A. & Chaudhury, S. (2019) A cadaveric study of ovarian veins: variations, measurements and clinical significance. *Anat Cell Biol 52* (4), 385–389.

Hildreth, A.G. (1942) *The Lengthening Shadow of Dr. Andrew Taylor Still,* 2nd edition. Paw Paw, MI: A.G. Hildreth & A.E. Van Vleck; p. 52.

Horton, K.M., Talamini, M.A., Fishman, E.K. (2005) Median arcuate ligament syndrome: evaluation with CT angiography. *Radiographics 25* (5), 1177–1182.

Kimura, B.J., Dalugdugan, R., Gilcrease, G.W., *et al.* (2011) The effect of breathing manner on inferior vena caval diameter. *Eur J Echocardiogr 12* (2), 120–123.

Konow, N., Thexton, A., Crompton, A.W., *et al.* (2010) Regional differences in length change and electromyographic heterogeneity in sternohyoid muscle during infant mammalian swallowing. *J App Physiol 109,* 439–448.

Lazareth, A., Deray, G., Cluzel, P., Bourry, E. & Izzedine, H. (2009). The case: an unusual cause of renovascular hypertension. *Kidney International 75* (11), 1239–1240.

Lippincott, H.A. (1949) The Osteopathic Technique of Wm. G. Sutherland, D.O. In: W.G. Sutherland (1990) *Teachings in the Science of Osteopathy.* A.L. Wales (ed.). Fort Worth, TX: Sutherland Cranial Teaching Foundation, Inc./Rudra Press.

Mayerl, C.J., Tobin, H.L., Chava, A.M., *et al.* (2020) Muscle function during feeding through infancy. *The FASEB Journal 34* (S1), 1.

Nassar S., Menias, C.O., Palmquist, S., *et al.* (2021) Ligament of Treitz: Anatomy, relevance of radiologic findings and radiologic-pathologic correlation. *Am J of Roengenology 216* (4), 927–934.

Patriquin, D.A. (1992) Viscerosomatic reflexes. In: M.M. Patterson and J.N. Howell (eds) *The Central Connection: Viscerosomatic and Somaticovisceral Interactions.* Athens, OH: University Classics Ltd.

Severino, R. & Severino, P. (2017) Surgery or not? A case of ventriculus terminalis in an adult patient. *J Spine Surg 3* (3), 475–480.

Still, A.T. (1899) *Philosophy of Osteopathy.* Kirksville, MO: A.T. Still; pp. 84, 36.

Still, A.T. (1902) *Philosophy and Mechanical Principles of Osteopathy.* Kansas City, MO: Hudson-Kimberly CC.; p. 44.

Sutherland, W.G. (1990) *Teachings in the Science of Osteopathy.* A.L. Wales (ed.). Fort Worth, TX: Sutherland Cranial Teaching Foundation, Inc./Rudra Press; pp. 143, 214, 250.

Sutherland, W.G. (1998) *Contributions of Thought,* 2nd edition. A.L. Wales and A.S. Sutherland (eds). Fort Worth, TX: Sutherland Cranial Teaching Foundation, Inc.; pp. 7–8, 260, 262, 270.

Wales, A.L. (1981) Lecture, British School of Osteopathy postgraduate course on Osteopathy in the Cranial Field.

Wales, A.L. (1988) Andrew Still Sutherland Study Group (ASSSG). Rhode Island, USA.

Wales, A.L. (1995, 1996) British tutorial group meeting. North Attleboro, MA, USA.

Wernham, J. (1975) Lectures at European School of Osteopathy drawn from notes of J.M. Littlejohn's lectures, BSO, 1935.

Willard, F., Vleeming, A., Schuenke, M.D., Danneels, L., Schleip, R. (2012) The thoracolumbar fascia: anatomy, function and clinical considerations. *J Anat 221,* 507–536.

Zheng, Z., Shang, Y., Wang, N., *et al.* (2021) Current advancement on the dynamic mechanism of gastroesophageal reflux disease. *Int J Biol Sci 17* (15), 4154–4164.

CHAPTER 5

The Fascia

SUSAN TURNER

'The fasciae envelop, separate, protect and support the various structures. Not the least important of their functions is to encourage and direct the movement of tissue fluids and to promote the flow of lymph through its channels. The various layers of fascia interconnect and present a continuity from head to foot. Dr. Still

recognised drags on the fascia which are caused by hypotonicity, the weight of viscera, strains and posture. Treatment to restore the normal tension, hence function, of the fascial system are extremely effective.'

(Sutherland 1990, TSO p. 274)

THE INTELLIGENCE OF FASCIA

It is only in the past few decades that the fascia has been seen as an organ with its own intelligence rather than something that anatomists discard in dissection in order to access the 'real' organs. After initial findings by Carre-Locke, a group of investigators around Benias assigned the title of an 'organ' to the interstitium as the fascial matrix and microenvironment of every cell and tissue (Benias *et al.* 2018). An organ is conventionally defined as any structure working as an organised whole, and this holds true of the fascial system. Oschman (2021) describes the fascia as a 'body-wide communication system' functioning as a unified whole, with the qualities of adaptability and responsiveness.

When we examine the dynamic constituents of fascia, it becomes possible to understand some of the mechanisms whereby gentle and intelligently applied manual procedures can awaken a powerful therapeutic response. Ahead of his time as ever, A.T. Still wrote:

'The fascia gives one of, if not the greatest, problems to solve as to the part it takes in life or death. It belts each muscle, vein, nerve and all organs of the body. It is almost a network of nerves, cells and tubes running to and from it. It is crossed and filled with, no doubt, millions of nerve centres and fibres to carry on the work of secreting and excreting fluid, vital and destructive. By its action we live and by its failure we shrink, swell or die.' (Still 1902)

In the words of Guimberteau, 'The fascia penetrates and intertwines with every nerve, muscle cell, lymphatic vessel, blood vessel, organ...' To illustrate its interconnectedness he continues, 'One gradually realises that the body is shaped by a fibrillar network at every level, from macroscopic to microscopic, from superficial to deep' (Guimberteau and Armstrong 2015). This very ubiquity means that wherever your hands contact the body, you are connected, through the fascia, to everywhere else. Very often you find therefore a total body response when treating the fascia, as is found through the fascial lifts described below.

During embryogenesis all structures develop in the mesodermal fascial envelopes within which they are embedded. Ligaments, tendons and aponeuroses are all adaptations of the same basic collagenous tissue, modified according to the developmental and continual functional demands placed upon them. Levin (2018) has pointed out that even bone is a fascial structure into which osteocytes and calcium crystals have integrated.

Throughout the body, the fascia forms an uninterrupted tensional network, connecting the gross structures with the tensegrity network of the extracellular matrix (Scarr 2018). The irregular weave and lack of distinct boundaries found in loose connective tissue meets functional needs for support and movement, while enabling the passage of fluids, nerves and blood vessels. A large part of the force from muscles is distributed and transmitted via the fascia to other muscles and to the whole limb. This function is made possible because fascial tissue is one of our richest sensory organs. Astonishingly, the fascia of muscle has six times as many sensory nerves as muscle itself (Schleip 2003a, 2003b).

Ho (2008) demonstrated in her research that the fascial system's ability to change and adapt to stimuli and functional demands also operates through quantum coherence. She likened this constant adaptation to 'quantum jazz', as 'the music of the organism dancing life into being'.

THE EXTRACELLULAR MATRIX (ECM)

The ECM contains protein polymers, i.e., collagen, elastin, fibronectin and laminin, forming a lattice-like structure to which all cells are attached. Fibroblasts are the most common cells in the ECM. They are responsible for secreting the precursors for all the constituents of the ECM. They have been likened to 'spiders fussing over a web' in that they constantly reshape the matrix, breaking it down in response to tension and compression forces or signals from other cells.

Fibroblasts are also capable of secreting more matrix where needed. Although they are attached to the matrix itself, they are capable of migrating to wherever required, changing their shape and function as necessary (Schleip 2012).

Fibroblasts play a key role in the immune system, secreting cytokines which activate and modulate immune response in wound healing (Kubo and Kuroyanagi 2005). Through their many surface and intracellular receptors, including those for oestrogen and relaxin, fibroblasts interplay dynamically with many other cells, and appear to play a role in the changes that hormone dysfunction exerts upon the fascia in women (Akey and O'Neil-Smith 2020). The responsiveness of fascial tissue to osteopathic treatment may, in part, be due to the dynamic responsiveness of the fibroblasts.

The proteoglycan molecules are another important component of the ECM. These are secreted by fibroblasts, have a 'bottle brush' appearance, and consist of proteins attached to sugars that exert a negative charge which causes them to be hydrophilic. Their capacity to attract water gives the ECM the consistency of a watery gel. The fluid gel-like matrix acts as a protective shock-absorber, providing resistance to compressive forces. The gel-like fascial matrix, with its ability to attract water, means that it can quickly shift its level of viscosity between a denser 'gel' state and the more fluid 'sol' state that permits freer diffusion of fluids. This shift is triggered by a variety of stimuli, be they chemical, neurological, mechanical or hormonal.

The fast responsiveness to biochemical signals and mechanical demands that initiates change in the configuration of the fibres and shifting between gel and sol may partly explain the response that we feel under our hands when treating a patient. The familiar sense of health returning under the hands, i.e., of tissue spaciousness, fluidity, flow, warmth, resiliency, rhythmic expression and more, coincide with a shift from gel to sol. To quote Littlejohn's student John Wernham: 'It never fails to delight me when I feel the vital force returning to the tissues under my fingers' (Wernham 1975).

A palpatory finding, familiar to many osteopaths in the process of developing a sensory vocabulary, is a revealing alteration of fascial density, related to levels of stress and hormonal change. Stress and increased activation of the sympathetic nervous system has been shown to promote the gel state, stiffening the matrix, giving it a denser quality. These responses are triggered, in part, by the growth factor TGF-β1, a powerful contractor of fibroblasts. This is also released during inflammatory processes by the immune system (Schleip 2012).

We may therefore find a different qualitative expression within the fascial tissues when a person has a balanced autonomic nervous system and is in a state of wellbeing, from one who is in an autonomic state that is altered, for example, by sadness, shock or fever. Drugs, alcohol and radiation therapy each have their unique qualitative expression within the tissues that can be palpated by the experienced practitioner.

All the molecules that the cells need for regulation of function, regeneration and growth are stored and circulated in the fascia and made accessible through it. The ECM and its encompassed cells are in continuous two-way communication, determining cellular migration, differentiation, proliferation and survival (Fede *et al.* 2021). It was not for nothing that A.T. Still called the fascia 'The hunting ground for health and disease' (Still 1902).

SPACE AND MOTION

In assessing the vitality and tissue quality of the patient under our hands, we may receive an impression of 'inner lift' and turgor similar to that of a healthy, vibrant, growing plant. Conversely there may be a sense of drag, as if the tissues were anchored by another area that is too fixed to move with the life dance of the unified fascial field.

In optimum health there should be no fixed fulcra anywhere in the body. Every part should be free to express the three-dimensional rhythmic shape change that provides an inherent physiological pump for the interchange of fluids, blood, lymph and cerebrospinal fluid, right down to the extracellular and intracellular levels. To quote W.G. Sutherland once again, 'Perfect health ensues when each part is in perfect adjustment and free to work' (Sutherland 1990, TSO p. 274).

Dr Wales' saying that 'Unwellness is an undesirable change of space' (Wales 1988) leads us to consider the reciprocal ever-changing balance of shape and pressure between the large cavities of the body, i.e., head, thorax, abdomen and pelvis, in thoracic respiration. The external shape and mobility of the 'containers' is inseparable from the spatial environment of the contents, be they the large body cavities, organ capsules, fine vascular channels, joint capsules or the intracellular structure (Ingber 1998).

In addition to the balance maintained between the body cavities, the posterior spinal sphere has been likened to a bow, balanced by the 'bowstring' of the anterior fascial chain of the body (Slijper 1946). These can be seen as two 'fascial columns'. The vertical relationships of the body are in balanced reciprocal tension with the transverse structures, i.e., the plantar fascia, knees, pelvic diaphragm, thoracic diaphragm, Sibson's fascia and, within the cranium, the tentorium cerebelli and sella turcica.

APPLIED ANATOMY OF THE FASCIA

Two interdependent fascial columns

The pelvic floor, viscera, thoracic diaphragm, manubrium sterni and anterior cervical fascia together form an anterior fascial column. The posterior fascial column consists of the ligaments and fascia of the neurospinal axis. The reciprocal influences between these anterior and posterior spheres can be distorted by restricted mobility, visceral sag or tissue tensions in any of their parts, as well as the upper and lower limbs. When functioning in balance however, with every part free to shift according to functional demands, the anterior fascial column assists the body in defying gravity and maintaining organ support. This applies especially to the spine.

This chapter describes Sutherland's approach to restoring a natural state of lift and tone, with the aim of enhancing both organ function and balance of the vertebral column. Fascial and visceral sag are implicated in impaired lymphatic and vascular circulation, drainage and neurotrophic flow, all of which are essential to optimum organ physiology.

The anterior (visceral) fascial column and the posterior (neurospinal) fascial column are functionally interdependent, both posturally and physiologically, through their neural, ligamentous and vascular connections.

The areas of the vertebral fascial column most affected by anterior fascial drag are the so-called 'transitional areas': the occipito-atlantal (OA), cervico-thoracic, thoraco-lumbar, lumbo-sacral (LS) and sacro-coccygeal junctions. This happens through drag on transverse structures where lymphatic and vascular flow may be impacted: the pelvic floor, thoracic diaphragm, supra pleural membrane and myodural bridges at the OA junction (Zheng *et al.* 2020) (see Chapter 2, Part 2: Transitional areas).

Regarding fascial suspension from the cranial base, in Sutherland's model the anterior fascial column interacts more with the sphenoid bone and the posterior (spinal) fascial column, primarily with the occiput, although there is reciprocal influence.

As described in Chapter 2, the anterior longitudinal spinal ligament (ALSL) is the front of a ligamentous 'spinal stocking' wrapping the vertebral bodies from the basiocciput to the sacrum. The posterior portion of the stocking is the posterior longitudinal spinal ligament (PLSL). Drag is often exerted on the vertebral column via the ALSL by the viscera and fascia of the anterior column.

In the neck, the prevertebral fascia (PVF) is suspended from the inferior surface of the basiocciput encircling the supraoccipital nuchal line. The PVF blends with the ALSL at the body of T3. This forms the front of the fascial 'tube' which overlies the longus colli (LC) muscle and wraps the deep muscles of the neck, cervical vertebrae, brachial plexus and cervical sympathetic ganglia. It connects posteriorly with the spinous processes via the nuchal ligament.

Sutherland observed the PVF to potentially drag on the basiocciput, disturbing the organisation of the intracranial dura and their cerebral venous drainage function (Sutherland 1998, COT p. 278). This is exacerbated when the anterior thoracic fasciae and manubrium sterni create downward drag on the cervico-thoracic junction.

The PVF lies posterior to the buccopharyngeal fascia with the thin alar fascia between them. The buccopharyngeal fascia forms a 'tube' with the pretracheal fascia (PTF) to contain the cervical viscera. These include the pharynx, trachea, thyroid and parathyroid glands, larynx, recurrent laryngeal nerves, oesophagus and infrahyoid muscles. Within the neck the only direct connection between these anterior and posterior fascial compartments is via the carotid sheaths laterally to them.

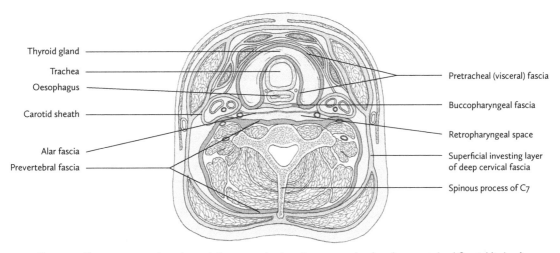

Figure 5.1 Transverse section through lower neck, showing pretracheal and prevertebral fascial 'tubes'.

The diaphragm's connection to the ALSL

'If the diaphragm is functioning, it acts as a piston in the cylinder of the trunk: the floor of the thorax and roof of the abdomen' (Wales 1997).

The crura of the diaphragm normally attach to the ALSL on the upper three lumbar vertebral bodies on the right and upper two on the left. The aorta and the cisterna chyli/thoracic duct pass between the two crura under the fascial bridge formed by the median arcuate ligament. This portal and its all-important cargo can be compressed by drag from sagging abdominal viscera. Tension in the crura both restricts diaphragmatic respiratory excursion and exerts fascial traction on the spine via the ALSL. This potentially influences everything up to the cranium above and the pelvis and legs below (Sutherland 1990, TSO p. 210). Crural tension can affect the healthy function of all the vital organs (see Chapter 4, Part 2 for a more detailed description of the posterior diaphragm).

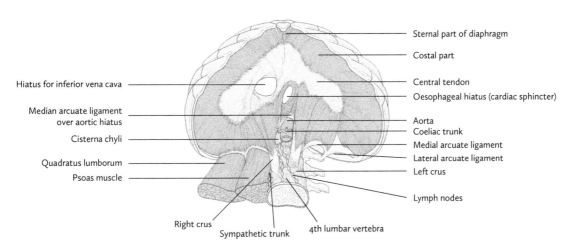

Figure 5.2 Diaphragm, crura and lumbocostal arches.

The ALSL also blends with the psoas muscles, the fascia of the posterior parietal peritoneum, renal fascia and fascia of the true pelvis. The uterosacral ligaments connect the uterus with the anterior periosteum of the sacrum.

THE THORACOLUMBAR FASCIA (TLF)

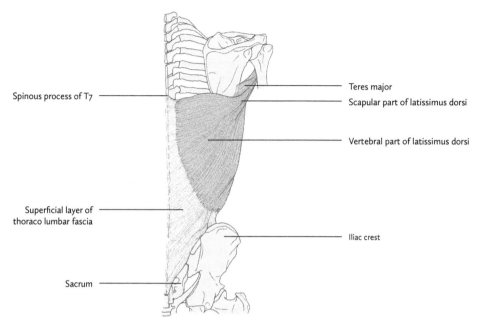

Spinous process of T7

Teres major

Scapular part of latissimus dorsi

Vertebral part of latissimus dorsi

Superficial layer of thoraco lumbar fascia

Iliac crest

Sacrum

Figure 5.3 Thoracolumbar fascia, posterior layer.

The TLF or 'thoracolumbar complex' plays a key stabilising role in counterbalancing the anterior fascial influences on the spinal column through its interaction with many muscles and ligaments. It transmits load and energy from the thorax to the pelvis and vice versa in running and walking and is crucial to the support of the lumbar spine and trunk (Willard *et al.* 2012).

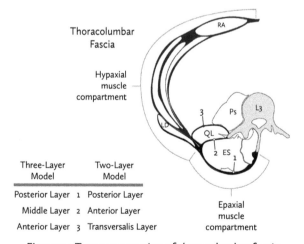

Thoracolumbar Fascia

Hypaxial muscle compartment

Epaxial muscle compartment

Three-Layer Model		Two-Layer Model
Posterior Layer	1	Posterior Layer
Middle Layer	2	Anterior Layer
Anterior Layer	3	Transversalis Layer

Figure 5.4 Transverse section of thoracolumbar fascia.

Used with permission of the Willard/Carreiro collection, University of New England, College of Osteopathic Medicine. Source: Willard, F.H, Vleeming, A., Schuenke, M.D., Danneels, L., Schleip, R. (2012) The thoracolumbar fascia: anatomy, function and clinical considerations. Journal of Anatomy 221 (6), 507–536. https://doi.org/10.1111/j.1469-7580.2012.01511.x.

Abbreviations used in this figure: L3 = 3rd lumbar vertebra, Ps = psoas muscle, Q = quadratus lumborum muscle, LD = latissimus dorsi muscle, ES = erector spinae muscle, RA = rectus abdominis muscle.

The TLF has three layers. Its superficial posterior layer attaches to the 12th ribs, interspinous ligaments, lower thoracic and lumbar spinous processes, posterior iliac crest and sacrum. It has a distinct connection with latissimus dorsi, trapezius and multifidus muscles above and with gluteus maximus and leg musculature below. In the lower lumbar region, it connects the multifidus, longissimus and iliocostalis muscles to the sacrum, ilium and spinous processes via a tendinous attachment within its dense aponeurosis (Willard *et al.* 2012).

Its middle layer separates the paraspinal musculature from quadratus lumborum through its thick aponeurosis. Laterally, together with the superficial layer, it connects with transversus abdominis and abdominal oblique muscles, forming the back of a 'corset'. This illustrates the importance of good abdominal tone in supporting the lumbar spine.

It attaches to the 12th ribs at its upper limit, and between T12 and L2 it is reinforced by the arcuate ligaments. At its lower border it connects with the iliac crests and forms the iliolumbar ligaments which are crucial to the suspension of L5 and the sacrum.

The thinner anterior layer is an extension of the transversalis fascia and, together with the middle layer, it surrounds quadratus lumborum. The quadratus lumborum forms a dynamic functional unit with the psoas muscles and diaphragm. The TLF, therefore, exerts a strong influence on the diaphragm. This has significance when addressing the diaphragm osteopathically.

The TLF has many free nerve endings that allow nociception (pain sensation), many of which communicate with the posterior horn of the spinal cord. The role of the TLF is thought to be proprioceptive, although not all studies confirm this (Mense 2019).

OVERVIEW OF ANTERIOR FASCIAL COLUMN

In the upper body, the 'tube' of the anterior fascial column extends from the cranial base to the diaphragm. This encompasses the fascia that contain the nasopharynx and cervical viscera, enlarging below to blend with the aortic arch, pericardium and central tendon of the diaphragm. From the diaphragm are suspended the liver capsule, stomach, descending colon, duodenum, etc.

The root of the mesenteries of the small intestine is suspended diagonally from the posterior abdominal wall between just left of L2 to anterior of the right sacroiliac (SI) joint. Although this is not directly attached to the ALSL, drag from the viscera can compress the crura with its vessels and weigh on the lumbar spine. Below, the peritoneum and mesenteries blend with the fascia of the false pelvis.

The anterior or 'visceral' fascial column is suspended from the pharyngeal tubercle of the basiocciput. It opens bilaterally to line the internal surface of the pharynx as the *pharyngo-basilar fascia*. This attaches to the sphenoid spines and undersurface of the petrous tips of the temporal bones; it extends to the medial pterygoid plates of the sphenoid, pterygomandibular raphe and mylohyoid line of the mandible. It also contributes to the sphenomandibular ligament.

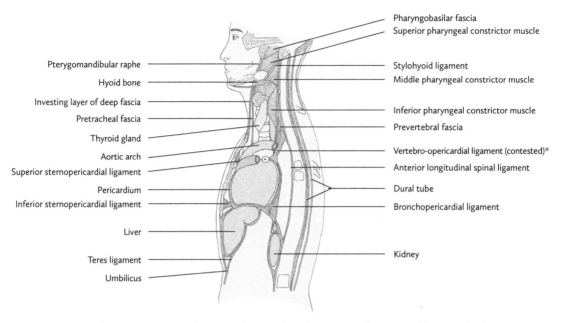

Figure 5.5 Schematic parasagittal section showing fascial continuity from cranial base to diaphragm.
The consistent existence of the vertebro-pericardial ligament is contested by some anatomists, based on repeated dissection findings. Professor F.H. Willard suggests that the mediastinal adventitia is mistakenly interpreted as this structure (Popa and Lucinescu 1932; Hollinshead 1956).

At this level, the tough pharyngobasilar fascia holds the nasopharynx open anteriorly. Just below, at the level of the hyoid bone, it closes anteriorly to form the tube composed of the PTF anteriorly and the buccopharyngeal fascia posteriorly to encompass the visceral organs of the neck.

The PTF is suspended from the hyoid bone. Through the infrahyoid muscles it is connected with the scapula, clavicle and sternum. Thus, the PTF directly influences lymphatic drainage of the head, neck, arms and chest into the subclavian veins. The cervical fasciae also blend with the superior, middle and inferior constrictor muscles of the pharynx. These relationships should therefore be examined thoroughly in such conditions as recurrent colds, laryngitis, otitis media, shoulder and arm pain, postural collapse, and brain fog.

The connection of the PTF (anterior tube) with the PVF (posterior tube) via the carotid sheaths implies a strong reciprocal influence between them. Strains between these anterior (visceral) and posterior (vertebral) columns may impact the function of the vagus nerve, carotid artery, jugular vein and ansa cervicalis within the carotid sheaths. The cervical spine, like the whole vertebral column, can be compromised by drag from the anterior structures.

The continuity of the PTF with the aortic arch, fibrous pericardium and central tendon of the diaphragm means that tension in the diaphragm and its crura may adversely affect arterial circulation and venous or lymphatic drainage of all structures up to and including the cranium.

FURTHER CLINICAL CONSIDERATIONS

The PVF will put inferior traction on the basiocciput when subjected to drag from the anterior fascial column. This may happen, for example, as a consequence of tight crura tugging on the ALSL or a sagged sacrum dragging on the intraspinal dura (see Chapter 3). This drag on the basiocciput may, in turn, be a potential cause of disturbance to intracranial dural balance and the brain's environment (Sutherland 1998, COT p. 278) (see also Chapter 3, Part 2: Anterior approach to the sacral alae).

Another such consideration is the effect of fascial drag on the delicate circulatory pathways of the thyroid gland. Because of its embryological 'descent' from the foramen cecum at the back of the tongue, an important component of its venous flow drains cephalad before joining the descending jugular vein. Likewise, much of its arterial supply ascends before flowing downward into the gland from the carotid artery. Being contained as it is within the PTF, drag from the thorax and below is likely to create further compromise to thyroid vascular flow.

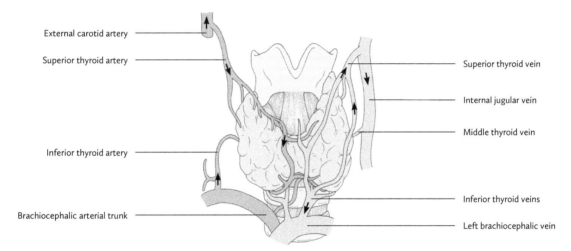

Figure 5.6 Vascular circulation of the thyroid gland.

The left recurrent laryngeal nerve, a branch of the vagus, loops under the aortic arch before ascending to the larynx. This arrangement can render the vasa nervorum of this nerve vulnerable to compression through fascial drag from below, and may be a consideration in some cases of vocal dysfunction (Titche 1976).

INTRATHORACIC INFLUENCES

Fascial strains, organ damage or scarring within the thorax can also exert their influence. The anterior pericardial ligaments attach to the internal surface of the sternum, and on palpation alterations in pericardial tension appear to adversely affect sternal respiratory excursion. In times of grief, the pericardium can give the impression, on palpation, of lying 'low' and 'heavy' in the thorax. This pattern is sometimes also associated with a tight diaphragm.

Following a respiratory illness, in the experience of the writer, tension can persist in the fan-shaped transversus thoracis muscle behind the sternum and anterior ribs. This is sometimes referred to as 'the coughing muscle', as its contractile action on the lower sternum can easily be palpated while coughing. This may be another cause of fascial drag on the anterior neck, clavicles and cervico-thoracic junction. In locking down the thoracic inlet and inhibiting the natural respiratory siphon action of lymphatic drainage, this pattern appears to be one of the contributing causative factors of repeated respiratory infections. Intrathoracic density in the lung and pleural tissues from past pneumonia or pneumothorax may create drag on the cervical vertebrae, fascia and temporal bones of the cranial base. This appears to compromise cranial venous drainage through the jugular foramen with resulting headaches and 'brain fog'.

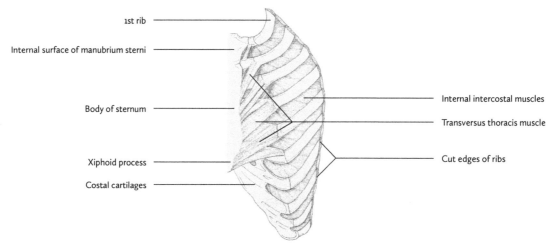

1st rib

Internal surface of manubrium sterni

Body of sternum

Xiphoid process

Costal cartilages

Internal intercostal muscles

Transversus thoracis muscle

Cut edges of ribs

Figure 5.7 Transversus thoracis muscle, viewed from internal surface of anterior ribcage.

In infants and young children, for the immune system to mature and develop discernment, it is crucial that the circulation within the thymus gland is free from manubriosternal compression. This pattern is sometimes associated with retained tensions in the diaphragm from insufficient expansion during the first breaths of life. Strains caused during delivery of the shoulders are also relevant since arterial circulation to the thymus is regulated by the stellate ganglion, which in turn may be compromised due to its close relation to the first and second ribs. (For further anatomy of diaphragmatic relationships see Chapter 4, Part 2.)

THERAPEUTIC ENGAGEMENT

Pelvic floor lift

'You can lift the fascias, with the aid of postural and respiratory co-operation from your patient. The pelvic lift is a fundamental place to begin. Then follow with lifting the diaphragm and anterior cervical fascia. The pelvic lift utilises the power of the diaphragm to do the lifting.' (Sutherland 1990, TSO p. 210)

Clinical considerations

The aim of the pelvic lift manoeuvre is to restore tone, resiliency, lift and balance to the levator ani muscles through the agency of the thoracic diaphragm. Where relevant, this may easily proceed to the release of obturator internus (see Chapter 16).

Tensions within the pelvic floor can inhibit the natural tone, movement and tensegrity of the fascia through the whole body. The pelvic organs may become congested and crowded by the sagging of the abdominal organs into the true pelvis, restricting venous and lymphatic drainage. This can often cause compensatory tension in the levator ani muscles. The author's experience suggests that constipation, recurrent cystitis, stress incontinence, local fungal infections, prostate problems and uterine prolapse can sometimes be associated with this situation. Diarrhoea that continues after an infection has resolved may be associated with an irritable gut lining and ptosis of the sigmoid colon (Wales 1995). As the muscles of the pelvic floor are interdigitated with the sphincters, the pelvic lift may also be helpful in cases of urinary incontinence (see Chapter 3).

The tone of the pelvic floor is crucial to the support of the pelvic and abdominal organs and is also important in restraining hyperextension or hypernutation of the sacrum. The following approach can help with restoration of normal pelvic floor tone and reorganisation of the perineum after episiotomy or tears in the process of childbirth. Because of the continuity of the fascial chain from pelvis to head, even the simple restoration of lift and tone to the levator ani can considerably relieve fascial drag from the whole body above it.

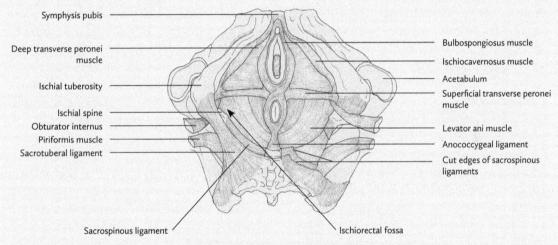

Symphysis pubis

Deep transverse peronei muscle

Ischial tuberosity

Ischial spine

Obturator internus

Piriformis muscle

Sacrotuberal ligament

Bulbospongiosus muscle

Ischiocavernosus muscle

Acetabulum

Superficial transverse peronei muscle

Levator ani muscle

Anococcygeal ligament

Cut edges of sacrospinous ligaments

Sacrospinous ligament

Ischiorectal fossa

Figure 5.8 Pelvic floor, inferior view.

The procedure

First explain to the patient what you intend to do. Ask permission, demonstrating your intended contact on the skeleton if possible. Take a moment to attune to the patient to be present to the quality of contact required.

The ischiorectal fossa is a fat-filled space between the anal canal and the ischium/obturator membrane and just behind the transverse perineal muscle. Each fossa is bordered posteriorly by the sacrotuberous ligaments and gluteus maximus.

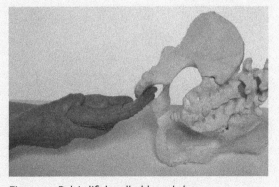

Figure 5.9 Pelvic lift handhold on skeleton.

1. HANDHOLD

To work with the right side, the patient lies on the left side with knees and hips flexed. First locate the right ischial tuberosity and gently advance two or three fingers along its medial surface to find the potential space of the ischiorectal fossa.

Using the medial surface of the tuberosity as a landmark will normally avoid any discomfort or embarrassment for the patient.

2. OPERATOR POSITION

Sit on the table caudally to the patient so that your forearm and hand are aligned in a cephalad direction in the ischiorectal fossa. It may be helpful to brace your straight wrist with the other hand and put your elbow against your own abdomen. This will enable you to put a little of your body weight behind it. Alternatively use the other hand to monitor the action of the patient's diaphragm.

3. ENGAGEMENT

Lean slightly into your fingertips just to the point where you meet the first hint of resistance in the tissues and then wait there, as you observe the levator ani descending and rising with each inhalation and exhalation. Throughout the procedure, maintain an awareness of the respiratory action of the thoracic diaphragm on the pelvic tissues under your hands. We are using the power of the diaphragm to do the lifting.

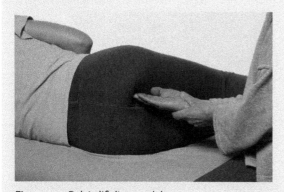

Figure 5.10 Pelvic lift live model.

4. SYNCHRONY WITH BREATHING

Ask the patient to deepen his or her breathing and imagine breathing into your hand contact. Steadily, but gently, match your weight to the tone in the tissues. Advance your straight index and third fingers cephalad with each exhalation, up to the first point of tension. Gently but firmly resist the tendency of the tissues to descend on each thoracic inhalation, holding the advance you have made on each out-breath. In this way you are working with maximum effectiveness because you are below the level of tissue resistance.

5. ADAPTING TO FASCIAL PLANES

As the tissues allow you to advance more deeply, you may become aware of the orientation of the fascial plane changing as the tissues seek a point of balanced tension. If this happens, adapt your hands to the direction of ease that the tissues dictate. By shifting your orientation a little, your contact can also be directed towards particular pelvic organs, e.g., bladder, prostate, uterus, as required.

6. LIFTING

After several respiratory cycles, the resistance will suddenly be felt to diminish and the tissues soften and 'draw' upwards as if a space were opening in advance of your contact. Note any effect through the rest of the body, and you may be surprised by a sense of lift right up to the cranium.

7. RESPIRATORY CO-OPERATION

It can be helpful also, in the final stage, to *ask the patient to hold the breath out to increase the 'drawing upward' effect on the pelvic floor. Hold your position as he or she inhales deeply again. On the next exhalation there is normally a still deeper tissue relaxation and lifting.*

8. ADDRESSING THE OTHER SIDE

Treatment on the patient's right side will have prepared the frequently more resistant left side, especially if the descending colon is impacted or the sigmoid flexure has dropped within the small pelvis.

Abdominal viscera lift

This can be useful to augment the sequence of fascial lifts, where ptosis of the abdominal viscera is dragging on the mesenteric root on the posterior abdominal wall and interfering with the rhythmic pumping of the crura. Anne Wales' advice for an initial treatment for patients with chronic stasis of the diaphragms was to 'give the patients uplift in their sag. The first change of space is from stasis, so this moves the condition from a chronic to an acute phase' (Wales 1988). Just enough stimulus for a small shift from a static state of the fascial and articular system makes the system accessible for more specific work possible in the following session.

1. HAND CONTACT

Stand to the right side of the patient who lies supine with hips and knees flexed and feet flat on the table. Contact the lower left abdominal quadrant and place the finger pads of your right hand in sensory (afferent) contact just above the inguinal ligament. Your left (motor) hand is placed over the right hand.

2. LIFTING

With your left hand, ease the finger pads of your right hand gently into the abdomen and gently lift towards the upper right abdominal quadrant. Your forces are directed to the viscera rather than just the abdominal wall. Pause at the first point of tissue resistance and hold there until a release is felt and the contents begin to lift. This may be repeated several times so that you progress in stages.

3. RESPIRATORY COOPERATION

This is helped by the patient partially inhaling and holding. When he or she has to breathe out, the abdominal contents are more amenable to lifting with you, releasing their drag on the mesenteric root. This may be repeated several times.

4. THE RIGHT SIDE

Then, when working on the patient's right, continue to stand on his or her right side. The lift is repeated but directed cephalad towards the upper right abdominal quadrant.

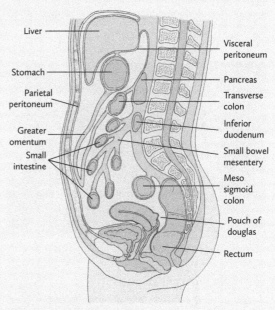

Figure 5.11 Mesenteries, schematic sagittal section.

Diaphragm lift

(See also Chapter 4, Part 2.)

The aim of this approach is 'to draw the diaphragm cranially, elevating the floor of the thorax, drawing upward on the abdominal contents, and promoting venous and lymphatic drainage in the lower half of the body. Visceroptosis and even haemorrhoids respond to it' (Sutherland 1990, TSO p. 276).

The diaphragm lift greatly eases the respiratory excursion of the ribcage, with benefit to its important contents. This is partly because the muscular portion of the diaphragm shares its sensory supply with that of the intercostal muscles of the lower six ribs. This is especially useful for diaphragmatic restriction, following a bad cough or depression. The diaphragm lift also stimulates the liver, increasing its activity. Patients often declare that they suddenly feel happy!

This is best rehearsed with the patient first.

1. HANDHOLD
With the patient supine and knees bent, stand at the head of the table and wrap your fingers around and under the cartilaginous lower costal border. If the patient is tender or ticklish here, your hands can be placed over his or her hands.

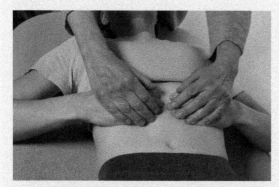

Figure 5.12 Diaphragm lift.

2. LIFTING WITH BREATHING
As the patient exhales, take advantage of the 'give' in the tissues by lifting the lower rim of the thorax cephalad and slightly laterally. As the patient inhales, hold the advancement you have made.

This is continued over several respiratory cycles, until there is no further upward progress. By this point there may be a perception of continuity between your hands and the whole undersurface of the diaphragm as far back as the crura.

3. RESPIRATORY COOPERATION
The patient is then asked to exhale fully and hold the breath out, locking the throat to prevent inhalation, while lifting the ribs to expand the chest as if inhaling. Continue to gently but consistently hold the 'upward and outward' lifting of the costal borders. In this way the diaphragm receives a double stretch as if for inhalation and exhalation simultaneously.

4. THE RELEASING BREATH
When the patient can hold the breath out no longer, he or she takes in a deep breath to complete the release of the whole diaphragm. This includes the posterior attachments and opens the aortic/lymphatic 'bunghole' under the median arcuate ligament and crura.

The liver's effect on the anterior column
The liver exerts considerable influence on the whole anterior fascial column, and where it loses its capacity to swing freely in its capsule this is a strong factor to be considered in cases of anterior fascial drag. A specific procedure for the liver, referred to as the 'liver turn', is described in Chapter 6.

Manubrial lift
Anne Wales often used the manubrial lift to relieve the PVF of anterior drag, where it blends with the ALSL at T3 and may cause a cervicothoracic flexion strain. Sutherland referred to this 'dowager's hump' as the 'old age centre'. Freeing the PVF also relieves its drag on the undersurface of the basiocciput. Sutherland made the observation that this strain can disturb the intracranial function of the Sutherland ('automatic shifting suspension') fulcrum, pineal gland, intracranial membranes and their cerebral venous drainage channels (Sutherland 1998, COT pp. 279–283). (See also Chapter 3, Part 2.)

Another consideration is the relationship of the manubrium to the superior sternopericardial ligament. Patients sometimes express a relieving sensation of lifting of the pericardium and pleura.

Effects may be perceived in the tissues of the anterior throat and nasopharynx including the larynx, thyroid gland, retropharyngeal fascia and palatine bones. Where relevant this can sometimes be helpful in otitis media. It may also have significant benefit to the circulation of the underlying thymus gland which is especially significant in the early years of childhood for the developing immune system.

Because the manubrium has a key position in the thoracic inlet, it is well to be sure it is free before addressing the clavicles and first ribs (see Chapters 4 and 7).

1. HAND CONTACT

Stand beside the supine patient, facing cephalad, and make a plastic (sensory) contact with the manubrium with the flat palmar surfaces of your distal phalanges. The contact should be with the manubrium only, avoiding the body of the sternum. The fingertips should be just below the sternal notch to avoid any pressure on the anterior throat when the lift is initiated.

This hand in contact is afferent, monitoring activity only. *The other (active) hand is placed over it, making a firm contact, but without posterior pressure on the manubrium.* The angle of this action has been likened to 'a plane coming in to land' (Chandler 2019).

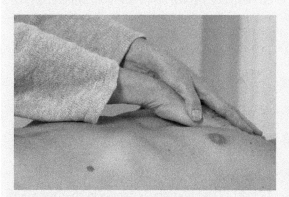

Figure 5.13 Manubrial lift contact on live model.

2. FASCIAL BALANCE

With the active (upper) hand, initiate a cephalad lift of the manubrium up to the first point of resistance, sensing how the retrosternal fascia is acting on the manubrium from behind it. Support any fascial movement towards a point of balanced tension for the manubrium if it deviates or rotates slightly to one side or the other.

3. LIFTING

Following the balance point, as the manubrium eases back to midline, the cephalad lift will normally proceed easily, meeting little resistance. Slowly release contact as the manubrium resettles.

Anterior cervical lift

'The anterior cervical fascia is attached to the base of the skull, mandible, hyoid, scapula, clavicle and sternum. Through the PTF it is connected to the fibrous pericardium, and thence with the diaphragm. It surrounds the pharynx, larynx and thyroid gland; it forms the carotid sheath; and by way of the PVF is continuous with that which surrounds the trachea and oesophagus. Therefore, the cervical fascia is concerned quite directly with lymphatic drainage of the head, neck, thorax and upper extremities.' (Sutherland 1990, TSO p. 275)

At the thoracic inlet, Sibson's fascia (suprapleural membrane) attaches to the transverse process of C7 and the posterior aspect of the 1st rib, maintaining intrathoracic pressure.

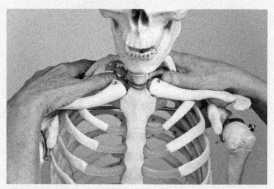

Figure 5.14 Anterior cervical lift handhold on skeleton.

1. POSITIONING

Stand facing the patient who sits on the treatment table. Place your thumbs softly along the posterior surface of the patient's clavicles, with the thumb tips beside the lateral heads of the sternocleidomastoid muscles. The contact needs to be medial enough to access the thoracic inlet but lateral enough not to compress the thyroid gland. Your palms and fingers softly wrap the trapezius muscles.

Ask the patient to rest his or her hands on your shoulders. If your arms are flexed at the elbows and pointing laterally, this supports the patient's arms, allowing them to relax.

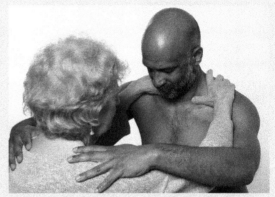

Figure 5.17 Anterior cervical fascia lift (3), patient sits up with head dropped.

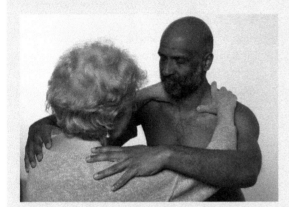

Figure 5.15 Anterior cervical fascia lift (1), initial contact.

2. POSTURAL COOPERATION AND ENGAGEMENT

The patient drops his or her head and slowly rolls the spine forward one vertebra at a time, slumping the lower back. This flexed position relaxes the PTF, creating a space as if your thumbs could gently advance towards the mediastinum just anterolateral to the trachea. *There should be no discomfort for the patient* as here we are using the principle of the '*glove settling over the thumb rather than the thumb being forced into the glove*'.

3. MATCHING BY LEANING

Quietly wait and 'get acquainted' with the tissues as they further relax, with the flow of respiration. *You and the patient lean towards each other slightly, equally and effortlessly matching each other's weight.*

4. GAINING DEEPER CONTACT

The patient's breathing is helpful in enabling your contact to advance towards the mediastinum. *Ask him or her to keep the head and neck dropped forward while inhaling and straightening the lumbar and thoracic spine so that the fasciae are suspended from your contact. Then, as the patient exhales, he or she again slumps, allowing the thoracic vertebrae to roll forward into a relaxed position.* This enables your afferent contact to comfortably move yet deeper into the mediastinum.

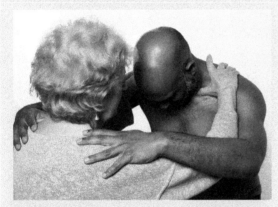

Figure 5.16 Anterior cervical fascia lift (2), patient slumps.

This alternate slow straightening and slumping may be repeated two or three times until there is no further advance into the opening space, but a quiet state of balance.

5. FINAL ACTION

Ask the patient to inhale and sit up tall, this time straightening the whole spine including the head and neck. The main corrective action here comes from the patient's action of sitting up and bringing the shoulders back. *You assist this by gently 'scooping up' the fascia as if 'peeling open' the thoracic inlet, to spread the patient's arms and shoulders posteriorly and laterally, reseating them over the scapulae. Finally replace the patient's arms at the side of the body.*

Balanced fascial tension of the anterior trunk

The following approaches are not fascial lifts as such, but ways of engaging a point of balance in the anterior fascial compartments. The aim is to improve the spatial environment of the thoracic and abdominal organs and free the energetic flow through the anterior midline, as expressed in the linea alba and midsternal line.

Release of umbilical torsion

This was taught by Robert Fulford DO (1984) and has been found especially useful where there has been umbilical trauma for the newborn, either by accidental traction on the umbilical cord or premature cutting before thoracic respiration was properly established. Dr Fulford observed such events to sometimes result in torsion of the umbilicus within its myofascial and ligamentous field. The continuity of the fascia means that this torsion is often reflected through the cranium, trunk, pelvis and legs.

On one occasion an overlap of the two hemi-frontal bones of a newborn resolved instantaneously when umbilical torsion was released. On another, an infant, whose very short umbilical cord had undergone inadvertent traction during delivery, looked as if she had grown 5 cm in length when her torsional umbilical strain released. Her mother and the osteopath both looked on with astonishment!

The umbilicus has wide-ranging myofascial and ligamentous connections. Centrally it is continuous with the linea alba between thoracic diaphragm and the pubis. It is related to the bladder via the median umbilical ligament (residual urachus) and to the pubic region bilaterally by the medial umbilical ligaments (residual umbilical veins). The teres ligament, a residue of the umbilical artery, connects it to the porta hepatis of the liver. The umbilicus sometimes appears to carry an emotional component associated with mother-infant bonding.

1. CONTACT

Make contact on the umbilical rim with both thumb tips. You will often find a tense spot on one side and a soft spot on the opposite side of the rim.

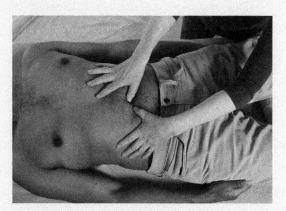

Figure 5.18 Hand contact for umbilicus.

2. MOTION TESTING

Test for the position of ease to see if the umbilicus moves more easily upwards, downwards, left, right, diagonally or is rotated clockwise or anticlockwise according to the tensional forces acting upon it. There may be a quality of either traction or recoil. Its point of balanced myofascial tension can express a combination of these components.

3. POINT OF BALANCE AND REORGANISATION

Find the composite position of ease and balanced tension and wait for spontaneous reversal of the tensions, and easing of all vectors.

4. REASSESS

Reassess the body as a whole, noting any changes that may indicate where your attention is next required.

Retrosternal influences and their relevance

The fan-shaped transversus thoracis muscle originates on the posterior surface of the xiphoid process and lower sternum, attaching to the costal cartilages of ribs 2–6. This contracts powerfully when coughing, and is often left hypertonic after respiratory infection. When contracted, this muscle pulls the sternum and anterior fascia inferiorly, exaggerating any thoracic kyphosis and diminishing thoracic respiratory excursion.

Full respiratory expression of thoracic 3D rhythmic shape change not only favours adequate oxygenation for the lungs, but assists the return of blood to the heart via the inferior vena cava (Kimura *et al*. 2011). It is also important for unrestricted aortic flow through the diaphragm. Limited thoracic excursion adversely affects lymphatic flow from the abdomen to the upper thorax (see Chapters 4 and 15) since thoracic respiration is the most powerful lymphatic pump in the body. It is therefore essential to release residual tensions in the transversus thoracis muscle after respiratory infection to ensure that diminished respiratory, cardiac and lymphatic function does not repeatedly expose the patient to further infections.

The pericardium attaches retrosternally via the superior and inferior sternopericardial ligaments. This makes the sternum a good 'handle' for 'reading' and supporting the positional state of the pericardium. Behind the heart, the bronchopericardial ligament/membrane connects the posterior pericardium, bifurcation of the trachea and bronchi with the diaphragm (Kozo *et al.* 2017; Popa and Lucinescu 1932; Hollinshead 1956).

The internal postures of the thorax have their own emotional language and metaphor (Schleip and Jäger 2021). For example, in grief there is often a palpatory impression of the heart and pericardium being 'heavy', as if being drawn down towards the diaphragm. In fear or shock, the tensions may be held high in the chest. In exhaustion there may be a literal sense of deflation. Past pneumonia or pneumothorax may leave a residual sense of density and contraction that needs to regain its natural spaciousness. These impressions are discernible, both through palpation, and the patient's subjective metaphoric description of an inner state.

If the maintaining cause of a physical tension pattern is an emotional or spiritual one, these subtler levels need to be met, acknowledged, and included in the way we read and support the tissues. The sternum is a sensitive and very personal area, so *to ensure an appropriate quality of contact, it may be helpful to bring to it the question 'If I were these tissues, how would I like to be held?'* When this is silently asked, it is often as if a clear instruction is communicated directly from the patient's tissues to the hands of the practitioner, independently of the mediation of thought (see Chapter 18).

The hands may then be 'invited' either to match the pattern by more compression or engage a lighter and more spacious contact. If the area is compressed, the hands sometimes feel as if they are being 'gathered up' around the area like a hug. In making oneself available, it can feel as if the very posture of one's body is being adjusted by the needs of the patient's system, so that we find ourselves leaning back to give more space or forward to enfold, as needed.

Intrathoracic fascia, transversus thoracis and pericardium supine approach

1. CONTACT

Sitting behind the head of the patient, contact the midthoracic spine with the middle ray of one hand, aligned along the spinous processes. The other hand contacts the whole sternum, aligned along its midline.

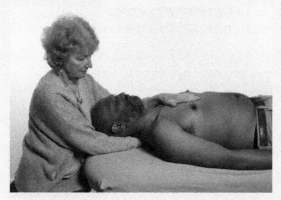

Figure 5.19 Retrosternal fascia, antero-posterior hold.

Anne Wales pointed out many times that the skeleton is a good handle 'on one side of the door' to sense what is acting on the 'handle' on the other side from within the body cavity (Wales 1981). In this case we are palpating not just the sternum under our hands, but the effect of the internal structures upon it.

Another piece of advice that she often gave was to *be aware of the shape and quality of the space between the hands* which can provide a sense of the spatial environment of the organs and vessels within (Wales 1988).

2. ENGAGEMENT

Holding the space between your hands, match and support the way the sternum tends to move more easily up, down, left, right, in rotation, etc. Acknowledge all that is contained in the space between the two hands. Hold that shape as it expresses the composite position of balanced tension in relation to the retrosternal fascia, pericardium, transversus thoracis, pleura, etc.

3. RESOLUTION

Match tissue tone and position with steady support until the space within the thorax unfolds, reverses its strain patterns and moves more freely.

Sitting release of the endothoracic and retrosternal fascia

This has also proved useful for releasing residual strains in the intrathoracic tissues following respiratory infections. These may involve the pleura, endothoracic fascia, transversus thoracic muscle, pericardium, etc.

1. HAND PLACEMENT

Stand facing the patient who is seated on the treatment table. Place your flat, crossed thumbs under the 'ledge' of the lateral parts of the manubriosternal angle. Your palms and fingers can be spread flat across the ribs.

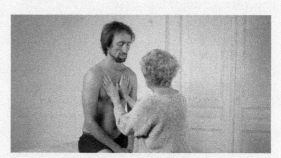

Figure 5.20 Handhold for retrosternal fascia and pleura.

2. LEANING LIKE A CARD HOUSE

Invite the patient to lean against you with a straight back and neck as you match his or her weight by your leaning. It should feel mutually supported and effortless for both so long as you remain firmly grounded throughout. *The patient will only be able to trust his or her weight to you if you communicate mountain-like stability and groundedness by being fully connected to the earth beneath your feet.*

3. ENGAGEMENT

Through your external contact, engage with the tissues within the thorax on the interior side of the sternum and ribs.

4. THE SEARCH FOR BALANCE
WITHIN THE PATTERN

Keeping your hand contact steady, observe the endothoracic fascia start to explore. You may feel them drawing into areas of tightness, left, right or medially, as the tissues seek a position of balance for the residual strain pattern they are revealing.

5. BALANCED FASCIAL TENSION

Steadily support whatever pattern is expressed, consciously keeping your contact with the ground as the tissues pause in balanced tension.

6. RESOLUTION

Following the moment of stillness and balance, continue to give support as the pattern resolves, returning to midline and symmetry. Increased thoracic spaciousness, often felt by both you and the patient, may give your hands the impression of being spread apart as if from a smile in the chest.

7. ESCORTING 'HOME'

As always, maintain your contact until the patient is back to vertical alignment and postural control.

VIDEOS FOR CHAPTER 5

Scan the QR code or visit https://www.youtube.com/playlist?list=PL3j_YuMBqigEFvdZYit79WES1sPHBTWBd to find a playlist of the videos that accompany this chapter.

REFERENCES

Akey, A.M. & O'Neil-Smith, K. (2020) Hormonal effects on fascia in women. In: D. Lesondak and A.M. Akey (eds) *Fascia, Function, and Medical Applications.* Boca Raton, FL: CRC Press.

Benias, P.C., Wells, R.G., Sackey-Aboagye, B., *et al.* (2018) Structure and distribution of an unrecognised interstitium in human tissues. *Sci Rep 8* (1), 4947. https://doi.org/10.1038/s41598-018-23062-6.

Chandler, P. (2019) Sutherland Cranial College of Osteopathy BLT course. Proitze, Germany.

Fede, C, Pirri, C., Fan, C., *et al.* (2021) A closer look at the cellular and molecular components of the deep/muscular fasciae. *Int J Mol Sci 22* (3), 1411. https://doi.org/10.3390/ijms22031411.

Fulford, R. (1984) British School of Osteopathy post-graduate course in Osteopathy in the Cranial Field.

Guimberteau, J-C. & Armstrong, C. (2015) *Architecture of Human Living Fascia: The Extracellular Matrix and Cells Revealed Through Endoscopy.* Edinburgh: Handspring Publishing; p. 19.

Ho, M.W. (2008) *The Rainbow and the Worm: The Physics of Organisms,* 3rd edition. Singapore: World Scientific Publishing.

Hollinshead, W.H. (1956) *Anatomy for surgeons: The thorax, abdomen and pelvis.* New York, NY: Hoeber-Harper; p. 101.

Ingber, D.E. (1998) The architecture of life. *Sci Am 278* (1), 48–57.

Kimura, B.J., Dalugdugan, R., Gilcrease, G.W., *et al.* (2011) The effect of breathing manner on inferior vena caval diameter. *Eur J Echocardiogr 12* (2), 120–123.

Kozo, N., Goto, H. & Ito, T. (2017) Fascial reinforcement fixing the bronchi to the heart: its anatomy and clinical significance. *Surgical and Radiological Anatomy 39* (12), 1301–1308. https://doi.org/10.1007/s00276-017-1880-5.

Kubo, K. & Kuroyanagi, Y. (2005) A study of cytokines released from fibroblasts in cultured dermal substitute. *Artificial Organs 29* (10), 845–849.

Levin, S.M. (2018) Bone is fascia. Accessed August 2023 at: https://www.researchgate.net/publication/327142198_Bone_is_fascia.

Mense, S. (2019) Innervation of the thoracolumbar fascia. *Eur J Transl Myol 29* (3), 8297.

Oschman, J.L. (2021) Fascia as a body-wide communication system. In: R. Schleip, C. Stecco, M. Driscoll, P.A. Huijing (eds) *Fascia: The Tensional Network of the Human Body,* 2nd edition. Edinburgh: Elsevier.

Popa, G.T. & Lucinescu, E. (1932) The Mechanostructure of the Pericardium. *J Anat. 67* (1), 78–107.

Scarr, G. (2018) *Biotensegrity: The Structural Basis of Life,* 2nd edition. Edinburgh: Handspring Publishing Ltd, p. 122.

Schleip, R. (2003a) Fascial plasticity – a new neurobiological explanation, Part 1. *J of Bodywork and Movement Therapies 7* (1), 11–19.

Schleip, R. (2003b) Fascial plasticity – a new neurobiological explanation, Part 2. *J of Bodywork and Movement Therapies 7* (2), 104–116.

Schleip, R. (2012) Fascia is alive. In: R. Schleip, C. Stecco, M. Driscoll, P.A. Huijing (eds) *Fascia: The Tensional Network of the Human Body,* 2nd edition. Edinburgh: Elsevier; pp. 157–164.

Schleip, R. & Jäger, H. (2021) Interoception. A new correlate for intricate connections between fascial receptors, emotion and self-regulation. In: R. Schleip, C. Stecco, M. Driscoll, P.A. Huijing (eds) *Fascia: The Tensional Network of the Human Body,* 2nd edition. Edinburgh: Elsevier.

Slijper, E.J. (1946) *Comparative Biologic-anatomical Investigations on the Vertebral Column and Spinal Musculature of Mammals.* Amsterdam: North-Holland Publishing Co.

Still, A.T. (1902) *The Philosophy and Mechanical Principles of Osteopathy.* Kansas City, MO: Hudson-Kimberly Co.; p. 60.

Sutherland, W.G. (1990) *Teachings in the Science of Osteopathy.* A.L. Wales (ed.). Fort Worth, TX: Sutherland Cranial Teaching Foundation, Inc./Rudra Press; pp. 210, 274, 275, 276.

Sutherland, W.G. (1998) *Contributions of Thought,* 2nd edition. A.L. Wales and A.S. Sutherland (eds). Fort Worth, TX: Sutherland Cranial Teaching Foundation, Inc.; pp. 278, 279–283, 287.

Titche, L.L. (1976) Causes of recurrent laryngeal nerve paralysis. *Arch Otolaryngol 102* (5), 259–261.

Wales, A.L. (1981) Lecture, British School of Osteopathy postgraduate course on Osteopathy in the Cranial Field.

Wales, A.L. (1988) Andrew Still Sutherland Study Group (ASSSG). Rhode Island, USA.

Wales, A.L. (1995) Personal communication.

Wales, A.L. (1997) Personal communication.

Wernham, J. (1975) Personal communication, European School of Osteopathy, Maidstone, Kent.

Willard, F., Vleeming, A., Schuenke, M.D., Danneels, L., Schleip, R. (2012) The thoracolumbar fascia: anatomy, function and clinical considerations. *J Anat 221,* 507–636.

Zheng, N., Chung, B.S., Li, Y.L., *et al.* (2020) The myodural bridge complex defined as a new functional structure. *Surgical and Radiologic Anatomy 42,* 143–153.

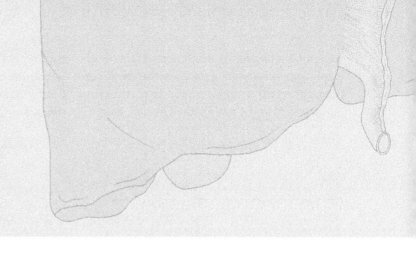

CHAPTER 6

The Liver Turn

KOK WENG LIM

'Following the release, the "liver can swing freely in its elastic capsule under the diaphragm".'

(Sutherland 1990)

The liver is the largest gland and the second largest organ in the body, representing 2–3 per cent of average body weight and exerting considerable influence on the anterior fascial column. It has a soft consistency and its edge is normally palpable only in children and thin adults. However, with deep inspiration the liver may be felt on superficial palpation in normal adults. Therapeutically,

this makes it possible for the operator's steady manual contact to form a fulcrum on the lower border of the capsule around which the liver may 'turn', restoring its freedom of movement.

A.T. Still described the liver as swinging in a 'hammock formed of five ligamentous ropes' (Still 1902). The hammock swings below the diaphragm between the anterior abdominal wall and the spine. Importantly the hammock has openings for blood vessels and lymphatic channels, so free movement of the liver within its hammock suspension is key to normal function.

THE LIVER'S 'LIGAMENTOUS ROPES'

There are actually seven peritoneal attachments of the liver to keep it in position in the right upper quadrant of the abdomen. These include the falciform, teres, coronary, triangular, hepatogastric and hepatoduodenal ligaments and the ligamentum venosum. These ligaments also serve as bridges for blood vessels to pass between the liver and adjacent structures (Ibukuro *et al.* 2016), again illustrating the importance of its free movement.

The *round ligament* or *ligamentum teres* is the fibrous remnant of the umbilical vein in foetal life. It runs between the umbilicus and the portal vein and is usually situated on the left side of the middle hepatic vein. It travels within the

double-layered peritoneal folds of the falciform ligament together with the paraumbilical veins, delineating the free edge of the falciform ligament (Yamaoka *et al.* 2019).

The *falciform ligament* is a fibrous sickle-shaped structure and is a remnant of the ventral mesentery within which the liver develops (from the junction of the foregut and midgut) in the 4th week of intrauterine life, also giving rise to its capsule and mesenteric ligaments. The falciform ligament anchors the anterior part of the liver to the ventral aspect of the abdominal wall and separates it into right and left lobes morphologically. It merges with the left and right *coronary ligaments* which surround the bare liver area and is attached to the inferior surface of the diaphragm. It runs along the posterior sheath of the right rectus abdominis muscle reaching as far inferiorly as the umbilicus. The bare area of the liver is attached to the diaphragm by delicate fibroareolar tissue. At the base of the liver, at the falciform ligament, the hepatic veins drain into the inferior vena cava (IVC).

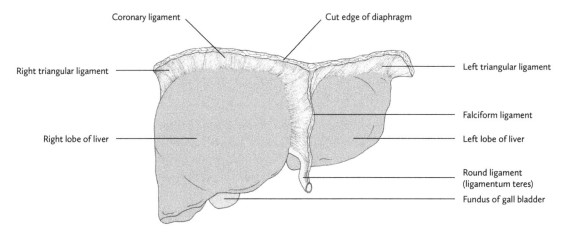

Figure 6.1 Liver, anterior view.

The coronary ligament suspends the liver from the undersurface of the diaphragm. The liver's attachment to the diaphragm resembles the outline of a crown, with an anterior and a posterior layer. The posterior layer of the coronary ligament is also attached to the right kidney and right adrenal gland by the *hepatorenal ligament.* The *right and left triangular ligaments* are the lateral union of the two layers of the coronary ligament.

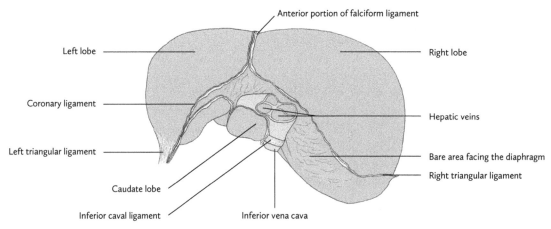

Figure 6.2 Liver, superior view.

The *hepatogastric* and *hepatoduodenal ligaments* form the double-layered lesser omentum which extends from the fissure for *ligamentum venosum* and porta hepatis to the lesser curvature of the stomach and the first part of the duodenum respectively. The hepatogastric ligament transmits the left and right gastric arteries and veins and the hepatic lymph node chain.

Contained in the free margin of the hepatoduodenal ligament are the common bile duct, the hepatic artery to its left and behind them the portal vein. The hepatic branch of the vagus nerve and sympathetic nerves to the liver and gall bladder also travel within the hepatoduodenal ligament. These neuromuscular structures enter and leave the liver at the porta hepatis.

The *inferior caval ligament* is a tissue bridge between the IVC and posterior surface of the right lobe and caudate lobe. It serves to anchor the IVC within the caval groove of the liver. It is a continuation of Glisson's capsule and may actually represent elements of hepatic tissue, including lymphocytes and hepatocytes (Kogure *et al.* 2007).

The *ligamentum venosum* is a fibrous remnant of the ductus venosus in foetal life, and this fibrous cord runs from the porta hepatis to the inferior vena cava. At the porta hepatis it is attached to the left branch of the portal vein. It is invested within the lesser omentum.

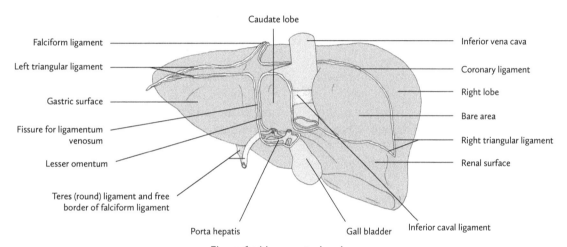

Figure 6.3 Liver, posterior view.

GLISSON'S CAPSULE

The liver capsule has an outer serous layer derived from peritoneum and an inner thick fibrous layer. The outer serous layer does not cover either the bare area of the liver, the porta hepatis or the space between the gall bladder and the liver. The capsule is thicker at the hilum where it wraps the portal vein, hepatic artery and bile duct. From the hilum, Glisson's capsule extends into the liver as sheaths around the branches of the hepatic duct, hepatic artery and portal vein forming 'the Glissonean pedicle tree'.

Further branches of the hepatic duct, hepatic arteries and portal veins remain together. These are invested by extensions of Glisson's capsule, the glissonian sheaths, deep into the substance of the liver. Superficial lymphatics are present within the capsule, pedicle tree and glissonian sheaths. The liver has a unique dual blood supply from the hepatic artery proper (25–30%) and from the portal vein (70–75%) (Abdel-Misih Sherif and Bloomston 2010).

The asymmetry of the body, for example the liver's right-sided position, may be a factor in frequently seen patterns of fascial bias in the common compensatory pattern (Zink and Lawson 1979). Fascial torsion in the trunk may compromise diaphragmatic excursion and therefore the suspension and drainage of the liver.

SURFACE ANATOMY

The liver is wedge-shaped and sits under the diaphragm, below the nipple on each side, covered on the right side by the 5th to 10th ribs.

Its upper surface extends between the 5th rib on the right towards the left 5th intercostal space between the midclavicular lines. The anteroinferior border follows the right costal cartilage from the tip of the 10th rib on the right to the left 5th intercostal space. This margin can be palpated at the right midclavicular line on deep inspiration.

The gall bladder is located at the tip of the 9th rib on the right. This isn't normally palpable, but the area can be tender if inflamed or when distended by bile, gallstones or a tumour.

It is a dense organ, dull to percussion, so its borders can also be percussed if palpation is difficult.

OSTEOPATHIC PALPATION OF THE LIVER

- Sitting to the right side of the supine patient, place your right hand on the patient's abdomen just lateral to the rectus muscle, and just below the costal margin.
- Place the left hand under the posterior lower right ribs.
- Ask the patient to take a deep breath in and feel the inferior edge of the liver as it descends, allowing it to pass under the fingers of your right hand. Sense its tissue quality, texture and quality of movement as it passes under your fingers. If the patient is asked to inhale deeply and hold that breath for as long as possible, the involuntary motion of the liver may be felt.

Liver reflex points

Chapman's point on the 5th intercostal space (between the mamillary line and the sternum) anteriorly is associated with liver dysfunction, and on the 6th intercostal space anteriorly with liver and gall bladder dysfunction (Owens 1963). Dr Frank Chapman's points represent hypercongestion of the deep intercostal fascia from increased sympathetic tone. This leads to lymphatic congestion and myofascial thickening that is felt as a painful nodule within deep fascia;

it is smooth, firm, discrete and around 2–3 mm in diameter. Paraspinal muscle changes or pain, felt at the level of T5–T9, may reflect abnormal visceral afferent activity from the liver (Chin *et al.* 2019) or gall bladder (Heineman 2014).

For consideration in treatment

In sensing the point of balance for the liver, it is desirable to place as much attention on Glisson's capsule as on the suspensory ligaments. As the capsule around the liver is engaged, appreciation of the glissonian pedicle at the hilum should enable the attention to be drawn into the deep substance of the liver and the internal connective tissue scaffolding (tensegrity) that is the glissonian sheaths. The internal scaffolding of the liver's extracellular matrix (ECM) is composed of reticular fibres which support hepatocytes, and this is useful to acknowledge in treatment (Wen *et al.* 2016). This reticular fibre arrangement which functions as a 'delicate' and thin supporting mesh for cells is very typical of lymphoid organs: spleen, lymph nodes, bone marrow and also the kidney.

When the liver rebalances, following the neutral point for the fascia and ligaments, it releases from within to without. Placement of attention in this way seems to bring Lippincott's words alive: 'the liver makes a turning movement probably attended by suction within its substance' (Lippincott 1949). If the lymphatics within the glissonian sheaths are acknowledged, this becomes, in essence, a lymphatic technique for the liver.

Before beginning this technique, it is helpful to place the finger pads of both hands along the linea alba between the xiphoid and umbilicus; 'listen' to the connection between the umbilicus, diaphragm and liver, via the ligamentum teres within the falciform ligament. In neonates who have had a difficult delivery with respiratory problems following the birth, tensions associated with the first breath may need to be released using this contact on the linea alba. This may help the diaphragm gain the full excursion that is required for the liver turn technique to be effective.

THERAPEUTIC ENGAGEMENT

The 'liver turn'

The aim of this approach is to access the physiology of the liver via its fascial envelope (Bordoni *et al.* 2019). In Dr Lippincott's words it is a treatment 'to stimulate the liver to increase activity' (Lippincott 1949). Dr Wales described this technique as 'establishing a fulcrum around which the diaphragm can free the liver from any static position it may have assumed. The diaphragm does the work, the operator merely establishes a fulcrum.' The principle of treatment is exaggeration to the point of balance, using respiratory cooperation to achieve the release.

1. HAND PLACEMENT AND PALPATION

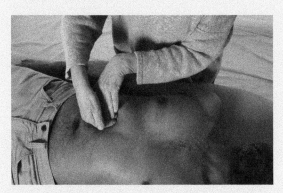

Figure 6.4 Handhold for liver turn.

Standing on the right side of the supine patient, place the dorsal surface of the fingers of your right hand over the liver capsule, below the inferior border of the right costal cartilages, inside the costal arch. This is a soft, listening contact with the anterior border of the liver. 'The fingernail is between the ribcage and the liver, you do not get on the liver. The liver just swings around the back of your fingernails' (Wales 1996).

2. ENGAGEMENT

Place the fingers of your left hand over the palmar surfaces of the fingers of your right hand; this is a reinforcement for stability and control.

Watch the patient's quiet breathing and sense the liver under your contacts. As it descends to meet your contact on the in-breath, engage it a little more with the left hand. Sense the position of ease for the suspension of the liver. This is often in an inferomedial direction towards the umbilicus.

Gently support this diagonal inferomedial tendency towards the midline and hold at the point of balance, being open to any other directions of ease.

3. MAINTAINING YOUR FULCRUM CONTACT

Keeping your contact steadily at the point of balance for the liver and its capsule, ask the patient to inhale deeply and hold the breath in for as long as possible. The diaphragm, at this point, holds the liver inferiorly against the back of your fingernails.

Maintain your contact, supporting the position of balance steadily throughout the inhalation.

When he or she must do so, the patient should breathe out forcefully.

As the diaphragm suddenly rises on strong exhalation, the liver rises too, but as *its capsule is still being held inferiorly by your finger contact, it makes a turning movement* 'probably attended by suction within its substance' (Lippincott 1949). 'As the diaphragm changes its position, the liver is swung on its ligaments around your finger contact as a fulcrum, it turns itself in any way that may be indicated.'

4. ALTERNATIVE USE OF EXHALATION

It is also possible to ask the patient to exhale and hold the breath out for as long as possible, while supporting the liver at the point of balance. When involuntary inhalation occurs, note how the liver turns when the diaphragm descends on the fulcrum of your fingers (Sutherland 1990). 'The important thing is to get the fulcrum established comfortably.'

Application in jaundice and infancy

This technique is very helpful for the jaundiced patient. It is particularly helpful in neonatal jaundice. In infants the liver edge is palpable one finger breadth (1.6 cm) below the costal margin at the midclavicular line. The palm of the right hand may be placed here along the costal margin and the left hand under the lower ribs. The natural breathing of the infant is used to guide the liver to the point of ligamentous and fascial balance on the in-breath. By supporting the direction of balance and gently providing a fulcrum with your contact during the baby's out-breath, the desired physiological outcome will be achieved.

Dr Wales recommended this approach for hyperemesis gravidarum (morning sickness).

VIDEO FOR CHAPTER 6

Scan the QR code or visit https://www.youtube.com/playlist?list=PL3j_YuMBqigEx6AlCJ-G8D3tNbXetvLF6 to find a playlist of the video that accompanies this chapter.

REFERENCES

Abdel-Misih Sherif, R.Z. & Bloomston, M. (2010) Liver anatomy. *Surg Clin North Am 90* (4), 643–653.

Bordoni, B., Varacallo, M., Morabito, B., *et al.* (2019) Biotensegrity or fascintegrity? *Cureus 11* (6), e4819. https://doi.org/10.7759/cureus.4819.

Chin, J., Francis, M., Lavallier, J., Lomiguen, C. (2019) Osteopathic physical exam findings in chronic hepatitis C: a case study. *Cureus 11* (1), e3939.

Heineman, K. (2014) Osteopathic manipulative treatment in the management of biliary dyskinesia. *J of Osteopathic Medicine 114* (2), 129–133.

Ibukuro, K., Fukuda, H., Tobe, K., Akita, K., Takeguchi, T. (2016) The vascular anatomy of the ligaments of the liver: gross anatomy, imaging and clinical applications. *Br J Radiol 89* (1064), 20150925. https://doi.org/10.1259/bjr.20150925.

Kogure, K., Ishizaki, M., Nemoto, M., *et al.* (2007) Close relation between the inferior vena cava ligament and the caudate lobe in the human liver. *J Hepatobiliary Pancreat Surg 14* (3), 297–301.

Lippincott, H.A. (1949) The Osteopathic Technique of Wm. G. Sutherland, D.O. In: W.G. Sutherland (1990) *Teachings in the Science of Osteopathy.* A.L. Wales (ed.). Fort Worth, TX: Sutherland Cranial Teaching Foundation, Inc./Rudra Press.

Owens, C. (1963) *An Endocrine Interpretation of Chapman's Reflexes,* 2nd edition. Colorado Springs, CO: American Academy of Osteopathy; p. 110.

Still, A.T. (1902) *The Philosophy and Mechanical Principles of Osteopathy.* Kansas City, MO: Hudson-Kimberly Co.; p. 182.

Sutherland, W.G. (1990) *Teachings in the Science of Osteopathy.* A.L. Wales (ed.). Fort Worth, TX: Sutherland Cranial Teaching Foundation, Inc./Rudra Press; p. 209.

Wales, A.L. (1996) British tutorial group meeting. North Attleboro, MA, USA.

Wen, S-L., Feng, S., Tang, S-H., *et al.* (2016) Collapsed reticular network and its possible mechanism during the initiation and/or progression of hepatic fibrosis. *Sci Rep 6,* 35426. https://doi.org/10.1038/srep35426.

Yamaoka, T., Kurihara, K., Kido, A., *et al.* (2019) Four 'fine' messages from four kinds of 'fine' forgotten ligaments of the anterior abdominal wall: have you heard their voices? *Jpn J Radiol 37,* 750–772.

Zink, G.J. & Lawson, W.B. (1979) An osteopathic structural examination and functional interpretation of the soma. *Osteopathic Annals 7,* 12–19.

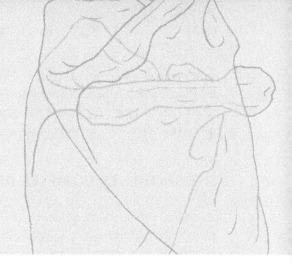

CHAPTER 7

The Shoulder Complex

SUSAN TURNER

'As the whole shoulder girdle and indeed the whole upper third of the ribcage are one functional unit, it is useful to check that the scapula is well-seated before treating the shoulder joint. The free function of the arms and the function of the shoulder joints depend on the position of the glenoid fossa. In patients with poor postural mechanics, where the shoulder "falls off the ribcage", this approach can "put the shoulder back where it belongs".'

(Wales 1997)

This statement by Anne Wales was revolutionary in our treatment of the shoulder complex. This approach, which has power and reliability without using force, teaches us to trust the body, making it possible to 'read its story' and support it in the extraordinary changes that it intelligently seeks to bring about. Dr Wales' emphasis on just how important postural factors are for the shoulder complex reminds us that it can only function harmoniously to the degree that it is well supported by the spine and ribcage.

Every change in posture influences the degree of scapular rotation possible on the trunk at the scapulothoracic joint. *The lateral facing position of the glenoid fossa is crucial to full rotation of the shoulder joint*, and this is greatly diminished, for example, by internally rotated or fixed clavicles. These are often associated with thoracic kyphosis and a slumped anterior thorax which turn the scapulae into winged internal rotation, causing the glenoid fossae to face anteriorly. The reader may try raising the outstretched forward-facing arms to vertical when slumped and then compare the range of motion of the shoulder joints when sitting upright with the clavicles well-seated on the top of the chest.

Painful shoulder restrictions and syndromes are a common presentation in osteopathic practice, especially in the over 50 age group. A study by Judge *et al.* (2014) found that 55 per cent of 60-year-olds have partial or complete tears of the supraspinatus tendon that are asymptomatic, as do 80 per cent of 80-year-olds. It is therefore possible that focus on tendon repair could be misleading in some cases.

Judge and colleagues found that between 2001 and 2010, subacromial decompression surgery had increased by 746 per cent, but the conclusion was that it was relatively unpredictable and ineffective, potentially creating as many problems as it sought to solve. There was also very little agreement about which pain-sensitive tissues are responsible for creating pain. A randomised surgical trial by Beard *et al.* (2018) also found that surgical decompression or arthroscopy do not appear to offer much clinical benefit as compared with no treatment.

Osteopathy has a role in improving mechanical function around the joint to reduce local overload and inflammation, to set up the best conditions for healing to progress, especially in cases where surgery offers no solution. The shoulder should not only be addressed when painful, but be a routine part of a general assessment and osteopathic diagnosis. Because of the reciprocal influence between the shoulder complex and the rest of the body, its treatment, where indicated, should ideally be part of a holistic approach to preventive care.

THE SHOULDER COMPLEX AS A UNIT OF FUNCTION

In terms of osteopathic treatment, the shoulder needs to be addressed as a complex, involving the clavicle, scapula and glenohumeral joint in the context of the postural balance and support afforded by the 'scaffolding' of the upper thorax. Optimum function of the shoulder joint is dependent on the apposition of the three bones in their reciprocal relationship to each other and to the ribcage.

The shallow glenoid fossa is barely a 'socket' in that only 10 per cent of the humeral head is in contact with it at any one time. As a tensegrity mechanism, it is dependent on the support of all the soft tissues around it to safely transfer the daily demands of weight, energy and power that it has to meet to avoid local overload.

The following areas will be considered as they each play an important role in shoulder function: the clavicles with the sternoclavicular and acromioclavicular joints, the coraco-clavicular ligaments, the scapulothoracic joint, the coraco-acromial ligaments, the subacromial space with its bursae, the rotator cuff and, last but not least, the glenohumeral joint proper.

The clavicles

The clavicles stabilise the shoulder girdle but also permit enough movement at the lateral end for the free movement of the arm. They provide a strut that allows the shoulders to suspend the arms from the side of the thorax by thrusting the scapulae, with their glenoid fossae, laterally and back. By permitting movement at both their sternal and acromial ends, they enable scapular rotation on the trunk.

Like the radius and the fibula, the clavicle needs to be free at both ends. It ossifies within the clavipectoral fascia which passes between its inferior proximal surface and the superior surface of pectoralis. In guiding and limiting the motion of the bone, W.G. Sutherland saw this as performing a similar function to the interosseous membranes in the forearm and leg. The coraco-clavicular ligaments (Wales 1988) and the clavipectoral fascia provide fulcra in various clavicular movements. Sutherland saw the clavipectoral fascia as performing a similar role to the interosseous membrane (IoM) in the upper and lower limbs (see Chapters 9 and 13). Thus, it can function as both a ligamentous and a membranous-articular mechanism.

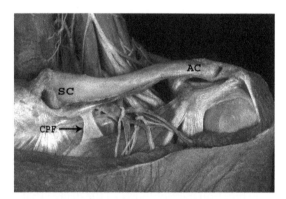

Figure 7.1 Dissection of clavipectoral fascia. AC, acromioclavicular; CPF, clavipectoral fascia; SC, sternoclavicular.

Used with permission of the Willard/Carreiro collection, University of New England, College of Osteopathic Medicine.

The sternoclavicular (SC) joint

The SC joint is the only articular connection of the shoulder girdle and upper limb with the trunk. Without articular movement of this joint, abduction of the arm above 90 degrees is not possible. Thus, it functions as an articular fulcrum for the movement of the upper limb.

The large medial head of the clavicle sits in the partial cartilaginous cup formed by the 1st manubriosternal segment and 1st costal cartilage. Strong ligaments merging with this articular disc prevent the clavicle from being driven medially by the sternum. These ligaments are continuous with the interclavicular ligament connecting the two clavicles and manubrium across the sternal notch. This arrangement has been likened to a reversed Dutch yoke used to carry milk churns.

The medial end of the clavicle is bound to the first rib cartilage on its inferior surface by costo clavicular ligaments which stabilise the clavicle in the action of lifting. The subclavius muscle connects the inferior surface of the clavicle to the costochondral area of the 1st rib and acts as a 'spring', protecting the vessels beneath it.

Loss of mobility of the SC joint can contribute to upper thoracic kyphosis if bilateral, or scoliosis if unilateral. This influence is even more marked if fascial drag from the intrathoracic fascia and diaphragm are acting on the manubrium and upper ribs.

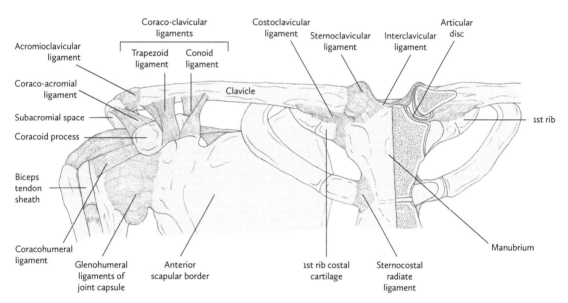

Figure 7.2 Clavicular ligaments.

Acromioclavicular (AC joint)

The AC joint enables the scapula to move vertically as in shrugging of the shoulder. It is made up of small oval facets on each bone, bevelled in relation to each other, with a small articular disc and strong parallel fibres forming the joint capsule. It is the stability provided by the strong coraco-acromial ligaments that protects the acromion from being driven medially in clavicular dislocation. This is assisted by the serratus anterior muscle.

Coraco-clavicular (CC) (conoid and trapezoid) ligaments

The clavicle and scapula are further stabilised to work as a functional unit by the coraco-clavicular ligaments which firmly bind the inferior surface of the clavicle to the coracoid process of the scapula. The trapezoid and conoid ligaments comprising them are positioned at the site of the embryological union between the lateral one third and medial two thirds of the clavicle (Ogata and Uhthoff 1990). These strong ligaments assist the sternoclavicular disc in providing the stability for the clavicle to hold the scapula and arm in their optimum lateral position on the ribcage.

The inferomedial direction of the cora-co-clavicular ligaments also assists in preventing the clavicles from being driven medially when a lateral force is applied to the upper humerus. Forces may also often be absorbed intraosseously by the clavicle, resulting in distortion patterns within the bone. Such intraosseous distortions can sometimes be felt to reorganise once the two ends of the clavicles are freed, taking the operator by surprise.

The scapulothoracic (ST) 'joint'

The scapulothoracic joint is not an anatomical joint as such, as it does not refer to two apposing bones; it is a physiological joint, holding the scapula against the thoracic wall with the help of many muscles, while the clavicle indirectly connects it with the manubrium. It allows complex scapular movements: elevation and depression, protraction and retraction, medial and lateral rotation. This enables and integrates the movements of the scapula with those of the upper limb.

When abducting and lifting the arms, the scapulothoracic joint allows glide and full rotation of the scapula on the ribcage. The wheel-like rotation of the scapula in relation to the body wall is made possible by the fact that it is balanced in a far-reaching multidirectional myofascial field. The fulcrum for scapular rotation is normally slightly inferomedial to the glenoid fossa below the root of the coracoid process. Its tensile suspension, within the myofascial field acting on the scapula, connects it to the occiput, upper limb and the anterior ribcage. Via the rhomboids, trapezius and latissimus dorsi also, it has a reciprocal relationship to the spinous processes of every vertebra from C1 to the sacrum and also the iliac crests via the thoracolumbar fascia (TLF). This is why Viola Frymann DO often used sidelying fascial unwinding of the scapula to treat the spine of young children via these ubiquitous connections (Frymann 1991). The rhomboid fasciae are often tender in respiratory infection.

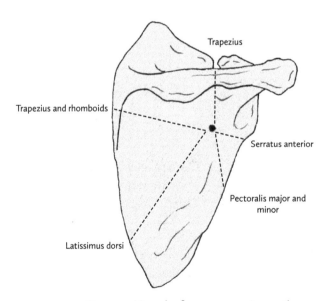

Figure 7.3 Muscular forces converging on the scapula.

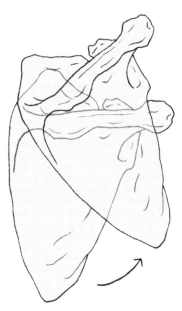

Figure 7.4 Scapular rotation on abduction of the arm.

The involved muscles acting on the rotational fulcrum of the scapula include:

1. Trapezius, superiorly, medially and inferiorly between the occiput and all spinous processes to T12.
2. The rhomboids, connecting to all spinous processes between C7 and T5. Their action balances the tendency of serratus anterior (SA) and pectoralis minor (PM) to rotate the glenoid fossa anteriorly.
3. The latissimus dorsi, connecting the inferior angle of the scapula with humerus, ribs, lower thoracic and lumbar spine and pelvis.
4. Serratus anterior (SA), originating on the anterolateral aspect of ribs 1–9 and inserting into the whole medial border of the scapula. Its action, which is to draw the scapula forward on the thorax, causes the glenoid fossa to face anteriorly. When SA is chronically tense, this position limits the range of motion of the glenohumeral joint.

5. Pectoralis minor, coraco-brachialis and the short head of biceps all insert into the scapular coracoid process. The action of pectoralis minor is internal and inferior rotation of the scapula which also tends to draw the glenoid fossa to face anteriorly.

The coraco-acromial (CA) ligament
The CA ligament spans the coracoid and acromial processes of the scapula, forming a 'roof' over the glenohumeral joint space. It protects the shoulder from upward dislocation of the humerus, especially in injuries from falling on an outstretched hand where the forces are transmitted up the arm to the humeral head. A study by Rothenberg *et al.* (2017) suggests that due to the high density of mechanoreceptors within the CA ligament, it serves as a sensory organ providing static and dynamic proprioception.

Studies examining the role of mechanoreceptors in the coraco-acromial ligament suggest that they also play a significant role in muscle coordination and functional stability of the shoulder (Diederichsen *et al.* 2004). Another study (Warner *et al.* 1996) suggests that the capsuloligamentous mechanism contributes to reflexive muscle contraction of the rotator cuff and biceps. As discussed in the introduction, this would explain why muscle tension appears to increase as a protective response to ligamentous imbalance.

The subacromial space
This is a potential space directly beneath the coracoid and coraco-acromial ligament and above the glenohumeral joint. It is especially vulnerable to compression as, packed into this limited area, are sensitive structures such as the long head of biceps, the subacromial bursa and the rotator cuff. Any friction within the subacromial space, leading to bursitis or inflammation and swelling of tendons, may create dysfunction and pain. Assessing and harmonising this spatial

relationship may be very important to enable the inflamed and irritated structures to calm and heal. We are, once again, 'changing the geometry of the space' (Wales 1988).

One of the structures traversing the subacromial space is the composite tendinous attachment of the four rotator cuff muscles, supraspinatus, infraspinatus, teres minor and subscapularis. These arise from the scapula and connect with the head of the humerus, forming a cuff at the shoulder joint. The tendon of supraspinatus fuses with the underlying fibrous capsule more extensively than the other three muscles. The rotator cuff is important, not only for shoulder movement, but also for maintaining glenohumeral joint stability, by grasping the head of the humerus and compressing it into the glenoid fossa during translations of the glenohumeral joint (Nicolozakes *et al.* 2022). The tendons of these four short muscles have been likened to 'accessory ligaments' which are 'active and alert' (Grant 1965). Their coordination is crucial to protection of the subacromial space from upward displacement of the humerus.

Bursae

The large subacromial bursa and its adjoining subdeltoid bursa also merit consideration. Both the subdeltoid bursa and the glenoid labrum are highly pain sensitive. They have free nerve endings as well as innervation from the suprascapular and lateral pectoral nerves (Vangsness *et al.* 1995). The subacromial bursa has the highest density of nociceptors in the shoulder (Kennedy *et al.* 2017). As the bursa is highly vascularised and contains stem cells, it may play a role in promoting the healing of rotator cuff injury or surgical repair (Klatte-Shulz *et al.* 2022).

The glenohumeral joint

The almost flat, pear-shaped glenoid cavity closely suspends the semilunar head of the humerus within a loose synovial membrane encapsulating the joint. The membrane is reinforced anteriorly by three bands of ligaments formed by thickenings in the folds of the capsule. The glenoid fossa is deepened by a labrum, and the lack of hyaline cartilage in this fibrous lip indicates that this joint is adapted for resisting tensional, rather than compressive, forces.

The wide range of movement of the joint is made possible by the balance of tension in the rotator cuff muscles with their blended tendinous attachment grasping the head of the humerus. Within the capsule, the intracapsular origin of the long head of biceps on the scapular supraglenoid tubercle can be prone to inflammation, giving rise to specific pain on the anterior arm in the bicipital groove.

As the arm is elevated or rotated, the fulcrum of the glenohumeral joint should be held in constant and finely balanced tension by the rotator cuff muscles, allowing gliding and translation of the humeral head in the glenoid fossa. Any unequal tension in the muscles disturbs the joint fulcrum and hence the positional relationship of the humeral head in the glenoid fossa. For example, in thoracic kyphosis the anteroposterior balance of the joint is affected by a tightening anteriorly and stretching posteriorly. This, in turn, may restrict the range of motion and cause compression or strain on the ligaments, tendons and capsule of the shoulder. This will adversely affect blood flow, nutrition and drainage and therefore healing processes within the joint.

Costovertebral and costochondral joints

Because of the interdependence of the shoulder girdle with the ribcage, we must include the *costovertebral* and *costochondral joints* in the essential articulations of the shoulder. Those relating to the 1st and 2nd ribs are of special importance. The whole shoulder girdle, together with the upper third of the thoracic spine and ribcage, need to be addressed as a functional unit because of their reciprocal influence.

FURTHER CLINICAL CONSIDERATIONS

Deltoid muscle pain

Sutherland observed that deltoid muscle pain could be associated with twisting of the muscle at its origin on the scapula and clavicle when they are misaligned at the AC joint. He saw changes in the distance between the origin and insertion of a muscle as affecting muscle function, with associated pain.

Thyroid function

A.T. Still, and W.G. Sutherland after him, made the observation that when the clavicles are pushed back in the 'Stand up straight and pull your shoulders back!' mode, the blood and nerve supply to the thyroid are altered, contributing to a tendency to goitre formation.

Neurovascular problems of the arms

The neurovascular bundle passes between the clavicle and the 1st rib, beneath the subclavius muscle, so where the clavicle is fixed low and the first rib elevated, the brachial plexus and vessels may be compromised.

Lymphatic drainage

Fixation of the clavicle(s) can interfere with the drainage of lymph into the subclavian veins, potentially slowing lymphatic flow in the whole body. The clavicles should be checked before addressing the lymphatic system osteopathically.

Greenstick fractures and intraosseous strains

Sutherland observed that greenstick fractures of the clavicle in children will often straighten out with the approach described below. Experience has shown that intraosseous strains and shape distortions from old fractures of the clavicle can often remould intraosseously once the two articular ends are free.

Subclavius and respiratory reflexes

The subclavius muscle carries filaments of the phrenic nerve so that ease of position of the clavicle may be relevant to important reflexes for respiration (Sharma *et al.* 2011).

Shoulder problems originating in the forearm

Injuries to the elbow, forearm or wrist can strain the shoulder by causing it to compensate for loss of the swivel action between ulna and radius in pronation and supination.

Whiplash or seatbelt injuries

These types of injury, which unilaterally fix the clavicle, upper ribs and retrosternal fascia, can alter sensory input, resulting in circulatory dysfunction in the shoulder girdle and neck.

THERAPEUTIC ENGAGEMENT

The clavicles and AC joint

Having examined the range of motion, tissue quality and relationships of the shoulder joint complex, each bone is attended to in turn.

1. STANCE

The patient sits on the treatment table while you face him or her with a well-grounded stance, feet apart and knees relaxed.

2. ASSESSMENT

Begin by diagnosing the clavicles to see if the manubriosternal ends are symmetrical and if they move freely with the patient's breathing.

3. HANDHOLD

Place your thumb pads under the inferior surface of each end of the strained clavicle. The lateral thumb contact should be just superolateral to the coracoid process with the fingers over the AC joint. The medial thumb contact should avoid the 1st rib which is tightly bound to the clavicle by the costo clavicular ligaments. The palms and fingers are also in comfortable proprioceptive contact.

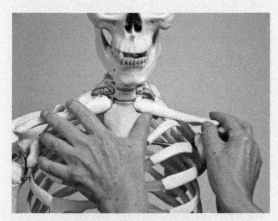

Figure 7.5 Clavicle handhold on skeleton.

4. MATCHING THE PATIENT'S WEIGHT

The patient is instructed to lean forward slightly onto your thumbs, moving from the hips with a straight spine 'like a tree', and head in line with the body. As you also lean forward slightly this will enable you to effortlessly match the patient's weight, supporting both ends of the clavicle from below. This allows the clavicle to lift slightly and engage the clavipectoral fascia and subclavius. The slight angle at which each person leans will be modified according to his or her relative size and weight, i.e., for each to match the other's weight, the slighter person will need to lean forward a little more than the heavier one.

5. ACROMIOCLAVICULAR JOINT

To engage the AC joint, counter the slight lifting of the lateral clavicle with a gentle downward pressure over the joint until you feel it soften slightly. (A more specific AC release is described below.)

6. POSTURAL COOPERATION

While you continue to stabilise the clavicle, ask the patient to turn the opposite shoulder back slightly, to move the manubrium away from the medial end. This alerts the sternoclavicular (SC) ligaments and also slightly disengages the SC joint. The patient should only turn up to the point where you feel the first point of tension in the SC ligaments. This is another example of 'holding the bolt as the patient turns the nut'.

7. LIGAMENTOUS REORGANISATION

Continue to support the clavicle steadily at its two ends. With the two articular ends now disengaged, it sometimes feels as if the fulcrum moves back and forth like a see-saw (teeter-totter) (Wales 1997) until a pause in stillness at the point of balanced tension is followed by resolution. There may be a sense of the clavicle reorganising intraosseously as the two articular ends are freed.

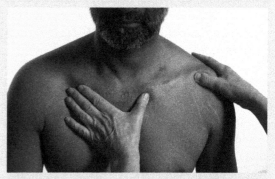

Figure 7.6 Handhold for suspension of the clavicle.

8. 'ESCORTING' THE PATIENT BACK TO POSTURAL CONTROL

Continue to support the patient as he or she moves the opposite shoulder back to symmetry again and sits up. Only when he or she has resumed full postural control do you withdraw contact.

9. BALANCING THE OTHER CLAVICLE

Check and rebalance the opposite clavicle as neces-sary. You may be surprised by an impression of the newly treated clavicle appearing wider than the untreated side. It is always advisable to address both sides when treating bilateral structures or at least engage with the second side to see if it is necessary. When one side of the body makes a therapeutic change, the opposite side will have to readjust to integrate the change.

A further variation for specific engagement of the AC joint

1. AC JOINT DISTRACTION

If the AC joint needs further specific attention, support and steady both ends of the clavicle as described above. In addition, *ask the patient to place his or her hand onto your shoulder, while resting that arm on your flexed and laterally held elbow. Gently draw your own shoulder back so that the patient's arm moves away with it.* Through this, the AC joint is subtly distracted, enabling it to reorganise through BLT.

2. ESCORTING HOME

On completion, 'escort' the patient back to postural control in the vertical position while guiding the patient's arm back to the side of his or her body.

The scapulothoracic 'joint'

The aim here is to rebalance and free scapular movement on the thoracic wall, within its myo-fascial field. This is enabled by springing the upper scapula outwards over the fulcrum of the practitioner's thumb. Dr Wales referred to one of the functions of this manoeuvre as 'opening up the top' to stretch the supraspinatus tendon and beneficially affect the fascia of the trapezius muscle across the shoulder.

Dr Sutherland observed that restoring the scapula to its functional position alters the origin and insertion of trapezius and supraspinatus. He observed that this helps to restore fluid inter-change within the muscles which, over time, will tend to break up fibrosis more efficiently than deep tissue work.

This procedure is also useful where serratus anterior (SA) has held the ribs in strain anterior to the scapula. When this is the case, rebalancing of the scapula is advisable before releasing the ribs. A hypertonic SA will tend to elevate and laterally displace the scapula.

1. HANDHOLD AND POSTURE

Stand beside the seated patient, facing the side to be addressed.

For the left scapula, wrap the fingers of your left hand around the patient's anterior upper ribs while slipping the thumb pad under the axilla as far supe-riorly as possible. Contacting the fascial space just anterior to latissimus dorsi and teres major will avoid compression of the neuromuscular bundle. *Place your left thumb parallel to the body wall.*

The palm of the right (back) hand holds the scapular blade, while the fingers hold the superior surface of the scapular spine. The heel of the right hand holds the scapular inferior angle.

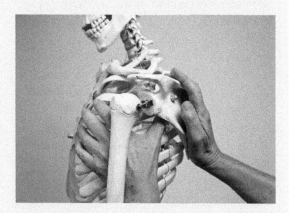

Figure 7.7 Scapular handhold on skeleton.

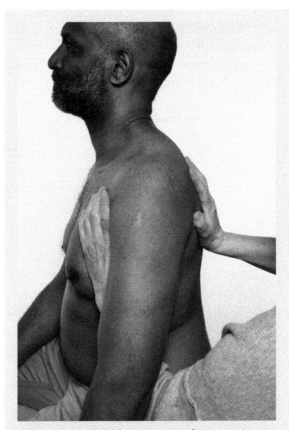

Figure 7.8 Handhold for treatment of the scapula.

2. CONTACTING THE ANTERIOR SCAPULA WITHOUT DISCOMFORT TO THE PATIENT

Ask the patient to shrug the left shoulder up towards the ear. As the shoulder lifts, this opens the space into which your thumb can advance superomedially along the posterior ribs. The thumb remains there as the patient slowly relaxes the shoulder down over your thumb. This may be repeated several times, progressively advancing along the anterior surface of the scapula until the thumb is as close as possible to the natural fulcrum of the scapula. From personal experience this appears to be just below the coracoid process. Resistance may be felt at serratus anterior.

Ask *the patient to lean sideways towards you without slumping, so that the shoulder is slightly suspended by the web of your anterior hand.* This helps to free the subacromial space.

You may also draw the scapula laterally towards you, with the posterior (right) hand. Dr Wales called this 'bringing it out in the open' to allow a still deeper contact on the anterior scapular surface.

This is an example of Sutherland's advice to 'put the glove over the thumb rather than the thumb into the glove'.

3. ENGAGEMENT

The left (anterior) thumb is then in position to form a fulcrum on the anterior surface of the scapula, pointing slightly posteriorly between the scapula and the body wall.

The heel of the right hand gently pushes the scapular apex anteriorly to bring focus to bear upon the thumb fulcrum. This is further enhanced by bringing the scapular spine inferiorly with the fingers.

4. POINT OF BALANCE AND REORGANISATION WITHIN THE SCAPULA'S MYOFASCIAL FIELD

As your right hand supports the scapula to seek its balance around the thumb fulcrum, its whole myofascial field engages and explores for a neutral point. The point of balance is followed by reorganisation and resettling of the scapula and its musculature. The whole shoulder may appear to drop as it relaxes. What is sought here is a sense of a scapula that is free to float and rotate on the thoracic wall, balanced in its wide-ranging tensional relationships.

5. PATIENT'S RESUMPTION OF POSTURAL CONTROL

In the final stage, *escort the patient to sit up and take back postural control.* The scapula may then be taken through its range of motion.

The glenohumeral joint

'This will permit you to find a position of balanced ligamentous tension in the shoulder joint and the ligaments will do the work.'

(Sutherland 1990, TSO p. 197)

This approach uses the principle of disengagement, enabling the ligaments to draw the humeral head back into its optimum position.

Diagnosis

An especially useful before-and-after screening for rotation of the humerus in the glenoid fossa involves holding the patient's humerus in abduction to 90 degrees in one hand and the wrist with the other hand. The patient's elbow is flexed to 90 degrees. An externally rotated glenohumeral joint will easily permit rotation of the forearm to vertical but may resist anteroinferior rotation of the forearm. If the glenohumeral joint is strained towards internal rotation, the reverse will be found where the forearm resists rotation to the vertical.

1. STANCE

Having examined the joint through all ranges of motion, *stand facing the affected side of the patient who sits on the treatment table.*

2. HANDHOLD

To treat the left shoulder, wrap both hands around the shoulder joint, with the thumbs providing an axillary fulcrum on which the joint can rest. This should be as close to the humeral head as possible between the inner arm and body wall. The fingers wrap the shoulder joint as if they were providing another set of ligaments. It can be helpful to imagine your thumbs as similar to 'snails' eyes', looking out from the centre of the floppy joint capsule to its periphery.

For extra support, the patient can lean slightly against you as you provide stability through your well-grounded stance.

3. POSTURAL COOPERATION

The patient is asked to place the left arm across the chest with the fingers on the distal third of the opposite clavicle. The patient's fingers should 'stick' to the clavicle, while leaving the shoulder joint as relaxed as possible. This action draws the arm over the fulcrum of your anterior hand providing slight distraction of the humeral head.

Remind the patient to relax the left shoulder so that your arm, supporting the elbow, can lift or lower it to find an approximate position of ease for the shoulder joint. Elevating the patient's elbow will tend to match internal rotation of the shoulder, and lowering it, external rotation.

Alternatively, using the same cooperation from the patient, your palms and fingers can support the upper humerus close to the axilla without supporting the elbow as shown here.

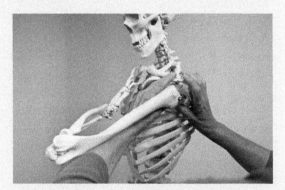

Figure 7.9 Shoulder joint handhold on skeleton.

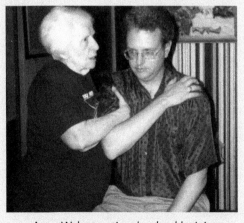

Figure 7.10 Anne Wales treating the shoulder joint.

4. ACTIVATION OF THE LIGAMENTS

To further disengage or 'give space' to the humeral head and increase leverage, *ask the patient to draw the uninvolved opposite shoulder back very slightly*. This draws the patient's hand, in contact with the right clavicle, back with it; this will draw the left glenohumeral ligaments over the fulcrum of the operator's hand, taking up the laxity in the capsule and engaging the ligaments so that they are activated to seek a position of BLT.

5. WAITING WITH THE POINT OF BALANCE FOR RESOLUTION

Continue to support the arm and shoulder at the point of balance until a shift is felt in the joint capsule and ligaments towards spontaneous reorganisation. The patient's natural breathing assists the shift in the joint fulcrum towards resolution of the strain.

6. INTEGRATION

In the final action, the patient is asked to let go of the arm, sit up and take back vertical postural control. You then take the shoulder joint through its range of motion and make a comparison with your original mobility findings. Note also any change in the quality of aliveness, spaciousness and fluid breathing in the tissues.

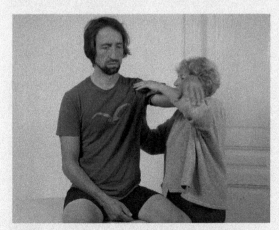

Figure 7.11 Taking the shoulder through range of motion.

Hand position should be modified to adapt to the size of the patient and the particular strain involved.

Alternative hold for the glenohumeral joint

1. HANDHOLD

Stand well-grounded, facing the side of the seated patient as above. For the left shoulder, ask the patient to grasp the left humerus with the right hand, locking it parallel to the ribcage.

Wrap the overlapping palmar surfaces of your hands around the medial surface of the upper left humerus.

2. ENGAGEMENT

Ask the patient to lean away from you very slightly as you resist, matching the tension to create subtle distraction of the glenohumeral joint. This will shift the articular fulcrum, enabling the ligaments to find a new fulcrum of equally balanced tension in relation to the strained joint.

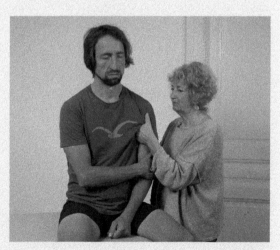

Figure 7.12 Shoulder BLT with patient's humerus held against ribcage.

3. BALANCE POINT AND RESOLUTION

As the whole joint mechanism becomes still at the balance point, *acknowledge the interior shape of the synovial space and wait until the patient's breathing subtly shifts ligamentous balance* towards resolution of the strain.

4. RESUMPTION OF POSTURAL CONTROL

The patient relaxes both arms and settles back into midline postural balance.

VIDEOS FOR CHAPTER 7

Scan the QR code or visit https://www.youtube.com/playlist?list=PL3j_YuMBqigEa8eDHHYz_c2a4H4EuSF9b to find a playlist of the videos that accompany this chapter.

REFERENCES

Beard, D.J., Rees, J.L., Cook, J.A., *et al.* (2018) Arthroscopic subacromial decompression for subacromial shoulder pain (CSAW): a multicentre, pragmatic, parallel group, placebo-controlled, three-group, randomised surgical trial. *Lancet 391* (10118), 329–338. https://doi.org/10.1016/S0140-6736(17)32457-1.

Diederichsen, L.P., Nørregaard, J., Krogsgaard, M., Fischer-Rasmussen, T., Dyhre-Poulsen, P. (2004) Reflexes in the shoulder muscles elicited from the human coracoacromial ligament. *Journal of Orthopaedic Research 22* (5), 976–983.

Frymann, V. (1991) College Atman Seminar, Paris.

Grant, J.C.B. (1965) *Grant's Method of Anatomy,* 7th edition. Baltimore, MD: Williams and Wilkins Co.; p. 178.

Judge, A., Murphy, R.J., Maxwell, R., Arden, N.K., Carr, A.J. (2014) Temporal trends and geographical variation in the use of subacromial decompression and rotator cuff repair of the shoulder in England. *Bone Joint J 96-B* (1), 70–74. https://doi.org/10.1302/0301-620X.96B1.32556.

Kennedy, M.S., Nicholson, H.D., Woodley, S.J. (2017) Clinical anatomy of the subacromial and related shoulder bursae: a review of the literature. *Clini Anat 30,* 213–226. https://doi.org/10.1002/ca.22823.

Klatte-Shulz, F., Thiele, K., Scheibel, M., *et al.* (2022) Subacromial bursa: a neglected tissue is gaining more and more attention in clinical and experimental research. *Cells 11,* 4, 663.

Nicolozakes, C.P., Coats-Thomas, S., Ludvig, D., *et al.* (2022) Translations of the humeral head elicit reflexes in rotator cuff muscles that are larger than those in the primary shoulder movers. *Frontiers in Integrative Neuroscience 15,* 796472. https://doi.org/10.3389/fnint.2021.796472.

Ogata, S. & Uhthoff, H.K. (1990) The early development and ossification of the human clavicle – an embryologic study. *Acta Orthop Scand 61* (4), 330–334. https://doi.org/10.3109/17453679008993529.

Rothenberg, A., Gasbarro, G., Chlebeck, J., Lin, A., *et al.* (2017) The coracoacromial ligament: anatomy, function and clinical significance. *Orthop J Sports Med 5* (4), 2325967117703398. https://doi.org/10.1177/2325967117703398.

Sharma, M.S., Loukas, M., Spinner, R.J. (2011) Accessory phrenic nerve: a rarely discussed common variation with clinical implications. *Clinical Anatomy 24* (5), 671–673.

Sutherland, W.G. (1990) *Teachings in the Science of Osteopathy.* A.L. Wales (ed.). Fort Worth, TX: Sutherland Cranial Teaching Foundation, Inc./Rudra Press; p. 197.

Vangsness, C.T. Jr, Ennis, M., Taylor, J.G., *et al.* (1995) Neural anatomy of the glenohumeral ligaments, labrum and subacromial brush. *Arthroscopy 11,* 180–184. https://dx.doi.org/10.1016/0749-8063(95)90064-0.

Wales, A.L. (1988) Andrew Still Sutherland Study Group (ASSSG). Rhode Island, USA.

Wales, A. L. (1997) Recorded conversation with Jayne Alexander DO. British tutorial group meeting. North Attleboro, MA, USA.

Warner, J.J., Lephart, S., Fu, F.H. (1996) Role of proprioception in pathoetiology of shoulder instability. *Clinical Orthopaedics and Related Research 330,* 35–39.

CHAPTER 8

The Elbow

KOK WENG LIM

Although the elbow is not a weight-bearing joint, it is subject to significant forces in everyday activities such as chores and exercises. Its complexity makes it the second most commonly injured joint in sports after the shoulder (Morris and Ozer 2017).

This chapter primarily explores the ligamentous relationships of the elbow. However, muscles such as the anconeus and brachioradialis are also crucial to the balance of pressures at the humero-ulnar joint surfaces. In reality these act together with all collagenous connective tissues including ligaments, fascia and aponeuroses to form a tensioned unit of function (Scarr 2012).

ANATOMY

The elbow is made up of three joints all within the same synovial capsule:

- Radiocapitellar: between the head of the radius and the capitulum on the lateral aspect of the distal end of the humerus.
- Ulnohumeral: between the trochlear notch on the proximal ulna and the trochlea on the medial aspect of distal end of the humerus.
- Proximal radioulnar: between the radial head and lesser sigmoid notch of the ulna.

The ulnohumeral joint allows for flexion and extension, being a hinge (ginglymus) joint. Pivoting or rotation into pronation and supination (trochoid movement) are allowed by the radiocapitellar and proximal radioulnar pivot joints (Tan *et al.* 2018).

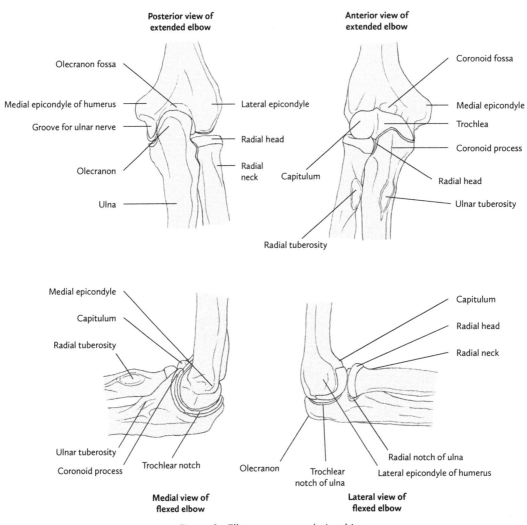

Figure 8.1 Elbow, osseous relationships.

The bony and soft tissue structures each contribute 50:50 to joint stability (Padron *et al.* 2020). The complexity of the ligamentous, fascial and osseous relationships of the elbow joint means that even slight positional alteration of the osseous relationships may impinge on the sensitive structures weaving through it. In treatment, 'our aim is to change the geometry of the space' (Wales 1988).

The joint capsule

The thin, transparent anterior part of the capsule is attached to the anterior margin of the coronoid and the annular ligament of the radius. The posterior part is attached to the articular margin of the sigmoid notch, and the superior part, to the upper border of the olecranon fossa.

The anconeus muscle stabilises both the posterior part of the capsule and also the ulna during forearm pronation. It abducts the ulna during rotatory movements.

The medial and lateral collateral ligaments are, in reality, thickened capsule and are considered primary stabilisers of the elbow. We see here how seamlessly continuous the ligaments of the elbow are with the capsule and its bursae.

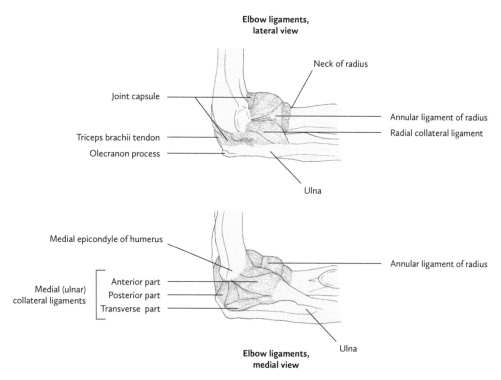

Elbow ligaments,
lateral view

Neck of radius

Joint capsule

Annular ligament of radius
Radial collateral ligament

Triceps brachii tendon
Olecranon process

Ulna

Medial epicondyle of humerus

Annular ligament of radius

Medial (ulnar)
collateral ligaments
- Anterior part
- Posterior part
- Transverse part

Ulna

Elbow ligaments,
medial view

Figure 8.2 Elbow, medial and lateral ligaments.

The medial collateral ligament (ligament of Cooper) is composed of anterior, posterior and transverse bundles. The anterior bundle is the strongest and resists valgus stress (Nazarian *et al.* 2003). Microtears can occur in the anterior bundle from repetitive valgus stress sustained from overhead movements such as in javelin throwing, tennis or cricket. The olecranon and humerus may also be twisted and forced into extension in this injury. Olecranon stress fractures are common in throwers and the ulnar nerve may be excessively and repeatedly stretched. Injury to this ligament should prompt an assessment of truncal core stability, shoulder girdle, scapular-thoracic motion and the degree of elbow pronation and carrying angle.

The lateral collateral ligament

This ligamentous complex has four parts: the radial collateral, annular, lateral ulnar collateral and accessory collateral ligaments. Injury to

this ligament may arise from supination stress from a fall on the outstretched hand and may be associated with elbow dislocation and fracture or posterolateral subluxation of the radial head. Entrapment of the ulnar nerve may often follow elbow dislocations or formation of scar tissue. Intra-articular entrapment of both the median and ulnar nerves has also been reported following dislocations in children (McCarthy *et al.* 2018; Petratos *et al.* 2012).

- The *radial collateral ligament* originates from the lateral epicondyle and gives origin to the supinator muscle.
- The *annular ligament* is an arch-shaped band. It holds the radial head against the ulna and resists lateral displacement of the radial head (Hayami *et al.* 2017).
- The *lateral ulnar collateral ligament* arises from the lateral epicondyle and blends with the annular ligament. It forms a

hammock behind the radial head to prevent varus and posterolateral shear (Edelmuth *et al.* 2021).

- The *accessory collateral ligament*, if present, also blends with the annular ligament and helps to stabilise the radial head. Both the lateral ulnar collateral and accessory collateral ligaments insert at the supinator crest of the ulna, forming the 'Y' ligament.

The quadrate ligament

This proximal radioulnar ligament is an inferior thickening of the elbow capsule. It extends from the neck of the radius and annular ligament to the inferior border of the ulnar notch. It is a separate structure from the annular ligament and serves to secure the neck of the radius to the ulna (Tubbs *et al.* 2006). It also resists posterior and lateral radial head displacement (Hayami *et al.* 2017).

The deep fascia of the elbow

The deep fascia of the elbow connects the forearm extensor muscles with the deltoid muscle and the posterior edge of the deltoid tendon, forming the lateral intermuscular septum (Dones *et al.* 2013). The septum inserts along the whole length of the lateral edge of the humerus including the lateral epicondyle. The interosseous membrane (IoM) between the radius and ulna can be considered continuous with the deep fascia of the elbow and indeed the periosteum of the radius and ulna. It is an important longitudinal stabiliser of the elbow joint as well as maintaining the relative position of the two bones during movement (Malik and Malik 2015).

Bursae

There are seven bursae associated with the elbow joint. Olecranon bursitis (student's elbow) is the most commonly presenting bursitis. The superficial olecranon bursa is situated between the subcutaneous tissue and the olecranon process;

if the bursa ruptures it may present as a triceps swelling.

The bicipital radial bursa is a deep bursa separating the biceps tendon from the tuberosity of the radius. Inflammation of this bursa can be confused with distal biceps tendinitis and impending biceps tendon rupture. Crepitus on pronation and supination may suggest a tendon pathology.

Median nerve compression: The median nerve passes under the bicipital aponeurosis (laceratus fibrosus), a sheet of ligamentous tissue *distal* to the elbow joint, which coordinates elbow flexion and supination of the forearm (Snoeck *et al.* 2021). The symptoms of acute or chronic median nerve compression from the lacertus tunnel syndrome are similar to that of carpal tunnel syndrome. Sensory disturbances may also be present (Lalonde 2015). Osteopathic stretching of the bicipital aponeurosis to a point of balance is helpful; simple stretching can also be helpful in carpal tunnel syndrome.

Ulnar nerve compression: The ulnar nerve may be affected by narrowing of the cubital tunnel as it passes through it. This is a tunnel of bone, muscle and ligaments, whose roof is the arcuate ligament. Its floor is the medial collateral ligament and it is bounded by the medial epicondyle, medial head of the triceps and the olecranon (Card and Lowe 2021). Osteopathic assessment and treatment of these ligamentous and bony boundaries can be helpful in improving the spatial dimensions of this tunnel and promoting nerve gliding.

Increased carrying angle and elbow instability: Axial alignment of the elbow joint is inspected visually by assessing the carrying angle which is formed by the long axis of the humerus and ulna with the elbow in full extension. On average, this angle is 10° in men and 13° in women and also 1° more on the dominant arm (Paraskevas *et al.* 2004). The angle increases with skeletal growth during childhood. The carrying angle allows the arms to swing during gait without contact on the hips. In full flexion these axes are aligned. Increased carrying angle of more than 15° may be associated with elbow instability and pain during sports, increased risk of a fracture from a fall onto an outstretched arm, or entrapment neuropathy of the ulnar nerve (Chang *et al.* 2008).

Fryette (1954) described an adduction ulnohumeral lesion from a sudden pull on the forearm or hand. More commonly an abduction lesion can result from a fall on the outstretched arm or from pushing vigorously while the elbow is extended. Both of these accentuate the carrying angle. An external or internal rotation lesion of the ulna, in relation to the humerus, can be produced by rotational forces in extreme radial supination or pronation.

There is a 6–8° valgus tilt of the distal humeral articulation in relation to the long axis of the humerus.

ELBOW PAIN

Lateral elbow pain and snapping

The anterior capsule has an internal fold, the plica synovalis, which crosses downward and medially over the radial head and neck to insert into the distal part of the anterior capsule. It envelops a portion of the radial head and may be a cause of snapping elbow if thickened. It may also mimic the symptoms of tennis elbow with lateral elbow pain (Kholinne *et al.* 2021).

Lateral elbow pain in children

Lateral elbow pain in children may be due to osteochondrosis of the capitellum (Panner's disease). It occurs most commonly in boys (90%) during the peak ossification period of the capitellar epiphysis, between 5 and 12 years of age.

Osteopathic treatment to reduce valgus stress on the elbow and improve the blood supply to the subchondral bone may be helpful during the growing phase.

Lateral elbow pain in early adolescence may be due to osteochondritis dissecans. This presents after the capitellum has almost completely ossified in early adolescence, and may result in a loose body in the joint, causing locking. There is loss of elbow extension and an effusion. The aetiology is often microtrauma with bone ischaemia and fragmentation (Ruchelsman *et al.* 2010). It can also affect the olecranon and trochlea. Panner's disease and osteochondritis dissecans probably represent a continuum of disrupted endochondral ossification (Kobayashi *et al.* 2004).

THERAPEUTIC ENGAGEMENT

The ulnohumeral joint

The primary movement between the humerus and ulna is flexion and extension. Complete extension of the arm is limited in strains affecting the position of the olecranon process within the olecranon fossa of the humerus (Lippincott 1949). Conversely flexion at the elbow is restricted when the position of the coronoid process within the coronoid fossa of the humerus is disturbed by strains.

1. HANDHOLD AND POSITIONING

To address the right elbow, *stand facing the seated patient with your right arm in front of the patient's right arm.*

With the patient's elbow initially flexed at 90 degrees, *support his or her forearm on your forearm, cupping your fingers around the olecranon process. Lock the palm of the patient's hand around your lower humerus so that the back of the hand is against your lower ribs.*

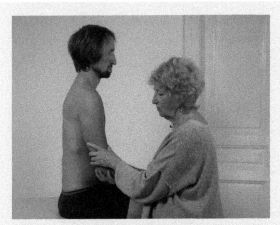
Figure 8.3 Handhold for BLT of the elbow.

2. REFINING THE DEGREE OF ELBOW FLEXION
With your second and third fingers on the ole-cranon process of the ulna, *explore for the point of ease in elbow flexion by shifting your body weight very slightly towards and away from the patient.* Make sure you are well grounded so that the *locking of the patient's hand against your trunk* allows your body to move as a unit with that of the patient as you sense for the point of ease.

3. LIGAMENTOUS ENGAGEMENT BY DISTRACTION
Wrap your left hand around the lower end of the patient's humerus. Ligamentous engagement at the ulnohumeral joint can be explored using dis-traction *by lifting the patient's humerus superiorly with your left hand while your right hand stabilises the olecranon process.* As the ligaments engage and activate, note subtle components of the strain revealing themselves as they seek a refinement of the point of balanced tension.

4. POSTURAL COOPERATION
Disengagement to the point of ligamentous bal-ance can be assisted by postural cooperation as *the patient very slightly raises the right shoulder to draw the humerus out of the trochlear notch of the ulna.* The advantage here is that your left hand is then free to sense the refinements in ligamen-tous balance at work within the joint in a purely afferent way.

5. OCCASIONAL USE OF APPROXIMATION
Sometimes rather than disengagement, approxima-tion may activate the ligaments more. This may be the case following a fall on the point of the elbow or on the outstretched hand where the absorbed compressive forces need to be matched before they can release.

6. POINT OF BALANCE
The distortions within the elbow joint become more apparent through engagement by either approximation or distraction. *Support the liga-mentous-articular arrangement as you find it in its seeking of the balance that neutralises the opposing forces of the strain pattern.*

7. SPONTANEOUS REORGANISATION
The resolution following a point of BLT can often be felt as a sense of spaciousness and improved congruence between the articular surfaces. The joint may appear to retrace the vectors of an old or new injury in the process of resolution.

8. RETEST
Re-check the elbow and compare.

Correction of the proximal radial head
The proximal end of the radius is relatively free of ligamentous attachments, allowing it to rotate freely within the annular ligament. 180° of pro-nation and supination is permitted, and lesions of the head of the radius (e.g., post-fracture of the radial head or neck following a fall onto an outstretched arm) will prevent free and full expression of movement.

Anterior or posterior radioulnar strain patterns can be tested and treated by holding the proximal head of the radius and gliding the ulna on it with the elbow in partial flexion.

1. POSITIONING
Sit opposite the patient who sits facing you with his or her forearm on the treatment table and elbow

only very slightly flexed. The patient's hand rests palm down on the table and the elbow is off the table.

2. ACTION

Stabilise the radial head with one hand. The other hand actively moves the proximal humerus around *it in a figure of eight or circular movements until an easing is felt in the annular ligament.* This is an example of 'holding the bolt and turning the nut around it'.

VIDEO FOR CHAPTER 8

Scan the QR code or visit https://www.youtube.com/playlist?list=PL3j_ YuMBqigFPagJE7BoYngxCbfjcDSKl to find a playlist of the video that accompanies this chapter.

REFERENCES

Card, R.K. & Lowe, J.B. (2021) Anatomy, Shoulder and Upper Limb, Elbow Joint. StatPearls [Internet]. Treasure Island, FL: StatPearls Publishing. https://www.ncbi.nlm.nih.gov/books/NBK532948.

Chang, C.W., Wang, Y.C., Chu, C.H. (2008) Increased carrying angle is a risk factor for non traumatic ulnar neuropathy at the elbow. *Clin Orthop Rel Research 466* (9), 2190–2195.

Dones III, V.C., Milanese, S., Worth, D., Grimmer-Somers, K. (2013) The anatomy of the forearm extensor muscles and the fascia in the lateral aspect of the elbow joint complex. *Anatomy & Physiology: Current Research 3,* 117. https://doi.org/10.4172/2161-0940.1000117.

Edelmuth, D.G.L., Hellito, P.V.P., Correa, M.F.P., Bordalo-Rodrigues, M. (2021) Acute ligament injuries of the elbow. *Seminars in Musculoskeletal Radiology 25* (4), 580–588.

Fryette, H.F. (1954) *Principles of Osteopathic Technic. A Harry L. Chiles Memorial Publication.* Carmel, CA: Academy of Applied Osteopathy.

Hayami, N., Omokawa, S., Iida, A., *et al.* (2017) Biomechanical study of isolated radial head dislocation. *BMC Musculoskeletal Disorders 18,* 470.

Kholinne, E., Nanda, A., Liu, H., *et al.* (2021) The elbow plica: a systematic review of terminology and characteristics. *J of Shoulder and Elbow Surgery 30* (5), e185–e198.

Kobayashi, K., Burton, K.J., Rodner, C., *et al.* (2004) Lateral compression injuries in the pediatric elbow: Panner's disease and osteochondritis dissecans of the capitellum. *J Am Acad Orthop Surg 12* (4), 246–254.

Lalonde, D. (2015) Lacertus syndrome: a commonly missed and misdiagnosed median nerve entrapment syndrome. *BMC Proc 9* (3), A74.

Lippincott, H.A. (1949) The Osteopathic Technique of Wm. G. Sutherland, D.O. In: W.G. Sutherland (1990) *Teachings in the Science of Osteopathy.* A.L. Wales (ed.). Fort Worth, TX: Sutherland Cranial Teaching Foundation, Inc./Rudra Press; p. 260.

Malik, S.S. & Malik, S.S. (2015) Elbow: functional anatomy. In: *Orthopaedic Biomechanics Made Easy.* Cambridge: Cambridge University Press; p. 136.

McCarthy, C.F., Kyriakedes, J.C., Mistovich, R.J. (2018) Type-V median nerve entrapment in a pediatric medial condyle fracture: a case report. *JBJS Case Connect 8* (4), e108.

Morris, M.S. & Ozer, K. (2017) Elbow dislocations in contact sports. *Hand Clin 33* (1), 63–72.

Nazarian, L.N., McShane, J.M., Ciccotti, M.G., *et al.* (2003) Dynamic US of the anterior band of the ulnar collateral ligament of the elbow in asymptomatic major league baseball pitchers. *Radiology 227,* 149.

Padron, M., Sanchez, E., Cassar-Pullicino, V.N. (2020) Elbow. In: *Musculoskeletal Radiology.* V.N. Cassar-Pullicino and A.M. Davies (eds). Berlin: Springer; pp. 301–330.

Paraskevas, G., Papadopoulos, A., Papaziogas, B., *et al.* (2004) Study of the carrying angle of the human elbow joint in full extension: a morphometric analysis. *Surg Radiol Anat 26,* 19.

Petratos, D.V., Stavropoulos, N.A., Emmanouil, A., Matsinos, G.S. (2012) Median nerve entrapment and ulnar nerve palsy following elbow dislocation in a child. *J of Surg Orthop Advances 21* (3), 157–161.

Ruchelsman, D.E., Hall, M.P., Youm, T. (2010) Osteochondritis dissecans of the capitellum: current concepts. *Am Acad of Orthop Surgeon 18* (9), 557–567.

Scarr, G. (2012) A consideration of the elbow as a tensegrity structure. *International J of Osteopathic Medicine 15*, 53–65.

Snoeck, O., Coupier, J., Beyer, B., *et al.* (2021) The biomechanical role of the lacertus fibrosus of the biceps brachii muscle. *Surg Radiol Anat 43* (10), 1587–1594.

Tan, Z., Ng, Y., Yew, A., *et al.* (2018) Geometric accuracy of elbow flexion extension (F-E) axis based on approximation to the epicondylar axis. *Orthopaed Proceedings 99B* (8).

Tubbs, R.S., Shoja, M.M., Khaki, A.A., *et al.* (2006) The morphology and function of the quadrate ligament. *Folia Morphol (Warsz) 65* (3), 225–227.

Wales, A.L. (1988) Andrew Still Sutherland Study Group (ASSSG). Rhode Island, USA.

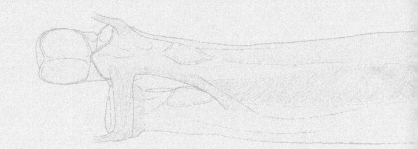

CHAPTER 9

The Forearm

ZENNA ZWIERZCHOWSKA

RADIOULNAR INTEROSSEOUS MEMBRANE (IoM)

In this approach to the forearm, the functional relationship between the ulna and radius is harmonised by balancing the IoM between them.

The elbow, forearm and wrist combined form a functional unit which gives strong support and mobility to the hand, while also allowing for load-bearing activities. In evolutionary development, the action of pronation and supination has permitted positioning of the hand in space in such a way that it has allowed apes to swing from tree to tree. Other mammals have a syndesmosis at the distal radioulnar joint. This ability to rotate the forearm together with a mobile wrist may be considered of equal importance to the opposable thumb in the development of manual skills (Lees 2009).

In pronation the proximal head of the radius rotates in the annular ligament while the distal head rotates around the end of the ulna. In supination (palms up) the two bones lie parallel. This double swivel action is stabilised by the IoM which also constrains the relative movement between these two bones. The IoM is continuous with the periosteum of the ulna and radius, which is one reason that optimum forearm function is so dependent on its balance. The key to restoring free pronation and supination often lies therefore in releasing strain in the membrane.

Strains through the radioulnar IoM affect the functional articular relationships of both the elbow above and the wrist below. Any treatment of either the elbow or wrist should include the IoM. Likewise, treatment of the IoM must include integration of the elbow and wrist.

Pronation strains are common, and limited capacity to supinate the wrist and forearm will tend to be compensated for by the shoulder complex, upper ribs and neck. In the experience of the author, compromise of the forearm's ability to swivel through full pronation and supination can, over time, also have a deleterious effect on the shoulder joint and cervicothoracic regions. This can result in wide-ranging compensatory postural patterns.

The IoM consists of proximal, distal and middle fibres in which there are areas of condensation to provide greater mechanical strength. These are the distal oblique band, central and accessory bands, dorsal oblique accessory cord and proximal oblique cord. With the forearm in the anatomical position, the central and accessory bands of the middle ligamentous complex run predominantly from the radius proximally to the ulna distally (Masouros *et al.* 2019). The distal oblique band and proximal oblique cord pass in the opposite direction (Lees 2009). Although the whole operates as an integrated mechanism, it may be necessary, in treatment, to specifically address different portions.

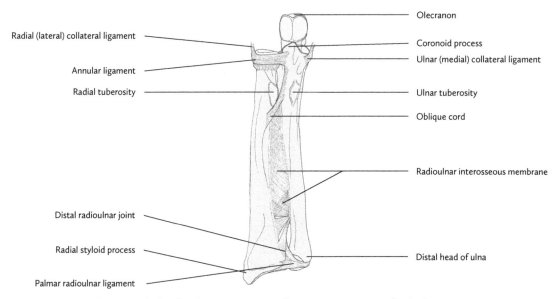

Radial (lateral) collateral ligament

Annular ligament

Radial tuberosity

Distal radioulnar joint

Radial styloid process

Palmar radioulnar ligament

Olecranon

Coronoid process

Ulnar (medial) collateral ligament

Ulnar tuberosity

Oblique cord

Radioulnar interosseous membrane

Distal head of ulna

Figure 9.1 Radioulnar interosseous membrane, anterior view of right forearm.

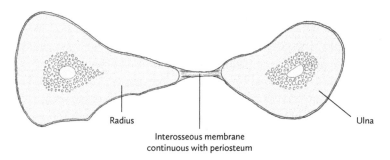

Radius

Ulna

Interosseous membrane
continuous with periosteum

Figure 9.2 Transverse section through mid forearm showing continuity of the
interosseous membrane with the periosteum of ulna and radius.

The forearm IoM also provides an expanded surface for forearm muscle attachment. In the anatomical position, its proximal anterior surface gives attachment for extensor pollicis longus on the radial side. On the ulnar side it provides attachment for flexor digitorum profundus and, more distally, pronator quadratus. Between these muscles it provides a highway for the interosseous vessels and nerve. On its posterior surface are attached supinator, abductor pollicis, extensor pollicis brevis and longus, and extensor indicis proprius. Near the wrist, the volar interosseous artery and dorsal interosseous nerve run along its surface. These are all significant in the function of the wrist and hand. Sutherland's observation merits consideration here, that ligamentous and membranous balance influence the distance between muscular origin and insertion and therefore muscle tone and coordination (Wales 1995).

It was previously believed that the forces absorbed by punching with a fist were transmitted, either through the middle of the wrist into the radius and then the humerus, or through to the ulna via the IoM. Studies now show however that forces actually transmit in a reciprocating manner between radius and ulna via the proximal and distal radioulnar joints and the IoM

(Wegmann *et al.* 2014). This suggests that load is transmitted in a dynamic manner, depending on the position of the forearm and wrist, and is varied by muscle action (Pfaeffle *et al.* 2000, 2006).

Integrity of this entire complex is essential to good function (Hagert 2010). The proprioceptive information from mechanoreceptors in the ligaments on the ulnar side of the wrist, centred on the triquetrum, are of particular importance in triggering the protective reflexes that are important for wrist stability (Hagert *et al.* 2016). This is fundamental to movement and load bearing of the forearm 'osseo-ligamentous' system (Hagert *et al.* 2007). Some of the problems that may arise within this system can be addressed with some very simple manoeuvres.

The natural anatomical position of the hand and wrist in relation to the forearm is in ulnar deviation. In this position the radioulnar articulation, via the IoM, is in easy neutral. Many everyday activities, such as using a small keyboard or hand-held device, may encourage use of the hand in radial deviation (Gholami *et al.* 2022). This takes the whole complex out of easy neutral and puts a strain through both the IoM and the hand flexor tendons, passing through the carpal tunnel. Osteopaths have found that such strains in the IoM can be a major contributing factor in problems such as repetitive strain injury (RSI) and carpal tunnel syndrome. Following treatment, it is important to give patients advice on improving ergonomic use of the forearm, hand and wrist.

THERAPEUTIC ENGAGEMENT

Balanced membranous tension (BMT) of the forearm IoM

1. IMPORTANCE OF GROUNDING
Greater depth of engagement with the connective tissues is made possible through grounding and sinking your weight. This uses the balance through your own connective tissues rather than engaging through muscle effort. Therefore, in this approach, make sure that by using your elbows as fulcra, you sink into your feet on the ground rather than use a lifting action of your hands and arms.

2. PRELIMINARY DIAGNOSIS
Check for radial and ulnar deviation at the wrist. Any excessive movement in the direction of radial deviation may indicate overuse of the hand in this position.

Look at both active and passive movement in pronation and supination, comparing both forearms.

The patient sits on the couch facing you while you stand on the side of the forearm to be treated. Alternatively, sit facing each other on either side of the treatment table with forearms and hands on its surface.

3. SUGGESTED HANDHOLD FOR PASSIVE EXAMINATION AND TREATMENT
For addressing the patient's right forearm, *cup the fingers of your right hand around the olecranon and hold the distal radial head and shaft with your left.* It is important to hold the elbow at a 90° angle. This ensures that the olecranon process is disengaged from the olecranon fossa posteriorly and the coronoid process from the coronoid fossa anteriorly.

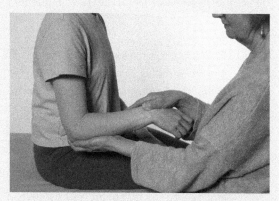

Figure 9.3 Forearm interosseous membrane BMT hold.

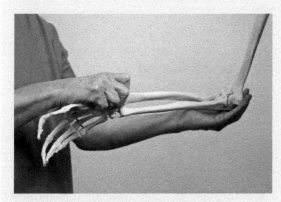

Figure 9.4 Forearm BMT hold on skeleton.

4. A HELPFUL MENTAL IMAGE IN ENGAGING THE IOM BALANCE POINT

Since the IoM is continuous with the periosteum of both ulna and radius, the bones 'go for the ride' on the membrane. *Remembering that microscopically bone is a fluid, think of the bones as secondary and adaptable to the command of the membrane.*

5. FINDING THE NEUTRAL POSITION OF THE IOM

To do this, *first assess the balance between supination/pronation and between proximal/distal shear.* Diagnostically, the fulcrum for the pivoting of the radius around the ulna should be two-thirds of the way down from the elbow within the IoM. This is also the point where the direction of fibres changes. *Find the neutral position in which the fibres of the membrane feel in easy balance for both components as follows:*

- Pronation/supination: *Slowly and gently move the radius towards supination and then pronation relative to the ulna.* Sense the point between them where the fibres of the IoM are in balanced neutral. Maintain this balance point as you then test to include the shearing component.

   Testing should involve taking the forearm only to the first point of resistance in each direction rather than the extreme of motion.

- Proximal/distal shear: *Gently move the radius and ulna proximally and distally in relation to each other, to the point where the fibres of the IoM are in balanced neutral.* The composite balance point now encompasses both components tested for.

6. ACTIVATION OF THE IOM

To activate the IoM, match the tone of the strain with your contact and observe a spontaneous process of refinement of BMT.

In matching the tone, *note whether a strain pattern is predominantly from excessive pulling or from compressive forces such as from a fall onto the hand.* If different bands within the membrane require particular attention, take these into the picture.

7. BALANCE POINT AND RESOLUTION

Maintain the composite balance point, position and tone of your hold until a release is felt as a spontaneous reversal of the strained forearm position. The patient's natural breathing will work on the balance point to shift the fulcrum towards the self-corrective phase. As the membranous-articular relationship resolves, the 'fluid' feel of intraosseous reorganisation can also sometimes be observed within the radius.

8. RETEST

Recheck for the normal fulcrum of movement before taking the forearm through its full range of motion.

Suspension of the IoM between radius and ulna

1. HANDHOLD

Stand or sit to the side of the seated patient. *With the patient's arm flexed at 90°, suspend the ulna on the IoM by taking a gentle 'clothes peg' hold of each end of the radius between your index finger and thumb.* It is more effective to sink your weight to achieve suspension rather than actively lifting.

The weight of the suspended ulna activates the IoM to seek a balance point for resolution of the strain pattern.

2. RELEASE

The resolution is often felt as a sense of lengthening and intraosseous breathing of the radius and a softening of the IoM. There is a sense of reseating of both ends of the radioulnar and radiocapitellar joints.

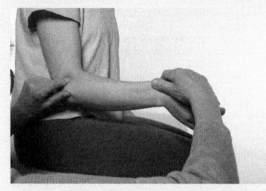

Figure 9.5 Engagement of interosseous membrane through suspension.

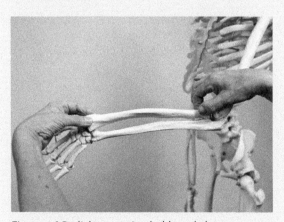

Figure 9.6 Radial suspension hold on skeleton.

Decompressing the distal radioulnar joint

The distal radioulnar joint may need specific attention (Aita *et al.* 2018).

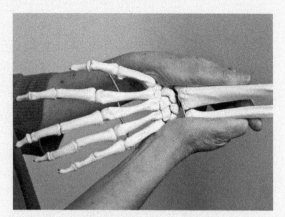

Figure 9.7 Distal radioulnar joint decompression.

1. HANDHOLD

Take hold of the distal head of the ulna with one hand and of the distal radius with the other. If necessary, squeeze to add a little compression to activate and engage the ligaments. Support the radioulnar ligaments as they seek a point of balanced tension and wait for resolution.

VIDEOS FOR CHAPTER 9

Scan the QR code or visit https://www.youtube.com/playlist?list=PL3j_YuMBqigGsE3ho1gobHAf2SSERwcWK to find a playlist of the videos that accompany this chapter.

REFERENCES

Aita, M.A., Mallos, R.C., Ozaki, W., *et al.* (2018) Ligamentous reconstruction of the interosseous membrane of the forearm in the treatment of instability of the distal radioulnar joint. *Rev Bras Ortop 53* (2), 184–191.

Gholami, M., Choobineh, A., Abdoli-Eramaki, M., *et al.* (2022) Investigating the effect of keyboard distance on the posture and 3D moments of wrist and elbow joints among males using OpenSim. *Applied Bionics and Biomechanics 2022.* https://doi.org/10.1155/2022/5751488.

Hagert, E. (2010) Proprioception of the wrist joint: a review of current concepts and possible implications on the rehabilitation of the wrist. *J Hand Ther 23,* 2–17.

Hagert, E., Garcia-Elias, M., Forsgren, S., *et al.* (2007) Immunohistochemical analysis of wrist ligament innervation in relation to their structural composition. *J Hand Surg Am 32* (1), 30–36.

Hagert, E., Lluch, A., Rein, S. (2016) The role of proprioception and neuromuscular stability in carpal instabilities. *J Hand Surgery (European Volume) 41* (1), 94–101.

Lees, V.C. (2009) The functional anatomy of forearm rotation. *J Hand Microsurg 1* (2), 92–99.

Masouros, P.T., Apergis, E.P., Babis, G.C., *et al.* (2019) Essex-Lopresti injuries: an update. *EFORT Open Reviews 4* (4), 143–150. https://doi.org/10.1302/2058-5241.4.180072.

Pfaeffle, H.J., Fischer, K.J., Manson, T.T., *et al.* (2000) Role of the forearm interosseous ligament: is it more than just longitudinal load transfer? *The Journal of Hand Surgery 25* (4), 683–688.

Pfaeffle, H.J., Fischer, K.J., Srinivasa, A., *et al.* (2006) Interosseous ligament of the forearm based on fiber network theory. *J Biomech Eng 128* (5), 725–732.

Wales, A.L. (1995) Personal communication. British tutorial group meeting. North Attleboro, MA, USA.

Wegmann, K., Engel, K., Burkhart, K.J. (2014) Sequence of the Essex-Lopresti lesion – a high-speed video documentation and kinematic analysis. *Acta Orthopaedica 85* (2), 177–180.

CHAPTER 10

The Wrist and Hand

ZENNA ZWIERZCHOWSKA

How often do we find in practice that at the end of a treatment the patient suddenly remembers that painful thumb or wrist? Time is needed for proper appraisal and treatment of the hand and wrist but much can also be done in just a few minutes. Still's wrist technique, described below, makes it possible to treat the whole wrist complex in a few easy movements.

In this chapter we will look systematically at the wrist and hand, working proximally to distally (Wales 1995, 1996, 1997). The wrist joint is a good example of a BLT mechanism with all the carpals bound together in the tensegrity of the ligamentous web, all sharing one synovial membrane except the thumb. No muscles attach to the proximal row and all the hand muscles bypass the carpals and attach to the metacarpals and phalanges.

It is important to assess the shoulder, elbow and forearm before addressing the wrist and hand as the upper limb operates as a unit and one area may have to compensate for lack of mobility in another part. It is especially crucial to look to the radioulnar articulation and its interosseous membrane (IoM) as any strains or restrictions here have a direct effect on the wrist. Also check that the wrist is not in radial deviation as this position tends to compromise wrist and forearm function (see Chapter 9).

ANATOMY

Twenty-seven bones comprise the hand and wrist: two rows of four carpals (eight in total), five metacarpals and fourteen phalanges. This allows great flexibility and dexterity in using the hands but also involves many articulations with all the possibilities for strains and restrictions between them.

The wrist

The proximal row of four carpal bones articulates with the radius and the disc of the ulna. The two rows articulate with each other at the midcarpal joint. The intercarpal joints connect each carpal bone to its neighbours via a network of ligaments.

The wrist joint or radiocarpal joint is an ellipsoid articulation. The concave surface of the distal end of the radius articulates with a triangular articular disc which stretches between the ulnar styloid process and the medial-distal surface of the radius. This articulates with the convex proximal surfaces of the scaphoid, lunate and triquetrum. Interosseous ligaments bind these three bones together (Eschweiler *et al.* 2022). There are, however, no ligamentous connections between the lunate and capitate. Palmar and dorsal radiocarpal ligaments link the radius to the front and back of the proximal row of carpals and the capitate. Radial and ulnar collateral ligaments (lateral and medial) extend from the styloid processes of the ulna and radius to the scaphoid and triquetrum respectively. Permitted movements at the wrist joint are flexion, extension, adduction and abduction, together creating circumduction.

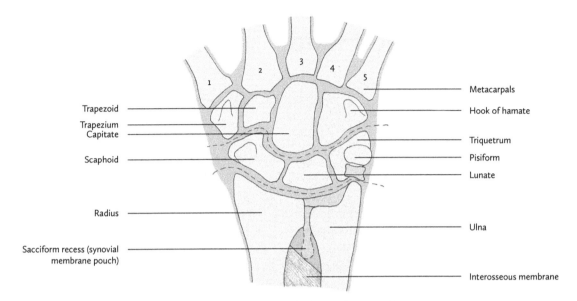

Figure 10.1 Schematic diagram of left wrist bones, palmar view.

The line of articulation between the two rows of carpals is sinuous. This acts as a hinge joint, accompanying the radiocarpal joint in flexion and extension, thus increasing the overall range of these movements. The greater part of flexion that appears to take place at the radiocarpal joint actually occurs at the midcarpal joint, as the capitate visibly moves up on the dorsum of the wrist (Kaufmann *et al.* 2005). However, there is more extension at the wrist than between the two rows of carpals (Sarrafian *et al.* 1977). Adduction occurs at the radiocarpal joint whereas abduction takes place almost entirely at the midcarpal joint (Cunningham *et al.* 2017).

The dorsal and palmar ligamentous bands, binding the carpal bones together, largely radiate from the capitate. Centrally located, this is the largest bone, around which the other bones are organised (Akhbari *et al.* 2020). The dorsum of the wrist is convex, forming an arch created by the shapes and alignment of the bones, but maintained by the tie beam of the flexor retinaculum. Proximally, this extends between two rounded prominences of the pisiform and the tubercle of the scaphoid. Distally, it extends between two crests: the hook of the hamate and the tubercle of the trapezium.

This creates the carpal tunnel, allowing passage for the tendons, nerves and blood vessels to the hand. Because of its shape, the lunate bone may dislocate anteriorly, which can compromise the arch of the tunnel (Nypaver and Liu 2021). In acute carpal tunnel syndrome, it is useful to look to the lunate specifically. It is the only bone to dislocate anteriorly except in severe injury, such as in a perilunar dislocation of a flexed wrist.

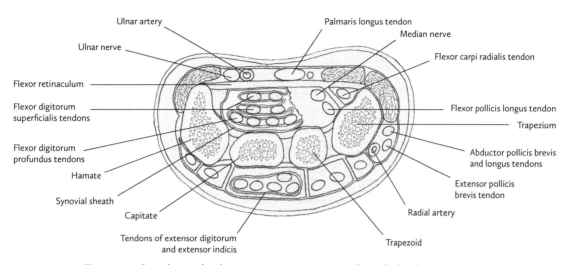

Figure 10.2 Carpal tunnel, schematic transverse section through distal carpal tunnel.

Wrist mechanoreceptors

Recent studies have shown an abundance of mechanoreceptors, in particular on the dorsal surfaces of the carpal ligaments. One of the most important areas is the scapholunate complex of ligaments. Information is transmitted from mechanoreceptors in the articular ligaments by means of local, segmental and suprasegmental pathways. This stimulates immediate local muscle responses as well as integration of movement in the higher centres (Hagert 2010). There is an ever-increasing amount of research on the importance of mechanoreceptors in ligaments and their important proprioceptive role in instructing muscles (see Chapter 1). This supports the emphasis Dr Sutherland placed on the ligamentous mechanisms in joint function for producing the greatest amount of therapeutic change (Crow 2006; Golden 1999; Sutherland 1990).

The palm

The five metacarpal bones of the palm of the hand are miniature long bones. Each has a fairly square base, a stout shaft and an expanded round head. The metacarpals do not run parallel to each other as the bases are close packed and the heads separated, forming a fan-shaped arrangement.

The deep transverse metacarpal ligaments link the metacarpal bases which articulate with each other. All the metacarpals are connected via articular capsules strengthened by dorsal, palmar and interosseous ligaments.

The 2nd to 5th carpo-metacarpal joints are complex sellar joints which share their synovial membrane with the intercarpal joints and the intermetacarpal joints. They articulate with the distal row of carpals and have articular facets at the side, to articulate with each other. The third metacarpal is supported by the large capitate. Together these form the axial midline of the hand, around which many fine movements of the hand are organised.

The 2nd metacarpal, belonging to the index finger, is the most fixed and is supported by three carpals: capitate, trapezoid and trapezium. The 2nd and 3rd metacarpals are in the most direct line of force transmission from a blow or a punch. The radiation of the surrounding intercarpal ligaments to and from the capitate directs forces into this largest of the carpal bones; these forces are then transmitted into the radius and through the arm. The 2nd and 3rd metacarpals have virtually no movement and are therefore very stable (Kollitz *et al.* 2014).

The 4th metacarpal is supported mainly,

and the 5th entirely, by the hamate. This allows a slight degree of movement which permits the cupping action of the palm.

Metacarpophalangeal joints

The 2nd to 5th metacarpophalangeal joints form the knuckle bones. The convex metacarpal heads articulate with the shallow concave phalangeal bases. The joint surface is prolonged at the front but does not reach the back, as its movement is predominantly flexion, a grasping action of the hand. The capsules are united at the front, each bound to its neighbour by short, strong, square ligaments that hold the knuckles together. The interphalangeal articulations are uniaxial hinge joints, arranged similarly to the metacarpophalangeal joints. Fingers can be flexed or extended with no other permitted movement and the joints are reinforced by collateral and palmar ligaments. The thinnest part of the capsule of both metacarpophalangeal and interphalangeal joints is at the dorsal surface. Here the extensor tendons flatten out and blend with the capsule for added stability.

The 1st metacarpal and thumb are unlike the other four in several ways. The metacarpal of the thumb is highly mobile because of the saddle-shaped joint surface in its articulation with the trapezium. It faces medially at 90° to the others, and is not bound by deep transverse metacarpal ligaments but has its own synovial membrane. The thumb has only two phalanges and its main purpose is opposition to the other digits. This movement occurs at the saddle-shaped joint between the 1st metacarpal and trapezium. The thumb is the most likely digit to get into trouble because of its greater flexibility (Komatsu and Lubahn 2018; Ladd *et al.* 2013).

THERAPEUTIC ENGAGEMENT

A.T. Still's wrist technique

Assessment

Examine the hand and wrist for tenderness, redness, swelling or deformity.

Check mobility with both active and passive movements.

Perform all the usual diagnostic tests, including those relating to the carpal tunnel and Guyon's canal where the ulnar nerve can suffer entrapment between the pisiform and the hook of the hamate.

Any treatment of the wrist and hand begins with an assessment of the radioulnar interosseous membrane which has a profound effect on wrist action.

Especially check ulnar and radial deviation. An increased movement in the direction of radial deviation may indicate that the patient's habitual use may not be in the optimal position.

This manoeuvre, credited to Still himself, takes into account the whole wrist in all its directions of movement in one procedure: a very useful 'shotgun' approach if pressed for time when the patient asks you to 'just have a quick look' at their wrist.

1. HANDHOLD

Sitting across the treatment table from the patient, wrap your palms around the dorsal and ventral surfaces of the patient's wrist, interlacing your fingers. Your hands firmly envelop the whole carpus to form a supportive and palpatory contact. *Ask the patient to extend the fingers and to keep them straight throughout.* This engages all of the ligaments in the wrist.

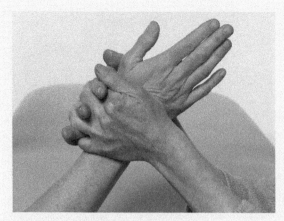

Figure 10.3 Hold for Still's wrist technique.

2. PATIENT COOPERATION

Active flexion: *Ask the patient to flex the wrist keeping the fingers straight.* As the patient gradually flexes the wrist joint, focus attention first on the proximal row of carpals where the flexion movement begins. As movement continues a little further, the midcarpal joint takes up the larger share of the movement. *If at any point any resistance is felt, retain a hold on that specific point until resistance melts.* Once the flexion movement feels free in all involved articulations, ask the patient to return to the neutral starting position. Throughout the procedure maintain a moulded supportive hold around the wrist.

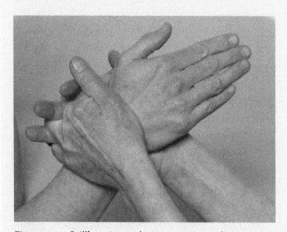

Figure 10.4 Still's wrist technique, active palmar flexion.

Active extension: *Maintain your hold and next ask the patient to repeat the procedure in extension, i.e., bending the wrist backwards.* The largest part of extension happens at the radiocarpal joint with only slight movement at the midcarpal joint. Again, follow the movement with subtle adjustments of the palms around the carpals until any resistance releases and the patient can return to neutral.

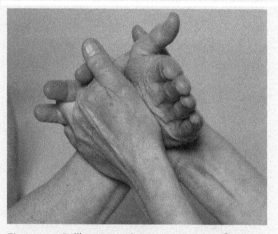

Figure 10.5 Still's wrist technique, active dorsiflexion.

Radial and ulnar deviation: Maintain the same hold, focussed now on the radiocarpal joint. *Ask the patient to move the wrist into radial and ulnar deviation or more simply in the direction of the thumb and then the direction of the little finger, returning to the neutral position in between the two directions.* At this point the proximal row of carpals should be felt to glide smoothly medially and laterally on the distal head of the radius and disc of the ulna. If resistance is felt at any point, maintain a firm but gentle hold until you feel a smooth glide.

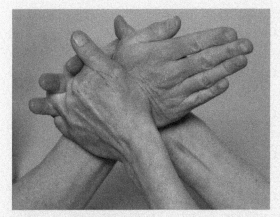

Figure 10.6 Still's wrist technique, active ulnar deviation.

Circumduction: *To integrate all the movements, ask the patient to circumduct, i.e., make a circle with the hand, while you follow and support all the little movements with the moulded palmar contact.*

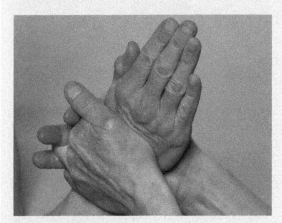

Figure 10.7 Still's wrist technique, active circumduction.

3. FINAL ACTION

For the final 'flourish' which spreads all the carpals in one action, *ask the patient to form a tight fist as you maintain a firm hold on the wrist.* Then ask the patient to spring open the hand, spreading the palm and fingers wide. Meanwhile you *maintain a firm hold until the end*, giving slight resistance to the lifting and spreading action of the 'exploding' fist.

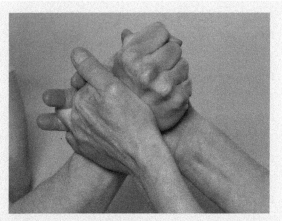

Figure 10.8 Patient makes a fist.

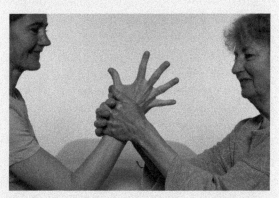

Figure 10.9 Active spread of the palm and fingers.

In this manoeuvre you are supporting the carpals in all their directions of movement, holding slightly at any point of resistance with a firm but gentle moulding action. This stimulates the ligaments to work and reorganise, with subsequent improvement in mobility.

Carpal lift using leverage with suspension

This is another very simple approach to the wrist. Sit across the treatment table from the patient. *Suspend the patient's wrist, allowing the carpal bones to reorganise, helped by the slight amount of traction introduced by the weight of the suspended arm.* This is most effective if the patient allows the forearm and elbow to hang off the edge of their side of the table.

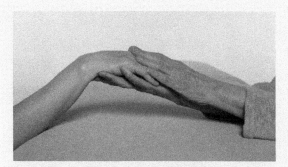

Figure 10.10 Carpal lift using leverage with suspension.

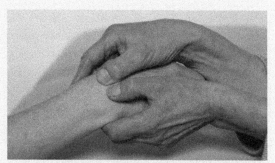

Figure 10.11 Handhold for BLT of individual carpal bones.

If you find that one of the carpal bones needs particular attention, a one-handed, one-finger contact under the pronated wrist can be used to focus on individual carpals within their interlocking web of ligaments. Two hands may also be used if preferred. This is assisted by the weight of the patient's suspended arm, acting on the fulcrum you are supplying with your finger. This can be especially useful for a dropped lunate which can sometimes dislocate anteriorly and may need to be lifted back into its position within the carpal arch.

An additional distraction may be engaged by asking the patient to lean away slightly.

Simple BLT of individual carpal bones

Where a more general approach has not re-established normal mobility, it may be necessary to work on the articulation between two individual carpal bones. Contact is made with a thumb and index finger on each of the two bones to be worked on. The normal steps for achieving BLT are taken, i.e., *first testing movement in each direction, looking for the ease until a point of approximate BLT is reached. At this stage it may be necessary to introduce slight distraction or compression, thus activating the ligaments to refine their position of balanced tension. Maintain your firm but gentle hold as you wait at the point of balance and then observe the ligaments reorganising the joint under your hands. Retest for improved articular balance and mobility.*

Carpal tunnel and retinacular spread

The retinacular spread is a useful procedure to re-establish the arch of the hand. The integrity of the transverse arch of the hand is lost if the lunate is forced anteriorly to the limit of its physiological range of motion. Carpal tunnel compression of vessels, nerves and tendons may result.

1. CONTACT
Use a crossed thumb contact across the attachments of the retinaculum with the fingers wrapped around the sides and back of the pronated wrist.

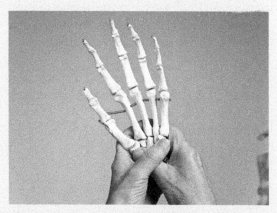

Figure 10.12 Handhold for carpal tunnel retinacular spread on skeleton.

2. PATIENT POSTURAL COOPERATION
Dorsiflexion: *Ask the patient to first dorsiflex the wrist as your crossed thumbs are spread between the retinacular attachments.*

Palmar flexion: *Then ask the patient to palmar flex the wrist, keeping the fingers straight. As the patient bends the wrist over your spreading crossed thumbs, resist this movement slightly.* At the same time the action of the hands, wrapped all the way around the wrist, contains the lateral borders of the wrist to encourage a spreading and opening of the arch. This action should make space for the lunate to glide posteriorly, re-establishing a functional arch to open the space for tendons, nerves and vessels to pass through the carpal tunnel.

For greater effectiveness this may be repeated several times.

Palmar fascia spread

1. CONTACT

Take a contact on the palmar fascia, either with thumbs crossed or side by side, spreading laterally.

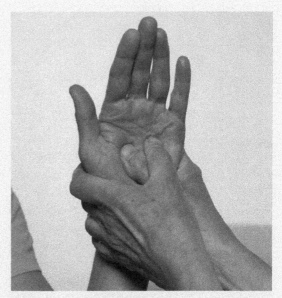

Figure 10.13 Crossed thumb handhold for palmar fascia (1).

2. PATIENT COOPERATION

The patient cooperates by alternately flexing and extending the pronated hand over this contact to assist the slow spread of the palmar fascia.

As the patient extends and spreads the fingers, follow with your thumbs across the palmar fascia, spreading outwards towards the sides of the hand. As the patient relaxes the hand, maintain the spread which was gained with the hand in full extension. As the patient repeats the action, attempt to increase the spread of the thumbs a little further each time.

This may be repeated several times until a release is felt in the palmar fascia.

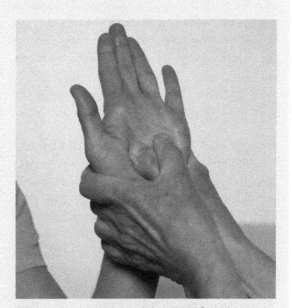

Figure 10.14 Crossed thumb handhold for palmar fascia (2).

Lift of proximal metacarpal head using leverage with suspension

1. HANDHOLD

Take a hold with the pad of your middle finger under the proximal end of the palmar surface of an individual metacarpal. Your thumb is over the dorsal surface of the distal head.

2. ACTION

Assisted by the weight of the patient's arm, *use leverage with suspension, gently lifting with the middle finger from underneath the proximal end. Apply slight downward pressure with the thumb from above the distal head.* The distraction and the spread that this creates helps to release each bone in relationship to its surroundings, both with its corresponding carpal and its neighbouring metacarpals.

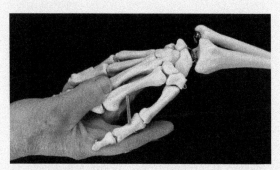

Figure 10.15 Lift of proximal metacarpal head, using leverage with suspension on skeleton.

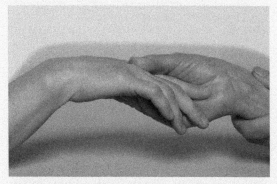

Figure 10.16 Lift of proximal metacarpal head, using leverage with suspension on live model.

The weight of the patient's arm is needed in the distraction, so remind the patient to relax the arm. In disengaging the proximal metacarpal head, the patient's wrist needs to be in a direct line with the shaft, neither too flexed nor extended, so that the angle of leverage directs the forces precisely to the articulation with the carpal bone. *To bring about a more precise focus, you may take hold of the corresponding carpal with the thumb and finger of the other hand.*

Interphalangeal joints

Specific interphalangeal joints may need to be addressed individually.

1. CONTACT

Take contact with thumb and index or middle finger on either side of the joint close to the articular surfaces. Apply the usual stages to find BLT, as described for the carpal bones above and for an interphalangeal joint in the 'What is BLT?' part of Chapter 1.

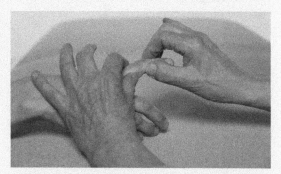

Figure 10.17 Handhold for BLT of interphalangeal joint.

The thumb, in particular, often requires individual attention as it can be overused, or used in a position of vulnerability in certain activities. It is much more mobile than the other fingers with its saddle joint and separate synovial membrane, and is used independently of the other fingers. In extension, for example, any axial force is received straight into the joint rather than being supported and absorbed as it is when lined up with the wrist and forearm.

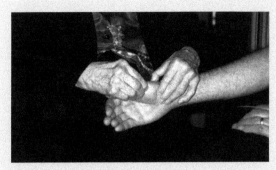

Figure 10.18 Dr Anne Wales treating the 1st carpometacarpal 'saddle' joint.

Finger suspension

Where appropriate, *the fingers can simply be suspended. The weight of the patient's hand and forearm engages any ligamentous-articular strains*

by just enough distraction to enliven ligamentous action. For example, torsional or axially compressive patterns in a finger or MCP joint will often exaggerate to the point of balanced tension and release.

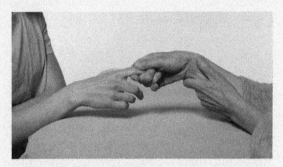

Figure 10.19 Finger suspension.

VIDEOS FOR CHAPTER 10

Scan the QR code or visit https://www.youtube.com/playlist?list=PL3j_YuMBqigHNBWNfc-laQT2B-hz7WcYh to find a playlist of the videos that accompany this chapter.

REFERENCES

Akhbari, B., Morton, A.M., Shah, K.N., *et al.* (2020) Proximal-distal shift of the centre of rotation in a total wrist arthroplasty is more than twice of the healthy wrist. *J Orthop Res 38,* 1575–1586.

Crow, W.T. (2006) The effects of manipulation on ligaments and fascia from a fluids model perspective. *AAO Journal,* 13–18.

Cunningham, C., Scheuer, L., Black, S. (2017) The upper limb. In: *Developmental Juvenile Osteology,* 2nd edition. Cambridge, MA: Academic Press; pp. 283–350.

Eschweiler, J., Li, J., Quak, V., *et al.* (2022) Anatomy, biomechanics and loads of the wrist joint. *Life 12,* 188.

Golden, W.J. (1999) A review of the principles of William G Sutherland's general techniques. *AAO Journal,* 32–34.

Hagert, E. (2010) Proprioception of the wrist joint: a review of current concepts and possible implications on the rehabilitation of the wrist. *J Hand Ther 23* (1), 2–17.

Kaufmann, R., Pfaeffle, J., Blankenhorn, B., *et al.* (2005) Kinematics of the mid carpal and radiocarpal joints in radioulnar deviation: an in vitro study. *The Journal of Hand Surgery 30* (5), 937–942.

Kollitz, K.M., Hammert, W.C., Vedder, N.B., Huang, J.I. (2014) Metacarpal fractures: treatment and complications. *Hand (NY) 9* (1), 16–23.

Komatsu, I. & Lubahn, J.D. (2018) Anatomy and biomechanics of the thumb carpometacarpal joint. *Operative Techniques in Orthopaedics 28* (1), 1–5.

Ladd, A.L., Weiss, A.C., Crisco, J.J., *et al.* (2013) The thumb carpometacarpal joint: anatomy, hormones and biomechanics. *Instr Course Lect 62,* 165–179.

Nypaver, C. & Liu, S. (2021) Perilunate injuries/lunate dislocations and radiocarpal dislocations. *Annals of Joint 6,* 36.

Sarrafian, S.K., Melamed, J.L., Goshgarian, G.M. (1977) Study of wrist motion in flexion and extension. *Clin Orthop Relat Res 126,* 153–159.

Sutherland, W.G. (1990) *Teachings in the Science of Osteopathy.* A.L. Wales (ed.). Fort Worth, TX: Sutherland Cranial Teaching Foundation, Inc./Rudra Press; pp. 191–217.

Wales, A.L. (1995, 1996, 1997) British tutorial group meeting. North Attleboro, MA, USA.

CHAPTER 11

The Hip

KOK WENG LIM

The hip both absorbs, and is affected by, strong forces from the lower extremity, pelvis and lumbar spine. If optimal function of the hip is lost, it in turn alters the distribution of forces around the pelvic bowl and beyond to the spine and feet. This is why osteopathic assessment of these reciprocal areas is important before beginning treatment of the hip.

Sutherland, for example, noted that twists in the ligamentous capsule of the hip joint, following bending and twisting movements, are not uncommon. He observed a causal association with iliopsoas contraction and suggested that this in turn can cause secondary rotation of the lumbar spine and sacroiliac (SI) joints. The patient then presents with low back pain (Sutherland 1990, TSO p. 200).

In the standing position, stability of the hip is assisted by the interaction of ground forces and gravity. The femoral head is pressed upward by ground forces, matching the weight of the body on the overhanging 'roof' of the acetabulum (Kapandji 1970). Harmonious apposition of the articular surfaces also depends on both the correct position of the femoral head and on atmospheric pressure.

FOUR LAYERS TO CONSIDER

Palpation, understanding and treatment of the hip are helped by acknowledging four layers (Hammond *et al.* 2012):

- the bony layer, including the femur, acetabulum and pelvis
- the soft tissue layer, including the joint capsule, ligaments, ligamentum teres and labrum
- the musculotendon structures of the hip and pelvis, responsible for dynamic stability and balance of the trunk, pelvis, hip and lower extremity
- the neuromuscular layer of the lumbosacral plexus, and the tissues and innervation of the trunk and lower extremity.

THE ANATOMY OF THE HIP

The acetabulum is formed by the ilium, pubis and ischium meeting at the triradiate cartilage. It is deepened by the circumferential labrum. In the upright posture, the acetabulum faces forward (anteverted) and more so in women (Maruyama *et al.* 2001). Femoral anteversion decreases from 30–40° at birth to 10.5° in the adult on average (Svenningsen *et al.* 1989). The normal neck-shaft angle of the femur is 125° (Kapandji 1970).

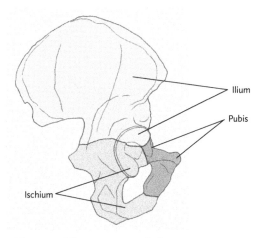

Figure 11.1 Three-part acetabulum.

SOFT TISSUES OF THE HIP: CAPSULE, LIGAMENTS AND LABRUM

The hip capsule

Three ligaments of the hip are actually thickenings of the joint capsule and are known as capsular ligaments. The capsule is thickest superiorly, but thinner posteriorly where it relates to the ischiofemoral ligament (Wagner *et al.* 2012). Anteriorly, longitudinal fibres relate to the iliofemoral ligament. Capsular laxity can lead to microinstability of the hip, resulting in joint degeneration (Han *et al.* 2018).

The hip ligaments

These are the iliofemoral, pubofemoral, ischiofemoral and teres ligaments. All hip ligaments are relaxed during flexion, and the spiral arrangement of the ligaments act in concert with the capsule and muscles to stabilise the hip in extension.

The *iliofemoral ligament* is the strongest and largest ligament in the body. It prevents excessive posterior tilt of the pelvis while upright, and it also resists anterior translation of the femoral head within the acetabulum. The importance of this ligament is illustrated by the fact that, in hip dislocation, if the iliofemoral ligament fails to heal, this leads to persistent anterior capsular weakness (D'Ambrosi *et al.* 2021). If it is damaged, e.g., in hip arthroscopy, this may lead to postoperative hip instability (Kho *et al.* 2020). As this ligament limits external rotation, advice to avoid external rotation should be given in these cases (Burkhart *et al.* 2020; Kain and Willier 2020).

The tendons of the gluteus minimus and the deep aponeurosis of the iliopsoas are continuous with the hip capsule and iliofemoral ligament. Collectively they ensure joint stability (Tsutsumi *et al.* 2020).

The *pubofemoral ligament* blends with the capsule and deep surface of the medial iliofemoral ligament. It prevents excessive extension and abduction and also external rotation, especially with the hip in extension.

The *ischiofemoral ligament* is a spiral-shaped ligament situated posteriorly, along the neck of the femur (Wagner *et al.* 2012). The ischiofemoral ligament is taut in extension. It also limits internal rotation and adduction.

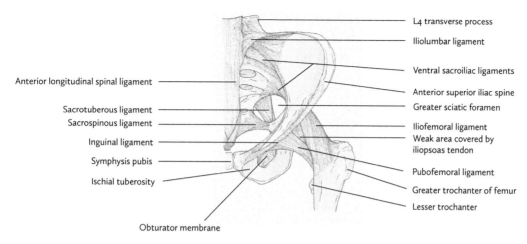

L4 transverse process

Iliolumbar ligament

Ventral sacroiliac ligaments

Anterior superior iliac spine

Greater sciatic foramen

Iliofemoral ligament

Weak area covered by iliopsoas tendon

Pubofemoral ligament

Greater trochanter of femur

Lesser trochanter

Anterior longitudinal spinal ligament

Sacrotuberous ligament

Sacrospinous ligament

Inguinal ligament

Symphysis pubis

Ischial tuberosity

Obturator membrane

Figure 11.2 Anterior ligaments of the left pelvis and hip.

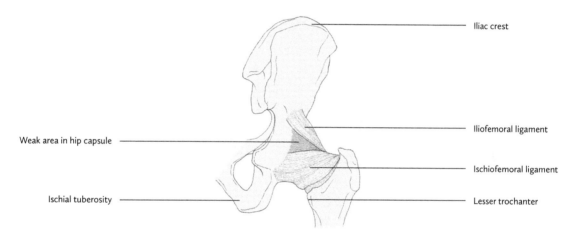

Iliac crest

Iliofemoral ligament

Ischiofemoral ligament

Lesser trochanter

Weak area in hip capsule

Ischial tuberosity

Figure 11.3 Posterior ligaments of the right hip.

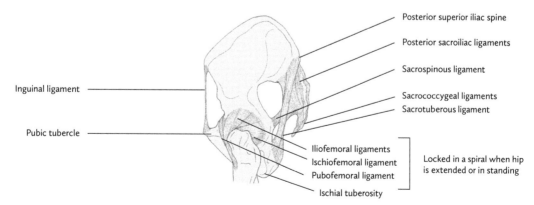

Posterior superior iliac spine

Posterior sacroiliac ligaments

Sacrospinous ligament

Sacrococcygeal ligaments

Sacrotuberous ligament

Inguinal ligament

Pubic tubercle

Iliofemoral ligaments

Ischiofemoral ligament

Pubofemoral ligament

Ischial tuberosity

Locked in a spiral when hip is extended or in standing

Figure 11.4 Lateral view of hip ligaments.

The *ligamentum teres* ('ligament of the head of the femur' or 'round' ligament of the hip) assists in maintaining the upright posture as it is tightest in this position. Clinically it is an important stabiliser in patients with hypermobility and dysplasia of the hip.

This intra-articular ligament within the pulvinar has a synovial covering and is attached to the transverse acetabular ligament, the periosteum of the ischium, the capsule and the fovea capitis of the femoral head.

Between the ligamentum teres and its synovial covering lies the acetabular branch of the obturator artery (medial circumflex femoral artery). Perumal *et al.* (2019) suggested a nutritive role of this artery to the head of the femur in the adult as well as in the developing femoral head in childhood. Mechanoreceptors have been noted in the ligament proper, and also in the walls of the larger blood vessels, implying that it plays a role in fine coordination of the hip joint (Lindner *et al.* 2013).

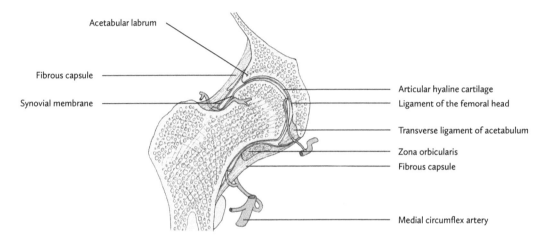

Figure 11.5 Longitudinal section through hip joint.

The ligamentum teres may be strained in a dislocation/subluxation and also from a sudden twist into external rotation. It may be torn from the fovea (most tears are from the femoral attachment site) or damaged in open surgical hip procedures. Acknowledgement of the integrity of this ligament and its relationship to the head of the femur is helpful during treatment.

Zona orbicularis (ZO)

The hip capsule has an annular ligament surrounding the distal part of the neck of the femur, the ZO. It wraps around the femoral neck in a spiral and functions as a locking ring around the neck of the femur, preventing the femoral head from slipping out of the acetabulum. It resists the forces of distraction at the hip joint when in

the neutral position (Ito *et al.* 2009). The capsule can therefore be viewed as an hourglass with the ZO sitting at the narrowest point of the femoral neck.

It has been proposed that a bellow-like movement of the ZO promotes the unilateral flow of synovial fluid in the joint during hip flexion and extension (Field and Rajakulendran 2011; Malagelada *et al.* 2014). Synovial tissue is located in the peripheral compartment of the hip joint, and synovial fluid that is produced there is directed towards the central compartment where the head of the femur articulates with the acetabulum.

In hip flexion, synovial fluid is forced from the distal to the proximal zone of the peripheral compartment. On extension, the fluid is directed over the articular surface of the joint. The fluid then pools adjacent to the labrum which functions to keep synovial fluid within the central compartment. This lubrication mechanism allows almost no wear in a normal hip despite a lifetime of mechanical motion. Disruption to the capsular ligament at the level of the intertrochanteric line can adversely affect synovial flow. Synovial fluid forms an adhesive hydraulic seal between the articular surfaces and therefore aids stability during everyday activities.

The labrum

The labrum surrounds 80 per cent of the acetabular rim and joins with the transverse acetabular ligament inferiorly to form a complete ring. Nerves and blood vessels are able to travel through the labrum. The key functions of the labrum (Bsat *et al.* 2016) are as follows:

1. It provides a seal around the femoral head to maintain the pressure of intra-articular fluid, which distributes and supports compressive load across the joint surfaces. This reduces wear by keeping the articular surfaces apart. Loss of the labral seal can lead to destabilisation of the hip.
2. It fits tightly around the femoral head, acting as a vacuum seal to resist the forces of distraction. This suction effect maintains hip stability. The seal restricts the flow of synovial fluid into and out of the joint space. It also provides a resistance to distraction of the femoral head and has a secondary role in resisting the forces of external rotation and translation.
3. It deepens the acetabulum by 21 per cent and increases the accommodation of the femoral head. It increases the articular contact area of the hip joint which reduces contact pressure on the cartilage. If the labrum becomes torn, this reduces the contact area and increases contact pressure, leading to degenerative changes in the cartilage.

It contains free nerve endings and nerve end organs which can potentially mediate pain as well as proprioception of the hip joint (Alzaharani *et al.* 2014). Abundant myofibroblasts scattered through the labrum may play a role in connective tissue repair.

The labrum may be crushed between the acetabular rim and the femoral neck. Labral tears are mostly traumatic in origin (e.g., repetitive trauma in dancers and athletes) and are particularly prevalent in ageing hips (McCarthy *et al.* 2001). Labral tears most commonly occur anterosuperiorly which is a largely avascular area.

Labral tears present as groin pain and clicking, locking and a sensation of giving way. Diminishing mobility of the hip may be apparent long before pain appears (Wyss *et al.* 2007). There may be an associated tear of the ligamentum teres.

In femoral acetabular impingement (FAI), the femoral head pinches against the acetabulum damaging the labrum. This can be due to an abnormality in the femoral head or bony spurs around the acetabular rim. Movements that aggravate the pain of FAI include squatting, twisting or turning. Osteopathic management may be helpful in small labral tears and in FAI, as a non-surgical approach is often first suggested.

SOFT TISSUES: THE MUSCLES OF THE HIP

The iliopsoas, iliocapsularis and rectus femoris muscles tension the hip capsule. They prevent anterior translation of the femoral head and aid stability in the standing position (Aguilera-Bohorquez *et al.* 2017; Lawrensen *et al.* 2019).

Iliocapsularis in particular has an origin on the

hip capsule as well as the anterior inferior iliac spine (AIIS) and inserts into the lesser trochanter with the iliopsoas (Elvan *et al.* 2019). The contraction of this muscle and consequent tightening of the capsule anteriorly prevents anterior translation of the head of the femur. In deep flexion of the hip, the iliocapsularis assists in retraction of the anterior capsule to prevent impingement.

Loss of tone, weakness or atrophy of the iliocapsularis may lead to pinching of the capsule between the joint surfaces. Osteophytic growth on the AIIS causes 'subspine impingement', as the AIIS and femoral neck makes abnormal contact on deep hip flexion (Sato *et al.* 2016).

Hypertrophy or spasticity of the iliocapsularis in patients with hip dysplasia may lead to iliopsoas impingement where it crosses the acetabular rim. This may also cause a traction injury of the anterior capsule. As the iliopsoas relates to the anterior capsule in the 3 o'clock position, this can sometimes lead to an atypical anterior labral tear (Andronic *et al.* 2019; Domb *et al.* 2011).

All the short external rotators of the hip, including the gemelli and obturators, have short fibre lengths which suggest that they play a joint stabilising role similar to ligaments, rather than a joint rotating role (Parvaresh *et al.* 2019; Retchford *et al.* 2013).

In palpation it is helpful to acknowledge that the rectus femoris, iliocapsularis, gluteus minimus muscles and external rotator tendons all attach to the capsule. The piriformis, however, has no capsular attachment (Cooper *et al.* 2015).

THE NEUROMUSCULAR LAYER

The neuromuscular (neurokinetic) layer of the hip is made up of the thoracolumbar and sacral plexi and also the lumbar, pelvic and lower extremity tissues and their innervation. The hip capsule is supplied by branches of the lumbosacral plexus, especially from the obturator and femoral nerves (L2, L3, L4) and also the nerve to quadratus femoris (L4, L5, S1) supplying the posterior capsule (Laumoneire *et al.* 2021; Tomlinson *et al.* 2021). All these spinal segments should be examined for restriction or facilitation.

The obturator nerve supplies both the hip and knee joint, providing a mechanism for referred pain. Crossing the legs is difficult with obturator nerve weakness, while walking is unaffected. Pelvic inflammation involving the obturator nerve can lead to pain in the groin and thigh with sensory loss on the inner aspect of the thigh. Clinically it is helpful to note that the sciatic nerve supplies the posterosuperior hip capsule.

DIAGNOSIS OF THE HIP JOINT

Diagnosis of the direction of ease of the hip can be made with the patient standing. With the weight on one foot, and without rotating the pelvis, the patient rotates the opposite non-weight-bearing leg into internal rotation with the toes pointing medially and then external rotation with toes pointing laterally. Look for the direction of greater movement and compare the two hips.

Resiliency at the end of the range can be palpated, and this may be useful for detecting bony abnormalities. This can also be done with the patient seated, with one leg resting over the other knee. The operator sits in front of the patient, holds the patient's knee and ankle and tests for internal and external rotation of the femur (Lippincott 1949). The direction of ease can be determined this way. External and internal rotation of the hip can also be tested with the patient seated.

Sutherland suggested checking to see if the head of the femur is twisted in the acetabulum because leverage from a twisted femur will transmit to the SI joint, psoas and iliac muscles. Then check to see if the lumbar spinal segments are also rotated or sidebent as a consequence (Sutherland 1990, TSO p. 203).

THERAPEUTIC ENGAGEMENT

Sitting BLT of the hip joint (1)

The following two manoeuvres use the principle of exaggeration and postural cooperation by the patient rotating the trunk around the midline, while the femur is held steady. This uses the principle of turning a nut on a stabilised bolt; turning the acetabulum (nut) is achieved by the patient turning or rotating the trunk, while the operator holds the head of the femur steady (bolt).

1. POSITIONING
Sit facing the patient who sits on the treatment table with both legs hanging over the edge. Double check the direction of ease on the strained side by rotating the femur into internal and external rotation.

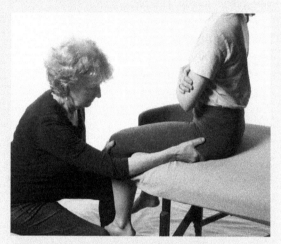

Figure 11.6 Sitting hip hold on live model.

2. HANDHOLD
Place the fingers of one hand curled just behind the greater trochanter, femoral neck and hip capsule. Place the other hand on the front of the patient's knee so that, without muscular effort, you will be able to lean in, proprioceptively, towards the hip.

3. ENGAGEMENT
Place the femur in the position of balance for the hip, i.e., towards either external or internal rotation. Then leaning into the hip with your body weight through the distal end of the femur to activate the hip ligaments, explore for the point of maximal involuntary ligamentous engagement. The capsule, ligaments and muscles of the hip will activate and begin to explore for the point of balance under your hands, as they exaggerate their internal or external rotation.

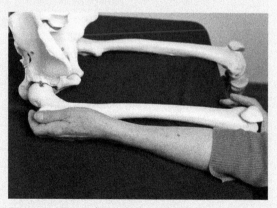

Figure 11.7 Sitting hip hold on skeleton.

4. POSTURAL COOPERATION
To augment the field of balance, postural cooperation from the patient is used. *Ask the patient to rotate the trunk around the midline, turning away from an externally rotated hip or towards the strained side for an internally rotated one.* The operator should maintain the point of balance

and the hold on the femur (bolt) steady during postural cooperation. Sense the ligamentum teres as a fulcrum for the joint.

5. RESOLUTION

At the point of ligamentous release, use respiratory cooperation by asking the patient to breathe in, sit tall and face forward while you continue to hold the femur steady. The patient's breathing, sitting tall and then de-rotating the trunk back to centre brings the acetabulum into correct apposition to the stabilised femur. You may feel a change in the quality of the soft tissues around the hip joint and a sense of alignment between the shaft/neck/head of the femur, ligamentum teres and the acetabulum.

6. RETEST

Re-check internal and external rotation of the femur.

Sitting BLT of the hip joint (2) using active rotation

This procedure uses postural cooperation and a slightly different hold, but with the same principles of treatment. It may be more suitable for hips that do not tolerate approximation or compression, e.g., painful hips with degenerative changes. This can be used either as a single manoeuvre, or after completing the technique above for further integration.

1. PREPARATION

Test the hip to confirm whether it is strained towards external or internal rotation by medially and laterally rotating the femur of the seated patient. This will enable you to determine which direction the patient will need to turn the body to exaggerate the lesion. *You may then find an approximate point of balance by taking the femur into the direction of ease as above, and holding this steady throughout the procedure.*

2. HAND CONTACT: STABILISING THE FEMUR

Using an antero-posterior (A/P) contact, firmly hold the whole upper surface of the femur with your forearm, with your fingers directed towards the groin.

Alternatively, create a strong stabilising fulcrum underneath the midfemoral shaft with the palm of one hand, while the other holds the distal end at the knee.

3. POSTURAL COOPERATION

As you hold the femur (bolt) steady, ask the patient to rotate the trunk in a circle around the hip joint, initially moving the acetabulum (nut) towards the direction of ease.

If the hip is strained towards external rotation, *ask the patient to lean forwards slightly, and then sidebend and rotate the trunk away from the lesioned side, then backwards, and continue to complete a full circle.* The patient should face forward throughout.

If it is strained towards internal rotation, the patient begins by rotating towards the strained side.

The strain pattern is most challenged as the patient's trunk rotation passes through the opposite side of the circle. This may need to be repeated a few times for a release to be felt.

The turning of the acetabulum on the head of the femur was described by Dr Sutherland (1990) as 'the patient furnishing the maximum effort and the physician the minimum, in fixating the bone and tendon while the physician is guiding with trained tactile skill'. In guiding the technique, the operator may indeed ask the patient to vary the speed and/or the amplitude of the turning of the acetabulum and using respiratory cooperation.

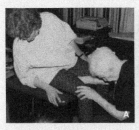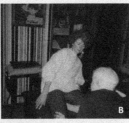

Figure 11.8A & B Dr Anne Wales treating the hip with active rotation of the patient's trunk on stabilised femur.

Occasionally Dr Wales asked the patient to rotate the opposite way, she didn't always ask the patient to turn in the direction of exaggerating the lesion: 'as long as you hold the femur (bolt), you don't have to worry about the direction of rotation, as the full circle of the nut should correct the strain'.

Supine BLT hip release through disengagement

This is performed bilaterally and is particularly useful in children with poor posture, due to hypertonicity or hypotonicity. This is typically seen in children with developmental problems, including learning difficulties.

1. POSITION
Sit to the side of the supine patient facing diagonally towards the feet.

2. CONTACT
Place one hand under the patient's sacrum. With the other hand, contact the lateral aspect of the hip joint with the greater trochanter in the palm of your hand and your fingers around the back of the femoral neck.

3. ENGAGEMENT
While stabilising the sacrum, gently disengage the hip laterally to the point of BLT. This is often a very minimal movement. Place your attention also on the short muscles of the hip as well as on the iliopsoas and glutei. The aim here is to release the soft tissues of the hip as well as providing a sense of increased joint space within.

4. RESOLUTION
The endpoint is felt as a sense of three-dimensional spaciousness and inherent tissue motion.

Alternative supine hip BLT

1. HANDHOLD
Sit beside the supine patient with the palm of one hand around the greater trochanter and your fingers around the back of the femoral neck to stabilise it.

2. TESTING FOR BALANCED TENSION
With the other hand on the anterior superior iliac spine (ASIS), test for the position of ease of the acetabulum by moving the innominate to the position where you feel the ligaments ease and balance in relation to the femur.

3. HOLDING AND RESOLUTION
Then simply hold that position of balanced tension with both hands, observing the tissue response to breathing until you feel the hip joint reorganising and releasing.

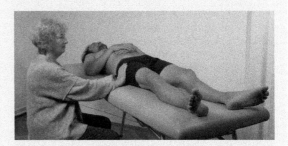

Figure 11.9 Supine hip BLT.

Further approaches relevant to the hip

The iliopsoas and obturator internus muscles exert strong influence on hip position and function. Procedures for releasing these are described in Chapter 16.

An approach to intraosseous strains of the acetabulum and hip joint is described in Chapter 17. This is especially applicable for hip problems in infants and children and also for resolving strains absorbed through traumatic impact.

VIDEOS FOR CHAPTER 11

Scan the QR code or visit https://www.youtube.com/playlist?list=PL3j_YuMBqigEyg26ehPsXqbxoYwq5ELJ9 to find a playlist of the video that accompany this chapter.

REFERENCES

Aguilera-Bohorquez, B., Gil, E., Fonseca, J., *et al.* (2017) Teno-suspension of the reflected head of the rectus femoris in hip arthroscopy: description of a portal and surgical maneuver. *Arthroscopy Tech 6* (4), e1015–e1019.

Alzaharani, A., Bali, K., Railton, P., *et al.* (2014) The innervation of the human acetabular labrum and hip joint: an anatomic study. *BMC Musculoskeletal Disord 15,* 41.

Andronic, O., Nakano, N., Daivajna, S. (2019) Non-arthroplasty iliospsoas impingement in athletes: a narrative literature review. *HIP International 29* (5), 460–467.

Bsat, S., Frei, H., Beaule, P.E. (2016) The acetabular labrum: a review of its function. *The Bone and Joint Journal 98b* (6), 730–735. https://doi.org/10.1302/0301-620X.98B6.37099.

Burkhart, T.A., Baha, P., Blokker, A., *et al.* (2020) Hip capsular strain varies between ligaments dependent on both hip position and applied rotational force. *Knee Surg Sports Traumatol Arthrosc 28* (10), 3393–3399.

Cooper, J., Walters, B., Rodriguez, J.A. (2015) Anatomy of the hip capsule and pericapsular structures: a cadaveric study. *Clinical Anatomy 25* (8), 665–671.

D'Ambrosi, R., Ursino, N., Messina, C., *et al.* (2021) The role of the iliofemoral ligament as a stabiliser of the hip joint. *EFORT Open Reviews 6* (7), 545–555.

Domb, B., Shindle, M., McArthur, B., *et al.* (2011) Iliopsoas impingement: a newly identified case of labral pathology in the hip. *HSS J 7* (2), 145–150.

Elvan, O., Aktekin, M., Sengezer, E., *et al.* (2019) Iliocapsularis in human fetuses. *Surg and Radiol Anat 41* (12), 1497–1503.

Field, R.E. & Rajakulendran, K. (2011) The labro-acetabular complex. *J Bone Joint Surg Am 93* (2), 22–27.

Hammond, S., Magennis, E., Voos, J.E., *et al.* (2012) Compensatory disorders around the hip. In: J.W.T. Byrd (ed.) *Operative Hip Arthroscopy,* 3rd edition. New York, NY: Springer.

Han, S., Alexander, J.W., Thomas, V.S., *et al.* (2018) Does capsular laxity lead to microinstability of the native hip? *Am J of Sports Medicine 46* (6), 1315–1323.

Ito, H., Song, Y., Lindsey, D.P., *et al.* (2009) The proximal hip joint capsule and the zone orbicularis contribute to hip joint stability in distraction. *J Orthop Res 27* (8), 989–995.

Kain, M.S. & Willier, D. (2020) Hemiarthroplasty through a direct anterior approach for femoral neck fractures. *J of Orthopaed Trauma Suppl 2* (34), S25–S26.

Kapandji, A.I. (1970) *The Physiology of Joints, Vol. 2,* 2nd edition. New York, NY: Churchill Livingstone; pp. 232–233.

Kho, J., Azzopardi, C., Davies, A.M., *et al.* (2020) MRI assessment of anatomy and pathology of the iliofemoral ligament. *Clin Radiol 75* (12), 960.e17–960.e22.

Laumonerie, P., Dalmas, Y., Tibbo, M.E., *et al.* (2021) Sensory innervation of the hip joint and referred pain: a systematic review of the literature. *Pain Medicine 22* (5), 1149–1157.

Lawrensen, P., Hodges, P., Crossley, K., *et al.* (2019) The effect of altered stride length on iliocapsularis and pericapsular muscles of the anterior hip: an electromyography investigation during asymptomatic gait. *Gait and Posture 71,* 26–31.

Lindner, D., Sharp, K.G., Trenga, A.P., *et al.* (2013) Arthroscopic ligamentum teres reconstruction. *Arthrosc Tech 2,* 21–25.

Lippincott, H.A. (1949) The Osteopathic Technique of Wm. G. Sutherland, D.O. In: W.G. Sutherland (1990) *Teachings in the Science of Osteopathy*. A.L. Wales (ed.). Fort Worth, TX: Sutherland Cranial Teaching Foundation, Inc./Rudra Press.

Malagelada, F., Tayar, R., Barke, S., Stafford, G.H., Field, R. (2014) Anatomy of the zona orbicularis of the hip: a magnetic resonance study. *Surgical and Radiologic Anatomy 37* (1), 11–18.

Maruyama, M., Feinberg, J.R., Capello, W.N., *et al.* (2001) The Frank Stinchfield Award: Morphologic features of the acetabulum and femur: anteversion angle and implant positioning. *Clin Orthop Relat Res 393*, 52–65.

McCarthy, J.C., Noble, P.C., Schuck, M.R., *et al.* (2001) The Otto E. Aufranc Award: The role of labral lesions to development of early degenerative hip disease. *Clin Orthop Relat Res 393*, 25–37.

Parvaresh, K.C., Chang, C., Patel, A., *et al.* (2019) Architecture of the short external rotator muscles of the hip. *Musculoskeletal Disorders 20*, 611. http://dx.doi.org/10.1186/s12891-019-2995-0

Perumal, V., Woodley, S.J., Nicholson, H.D. (2019) Neurovascular structures of the ligament of the head of the femur. *J of Anat 234* (6), 778–786.

Retchford, T., Crossley, K.M., Grimaldi, A. (2013) Can local muscles augment stability in the hip? A narrative literature review. *J of Musculoskeletal Neuronal Interactions 13* (1), 1–12.

Sato, T., Sato, N., Sato, K. (2016) Review of the iliocapsularis muscle and its clinical relevance. *Anat and Physiol: Current Research 6,* 5.

Sutherland, W.G. (1990) *Teachings in the Science of Osteopathy.* A.L. Wales (ed.). Fort Worth, TX: Sutherland Cranial Teaching Foundation, Inc./Rudra Press; pp. 200, 203.

Svenningsen, S., Apalset, K., Terjesen, T., *et al.* (1989) Regression of femoral anteversion. A prospective study of in-toeing children. *Acta Orthop Scand 60,* 170–173.

Tomlinson, J., Ondrushka, B., Prietzel, T., *et al.* (2021) A systematic review and meta-analysis of hip capsule innervation and its clinical implications. *Sci Reports 11* (1), 5299.

Tsutsumi, M., Nimura, A., Akita, K. (2020) New insights into the iliofemoral ligament based on the anatomical study of the hip joint capsule. *J of Anat 236* (5), 946–953.

Wagner, F.V., Negrao, J.R., Campos, J., *et al.* (2012) Capsular ligaments of the hip: anatomic, histologic, and positional study in cadaveric specimens with MR arthrography. *Radiology 263* (1), 189–198.

Wyss, T.F., Clark, J.M., Weishaupt, D., Notzli, H.P. (2007) Correlation between internal rotation and bony anatomy of the hip. *Clin Orthop Relat Res 460,* 152–158.

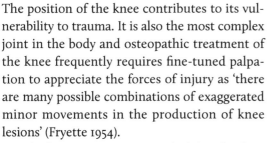

CHAPTER 12

The Knee

KOK WENG LIM

The position of the knee contributes to its vulnerability to trauma. It is also the most complex joint in the body and osteopathic treatment of the knee frequently requires fine-tuned palpation to appreciate the forces of injury as 'there are many possible combinations of exaggerated minor movements in the production of knee lesions' (Fryette 1954).

The knee joint is comprised of the tibiofemoral and patellofemoral joints. While the quadriceps, biceps femoris and pes anserine muscle group provide dynamic alignment, the capsule, ligaments and patella tendon are crucial to providing static stability. It is the mechanoreceptors present in the ligaments that provide dynamic stability.

Ligamentous injury is more common than any other type of knee injury (Bollen 2000). This can have serious implications, in that weight-bearing function and recovery of the knee, post-injury, are dependent on the sensory proprioceptive feedback loop from the ligaments to the muscles.

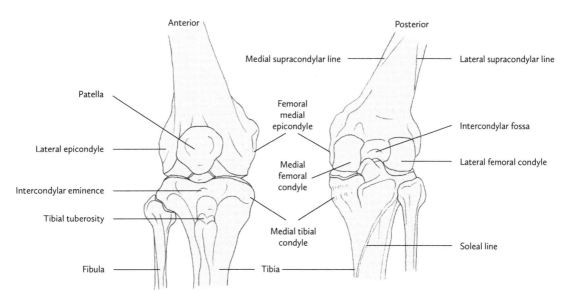

Figure 12.1 Knee bones, anterior and posterior view.

THE CAPSULE OF THE KNEE

The capsule attaches the menisci to the femur and the tibia, by what are known as coronary ligaments. The posterior capsule is related to the popliteal artery and vein, and openings in the posterior capsule allow blood vessels and veins to access the knee joint. From an osteopathic viewpoint, while the anterior and lateral aspects of the knee are key areas in assessing articular dysfunction, accessing the posterior aspect of the knee is important in promoting blood supply, and venous and lymphatic drainage.

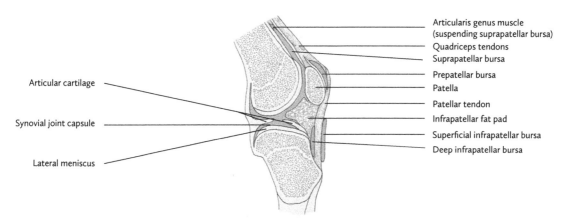

Figure 12.2 Parasagittal section through the right knee joint showing continuity of suprapatellar bursa with synovial capsule.

THE POSTEROLATERAL STRUCTURES OF THE KNEE

Lateral collateral ligament

The lateral (or fibular) collateral ligament is a readily palpable rounded ligament on the lateral epicondyle of the femur, attaching to the head of the fibula with the long head of the biceps femoris, to form the conjoint tendon. It resists varus stress and external rotation at the knee joint (Branch and Anz 2015; Wroble *et al.* 1993).

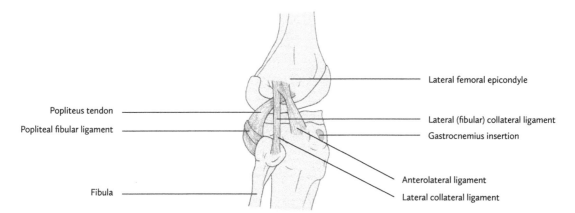

Figure 12.3 Lateral ligaments of the right knee, schematic view.

Popliteus muscle and tendon, popliteal fibular ligament, and posterior cruciate ligament (PCL)

Clinically, it is very important to assess the popliteus muscle as this provides dynamic stability at the knee in three ways (Barker *et al.* 2009). First, the lateral meniscus is stabilised by the popliteus tendon. Lateral knee pain can be the result of weakness of the popliteus muscles or tears to the meniscal attachment to the popliteus, resulting in instability of the lateral meniscus.

Second, the popliteus is attached to and stabilises the posterior capsule, resisting excessive tibial external rotation (LaPrade *et al.* 2007). Third, the popliteus gives rise to the popliteofibular ligament which is attached to the head of the fibula. This ligament is the main stabiliser of the knee in external rotation and flexion.

The PCL is reinforced by four 'posterolateral structures':

- popliteus tendon
- popliteofibular ligament
- posterior knee capsule
- lateral collateral ligament.

Together these function as a unit to restrict excessive external rotation of the knee, posterior translation and varus angulation (Bolog and Hodler 2007). This combined reinforcement is the reason why PCL injury does not cause significant pain and knee instability.

The PCL limits posterior tibial translation throughout the range of knee flexion. PCL injury is suspected if, on passive testing, there is increased posterior translation at 30–45° of flexion.

Fabellofibular ligament

The fabella is a sesamoid bone and often articulates with the lateral femoral condyle. Irritation at this articulation leads to fabella impingement syndrome (Weng *et al.* 2021). The fabella can be palpated within the lateral head of the gastrocnemius. Posterolateral knee pain may be caused by:

- cartilage softening of the fabella articular surface
- fabella syndrome due to repetitive strain in athletes and bikers which is worse on full extension of the knee
- fracture of the fabella
- common fibular nerve irritation and popliteal artery compression impingement after total knee replacement (Provencher *et al.* 2017).

ANTEROLATERAL LIGAMENT AND ILIOTIBIAL BAND

The anterolateral ligament is on the lateral aspect of the knee anterior to the fibular collateral ligament. It acts in concert with the anterior cruciate ligament (ACL) to reinforce knee stability in rotation (Ahn *et al.* 2019).

The iliotibial band (ITB) and the vastus lateralis together form the lateral retinaculum attaching to the lateral aspect of the patella. The lateral retinaculum aids in resisting medial glide of the patella, guiding the lateral tracking and tilt of the patella on the femur.

The iliotibial band and the anterolateral ligament together reinforce the function of the anterior cruciate ligament in preventing excessive internal tibial rotation and anterior tibial translation (Grassi *et al.* 2021; Lovse and Getgood). Avulsion of its insertion on the lateral tibia results in a Segond fracture (Kushare *et al.* 2021; Wei *et al.* 2021).

Direct contact on the lateral femoral epicondyle, while moving the tibia into flexion or extension, can reproduce the pain felt in running or cycling in ITB syndrome. It is due to bursitis over the lateral femoral epicondyle, a cause of pain in runner's knee.

MEDIAL KNEE LIGAMENTOUS ANATOMY

The ligaments of the medial side of the knee are not discrete. They are fascial condensations within tissue planes or layers (Warren and Marshall 1979). The most superficial layer is the deep investing fascia of the thigh, enclosing the sartorius within. The deepest layer includes the deep medial collateral ligament.

Medial collateral ligament

The deep medial collateral ligament (MCL) is part of the capsule of the joint and is attached to the medial meniscus (LaPrade 2007). The medial meniscus is relatively more fixed, due to its intimate connection with the medial collateral ligament and joint capsule and therefore is more prone to injury than the lateral meniscus.

Valgus stress on a stationary knee is the most common cause of injury to the medial collateral ligament. If severe, Stieda avulsion fractures of the medial femoral condyle can occur (Stevens *et al.* 2021). A valgus force to the knee passively flexed at 30° will detect MCL injury. A 5–8 mm medial joint opening on performing this test is indicative of significant MCL damage (Chen *et al.* 2007).

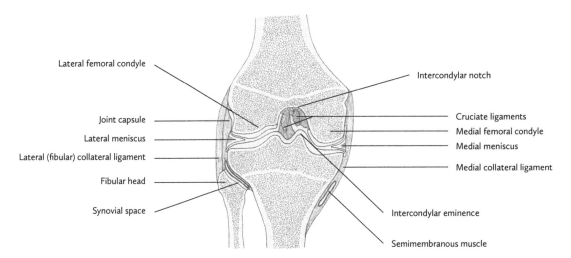

Figure 12.4 Coronal section through knee joint, anterior view.

Medial patellofemoral ligament

The medial patellofemoral ligament (MPFL) acts to prevent lateral patellar subluxation. The blending of MPFL with vastus medialis makes up the 'medial retinaculum' of the knee (Felli *et al.* 2021). The patella tends towards a lateral position during full extension of the knee. The medial retinaculum counterbalances this by drawing the patella more medially toward the trochlea in full extension, enabling the patella to enter the trochlea at the start of knee flexion (Bicos *et al.* 2007).

Commonly in young adults the MPFL can be ruptured following lateral patellar dislocation. The highest incidence of strain occurs at about 25–30° of knee flexion. The patella enters the trochlear notch from 15 to 25° of knee flexion, and the increasing bony congruence as it moves further into flexion is protective (McCulloch *et al.* 2014).

PATELLA TENDON

The patella has been described as a balance beam, mediating tensions between the quadriceps and patella tendons in varying degrees of knee flexion. In the first 20° of knee flexion, stability is dependent on the medial and lateral soft tissue structures and the joint capsule, as there is no bony support for the patella. During this initial range of flexion, the tibia derotates and the patella enters the trochlear notch. Between 0 and 30° of extension, the patella has a tendency towards a lateral glide of 2 mm.

Patellofemoral stability is provided medially by the medial patellofemoral ligament merging with the vastus medialis. Laterally, stability is provided by the tone of the tensor fascia lata and gluteus maximus via the iliotibial band.

Anatomical and structural factors that should be assessed in patella dysfunction include:

- ligamentous laxity
- hypotonia
- patella alta (high sitting patella)
- increased quadriceps angle, e.g., from genu valgum which increases the obliquity of the femur and the obliquity of the pull of the quadriceps
- the trochlear groove of the femur for the patella being concave; in trochlear dysplasia it is flat or convex leading to recurrent dislocations
- external tibial torsion around a longitudinal axis beyond the normal range of 24–30°, seen in children, which may be due to intrauterine moulding or genetic factors (Snow 2021). It usually resolves with age. It results in an inwardly pointing knee with a valgus vector on the patella.

- excessive distance between the tibial tubercle and trochlear groove, which increases the lateral pull from the knee extensors. A distance of more than 15 mm on MRI scan is considered pathological (Ho *et al.* 2015).

Wider influences on the patella

Looking beyond the knee, structural factors such as pronated feet, internal rotation of the hip and the resulting increased Q angle (line of pull of the rectus femoris muscle) can affect patellofemoral stability. Correct positioning of the femur determines the orientation of the trochlea. Because of this, the possibility of femoral anteversion should also be kept in mind since this results in the patella being positioned more laterally. The gluteal muscles function as proximal stabilisers, and weakness of hip abduction and external rotation is often present in patellofemoral pain.

The knee should be assessed in the context of the spine, pelvis, hip and feet. The pelvis, for example, can be rotated as a result of tibial torsion, e.g., an intraosseous twist along the long axis of the tibia. The hip is where maximal compensation to tibial torsion occurs, resulting in internal rotation of the hip, coupled with either abduction or adduction (Snow 2021). The foot, in turn, can compensate by pronation of the midfoot (Paulos *et al.* 2009). The knee has to adapt to these conflicting influences from above and below. Osteopathic treatment should aim to improve internal and external hip rotation equally, for optimum adaptation to any abnormal lower limb alignment.

CRUCIATE LIGAMENTS

The two cruciate ligaments are outside the synovial capsule. They form a cross (X) within the knee, preventing excessive forward or backward translation of the tibia on the femur during flexion and extension movements. The anterior cruciate ligament (ACL) provides 85 per cent of the resistance against anterior tibial translation. Both cruciate ligaments, acting together, guide the centre of rotation of the knee.

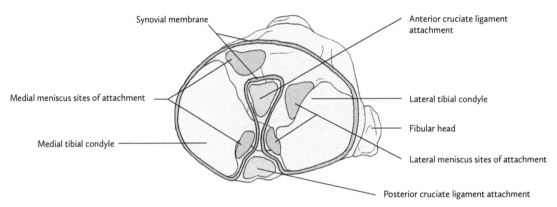

Figure 12.5 Tibial surface of the knee, showing extrasynovial attachment of cruciate ligaments.

The PCL is wider and stronger than the ACL, making it less susceptible to injury. It primarily restricts posterior translation. Its function is supported by the meniscofemoral ligament (MFL). The MFL reduces contact stress by 10 per cent under axial compression in the knee (Chahla *et al.* 2021; Pekala *et al.* 2021).

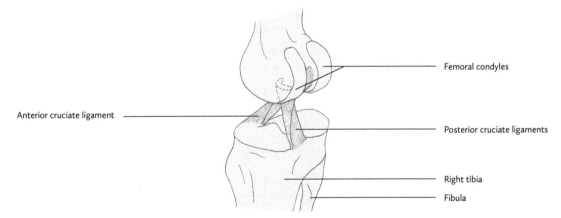

Figure 12.6 Schematic view of cruciate ligament attachment (joint separated for clarity).

The cruciate ligaments are crucial to controlling anteroposterior translation when the knee is at 30–90° of flexion. The ACL limits anterior tibial translation, but more importantly, internal tibial rotation during flexion and extension. From 20° of flexion towards full extension, the screw home mechanism with internal rotation of the femur against the tibia involves the cruciate ligaments tightening to lock the knee. The knee is unlocked by the action of the popliteus. The cruciate ligaments pivot about their insertion points, and the centre of rotation is at the crossover point of the cruciate ligaments. The cruciate ligaments also are able to change in length slightly in order to allow internal-external rotation of the joint.

During walking, the tibia rotates because of the difference in the curvature of the condyles. The medial femoral condyle is larger and more curved and moves against the concave medial tibial plateau (Anetzberger *et al.* 2014). The curvature of the lateral condyle is spiral shaped against the convexity of the lateral tibial plateau. Internal rotation of the femur and tibia occurs during the swing phase of gait. External rotation occurs as the leg reaches full extension.

Both cruciate ligaments and the MFL have proprioceptive nerve endings, mechanoreceptors being present on the ligament surface (Gupte *et al.* 2014). Mechanoreceptors contribute to joint position sense and are part of the afferent spinal arc, controlling muscle and postural tone at the knee, the *ACL reflex*. The cruciate ligaments, in effect, function as active stabilisers of the knee via this proprioceptive feedback. It is this loss of the reflex sensory feedback arc, in ligamentous injury, that leads to loss of quadriceps function and weakness. During treatment, attention can be paid to the *ACL reflex* in modulating postural control at the knee.

THE MENISCI

Because of the differences in the curvature of the femoral condyles and the tibial plateau described above, the menisci function primarily to enlarge the contact surface and allow a closer fit between the tibial and femoral surfaces. They also help to distribute the forces at the knee joint and carry 70 per cent of the load across it. Being viscoelastic, the menisci are able to dissipate loading and unloading forces by changing shape. This contributes to their ability to act as shock absorbers (Seitz *et al.* 2022).

CLINICAL EXAMINATION OF THE KNEE

Dynamic tests of the knee should ideally include squatting and 'duck waddling' as a full squat is not possible with a meniscal injury. Motion testing is a key component of the osteopathic examination, and loss of movement implies meniscal or obstructive lesions. Laxity implies ligamentous tears or hypermobility. Loss of extension may suggest intra-articular pathology or be the result of a pseudo-locked knee after an acute injury, with severe pain, e.g., arthrogenic muscle inhibition (Rice and McNair 2010). Normal flexion of the knee is limited at 160° by the compression of the posterior horn of the medial meniscus between the femur and tibia (Pinskerova *et al.* 2009). Small secondary motion in other planes can be assessed with the knee in flexion. Osteopathic assessment should include the palpatory sense of ease and quality of motion at the knee.

A full examination of the knee should include assessment of its blood supply, lymphatic and venous drainage of the lower extremity and fascial tension from the feet to the trunk (Altinbilek *et al.* 2018). The nerve supply is from the femoral, obturator and sciatic nerves; therefore vertebral levels L2–L4 should be examined closely for restrictions (Tran *et al.* 2021). L2–L4 may also be involved in sympathetic disturbances around the knee contributing to chronic inflammation (Widenfalk and Wiberg 1989).

Synovial folds or plicae are vestigial folds of synovium in the joint and are persisting remnants from embryological development that ordinarily do not cause symptoms. In plica syndrome they can be palpable if inflamed or fibrosed (Wong and Lalam 2019). This condition can be seen particularly in children, adolescents and cyclists and is a diagnosis of exclusion (Hoehmann 2017). Pain is experienced in sustained flexed positions. Clicking may be present and the tenderness may be palpable over the medial patellar, lateral patellar, suprapatellar and infrapatellar plicae.

The medial patellar plica is the most common source of pain. This mimics patellofemoral syndrome, showing tenderness on palpating the medial side of the patella with the knee flexed and tibia in medial rotation. It is not uncommon for the infrapatellar plica (ligamentum mucosum) fat pad to be scarred and fibrosed after arthroscopic surgery.

The folds span the synovium of the patella to the tibiofemoral joint. The patella lift technique may be performed with attention placed on the plicae and an appreciation of the elastic nature of the tissue. Inflammatory changes can be sensed.

THERAPEUTIC ENGAGEMENT

Sitting BLT of the knee joint

The aim of this seated BLT approach is to restore tibiofemoral joint integrity and alignment. Tibiofemoral strains are caused by sudden or forceful rotation of the tibia relative to the femur with a valgus strain. This causes the lateral articulation to act as a fulcrum for the external rotation of the tibia and the tibial medial condyle to be directed anteriorly (Lippincott 1949).

Have the patient seated on the table in front of you with the edge of the table well behind the knees so that there is no weight bearing on the back of the knees. Alternatively, the lower thighs may rest on a soft cushion. The knee is suspended at 90° of flexion.

1. CONTACT

Sit facing the patient who is seated on the treatment table. Wrap your fingers around the medial and lateral tibial condyles with your thumbs crossed under the tibial tuberosity. This provides a short lever in relation to the femur. The intention is to allow your contacts to blend with the periosteum. The crossed thumbs provide a fulcrum for the inherent motions of the knee at the point of balanced tension.

The joint space may also be monitored with the index fingers of both hands placed over the medial and lateral joint lines.

Use your knees to support the patient's leg on the medial and lateral sides.

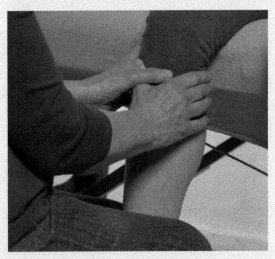

Figure 12.7 Sitting tibiofemoral joint contact.

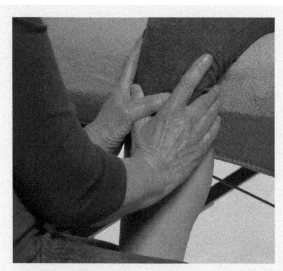

Figure 12.8 Alternative contact for sitting BLT of the knee.

2. MOTION TESTING

Find the direction of ease within the strain by sensing, through your legs, any tendency towards valgus or varus deviation. With your hands, test any preference for internal or external rotation or for anteroposterior translation of the tibia, as you monitor the three-dimensional joint space for a sense of balance. Motion testing in these directions may use both exaggeration towards the direction of ease and direct action to discern the point of restriction.

3. ACTIVATION

To activate the ligaments, approximate the joint by minimally lifting the tibia towards the femur with your knees, but without lifting the patient's femur. This leaves your hands more available in a sensory (afferent) capacity, for attending to subtle refinements of the state of balance. Be sure that the patient does not take this as a signal to lift his or her thighs or approximation will be lost.

4. BALANCE POINT

Place the joint in a position of composite balanced tension for all the components discerned, supporting it as the ligaments explore for further refinement.

At the point of BLT, the inherent self-correcting action may pivot around the fulcrum at the crossover point of the cruciate ligaments; attention should be placed here as this represents the centre of rotation of the knee. Wait with the stillness of the state of balance.

5. RESOLUTION

As the ligamentous-articular mechanism begins to reorganise, it may go through various motions, even exaggerating its strain pattern before returning to centred alignment. As the strain reverses there may be an impression of greater joint space, restoration of midline organisation of the entire limb, warmth and three-dimensional expression of rhythmic shape change between the hands.

Retest the movements of the knee before removing your contacts.

Sitting patella lift

The aim here is to restore balance at the patellofemoral joint to reseat the patella in its femoral sulcus. It is also effective in engaging all the intra-articular joint components through the continuity between the suprapatellar synovial bursa and the synovial capsule (Perdikakis and Skiades 2013). This approach may be considered, either as part two of the manoeuvre described above, or as sufficient in itself. It is especially helpful for painful and arthritic knees with very limited movement, as part of a regular treatment programme. (See Figure 12.8.)

This seated patella technique allows visual examination of the patella from the front and the sides. In patella alta, the patella will be sitting high and more laterally in the 'grasshopper's eyes' position. The relative positions of the patellar tubercle and the centre of the patella can be visually assessed: the tibial tubercle should ideally be within the femoral trochlea when the knees are at 90° of flexion.

In addition to the orthopaedic tests for the

patella and assessment of passive and active tracking, osteopathic assessment of the patella includes sensing the following:

- the quality of medial and lateral glide
- the degree of patellar tilt: is the medial border anterior due to tightness of the lateral retinaculum or cartilage/bone loss?
- medial or lateral patellar rotation in relation to the long axis of the femur: again, due to a tight retinaculum
- the inferior pole of the patella may be felt to be posterior and pain may be elicited by compressing the highly nociceptive infrapatellar fat pad: especially in hyperextended knees
- palpation of the tibial tubercle (Osgood-Schlatter disease) or inferior pole (Sinding-Larsen-Johansson syndrome) of the patella can be tender in adolescent patients.

1. POSITIONING

The patient is seated as before, with the operator sitting and facing the side of the leg to be addressed. Straighten the patient's leg to the degree possible, and place the ankle on your thigh, with the heel dropping off its lateral edge.

This contact on the thigh enables you to either approximate or introduce traction to the patient's tibiofemoral joint, with varying degrees of flexion or extension as appropriate.

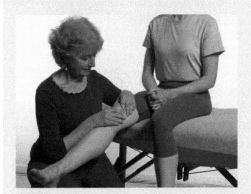

Figure 12.9 Sitting patellar lift hold on live model.

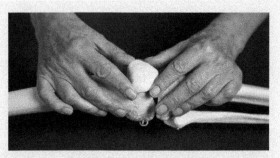

Figure 12.10 Patellar lift hold on skeleton.

2. HANDHOLD

Place the thumb and index fingers of each hand on the medial and lateral sides of the patella, with the heels of your hands resting on the tibia and femur above and below the knee joint.

3. MOTION TESTING

Gently test for any tendency towards translation longitudinally or sideways, tilting or rotation. Sense the quality of fluidity at the patellofemoral joint.

4. LIFTING

Place the patella in its position of ease for all the components perceived and then introduce a gentle lift superiorly (anteriorly to the patient's leg) away from the femoral trochlea. This will engage the capsule, ligaments and synovial plicae towards a point of balance and awaken fluid activity.

Keep in mind the continuity between the synovial suprapatellar bursa and the synovial capsule of the tibiofibular joint. This continuity is what makes the patella lift so effective in stimulating self-organising activity throughout the interior joint space. If the inertial forces are great, it is helpful to slightly exaggerate the direction of ease, to shift the joint fulcrum and facilitate ligamentous action.

5. BALANCE POINT

Support the patella as the inherent fluid and connective tissue forces tune the balance point.

The resolution is felt as improved balance in all directions, so that the patella 'reseats' and its function as a sesamoid bone is restored. The long axis of the patella may then be better aligned with the long axis of the femur. Its intraosseous breathing and 'floating' can often be perceptible.

Reassess the quality of patella motion.

Supine patella and tibiofibular joint

The patella lift may also be performed with the patient in the supine position with hand contact as above, on tibia, patella and femur.

This has the advantage of making it possible for the operator to engage BLT of the patella, femur and tibia simultaneously, bringing the entire knee joint into balance.

Supine approach to the tibiofemoral joint

This can also be accomplished with the patient supine. A small pillow may be placed under the knee as necessary. *The hands are placed on the femoral epicondyles and tibial condyles, above and below the joint line. Approximate the two bones to engage the ligaments and motion test as necessary to bring the articulation to the point of BLT.* This approach is especially helpful if compression is required to match the internal vectorial forces absorbed by the joint, to achieve a point of balance.

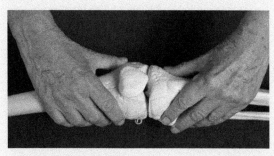

Figure 12.11 Handhold for supine BLT of tibiofemoral joint.

Popliteal drainage

Lymphatic congestion and effusion may be drained by addressing the posterior tissues of the knee.

1. POSITIONING AND HANDHOLD

The patient is supine with the knees slightly flexed and the heels resting on the table.

Place your fingers medial to the tendons of the biceps femoris and semitendinosus muscles in the upper part of the popliteal fossa.

2. ACTION

Alternately separate and relax these tendons with your fingers. This will act as a pump for drainage of the popliteal fossa.

3. POSTURAL COOPERATION

Alternatively, *with your finger contacts firmly on the tendons of the biceps and semitendinosus muscles,* use patient postural cooperation: *ask the patient to alternately press against, or into, the table with the heel to flex the knee, against your resistance and then relax it* (Lippincott 1949). This is isometric knee flexion. Compression of the tissue spaces of the popliteal fossa during flexion will squeeze fluids upwards.

The same hold may be applied with the supine patient rhythmically straightening and relaxing the knee against the operator's slight resistance.

VIDEOS FOR CHAPTER 12

Scan the QR code or visit https://www.youtube.com/playlist?list=PL3j_ YuMBqigH_J4PZ8DMA4CeoF8mcJpHn to find a playlist of the videos that accompany this chapter.

REFERENCES

Ahn, J.H., Patel, N.A., Lin, C.C., Lee, T.Q. (2019) The anterolateral ligament of the knee joint: a review of the anatomy, biomechanics, and anterolateral ligament surgery. *Knee Surg & Related Research, 31* (12). https://doi.org/10.1186/s43019-019-0012-4.

Altinbilek, T., Murat, S., Yumusakhuylu, Y., *et al.* (2018) Osteopathic manipulative treatment improves function and relieves pain in knee osteoarthritis: a single-blind, randomised-controlled trial. *Turk J Phys Med Rehabil 64* (2), 114–120.

Anetzberger, H., Biorkenmaier, C., Lorenz, S.G.F. (2014) Meniscectomy: indications, procedure, outcomes and rehabilitation. *Orthopaedic Research and Reviews 6, 1–9.*

Barker, R.P., Lee, J.C., Healy, J.C. (2009) Normal sonographic anatomy of the posterolateral corner of the knee. *Am J Roentgenol 192, 73–79.*

Bicos, J., Fulkerson, J.P., Amis, A. (2007) The medial patellofemoral ligament. *Am J Sports Med 35* (3), 484–492.

Bollen, S. (2000) Epidemiology of knee injuries: diagnosis and triage. *Br J Sports Med 34* (3), 227–228.

Bolog, N. & Hodler, J. (2007) MR imaging of the posterolateral corner of the knee. *Skeletal Radiol 36, 715–728.*

Branch, E.A. & Anz, A.W. (2015) Distal insertions of the biceps femoris. A quantitative analysis. *Orthop J Sports Med 3* (9), 2325967115602255. https://doi.org/10.1177/2325967115602255.

Chahla, J., Beletsky, A., Smigielski, R., *et al.* (2021) Meniscal pathology. In: R.F. LaPrade and J. Chahla (eds) *Evidence-Based Management of Complex Knee Injuries.* Amsterdam: Elsevier; pp. 157–175.

Chen, L., Kim, P.D., Ahmad, C.S., Levine, W.N. (2007) Medial collateral ligament of the knee: current treatment concepts. *Curr Rev Musculoskeletal Med 1* (2), 108–113.

Felli, L., Alessio-Mazzola, M., Lovisolo, S., *et al.* (2021) Anatomy and biomechanics of the medial patellatibial ligament: a systematic review. *The Surgeon 19* (5), e168–e174.

Fryette, H.H. (1954) *Principles of Osteopathic Technique. A Harry L Chiles Memorial Publication.* Carmel, CA: The Academy of Applied Osteopathy; p. 205.

Grassi, A., Roberto di Sarsina, T., Di Paolo, S., *et al.* (2021) Increased rotational laxity after anterolateral ligament lesion in anterior cruciate ligament (ACL) deficient knees: a cadaveric study with noninvasive inertial sensors. *BioMed Research International, 7549750.*

Gupte, C.M., Shaerf, D.A., Sandison, A. (2014) Neural structures within human meniscofemoral ligaments: a cadaveric study. *Int Scholarly Res Notices.* https://doi.org/10.1155/2014/719851.

Ho, C.P., James, E.W., Surowiec, R.K., *et al.* (2015) Technique-dependent differences in CT versus MRI measurement of the tibial tubercle-trochlear groove distance. *Am J Sports Med 43* (3), 675–682.

Hoehmann, C.L. (2017) Plica syndrome and its embryological origins. *Edorium J Orthop 3, 1–12.*

Kushare, I., McHorse, G., Ghanta, R., *et al.* (2021) High incidence of intra-articular injuries with Segund fractures of the tibia in paediatric and adolescent populations. *J of Ped Orthopedics 41* (8), 514–519.

LaPrade, R.F. (2007) The anatomy of the medial part of the knee. *J Bone Joint Surg (Am) 89* (9), 2000.

LaPrade, R.F., Morgan, P.M., Wentorf, F.A., *et al.* (2007) The anatomy of the posterior aspect of the knee. An anatomic study. *J Bone Joint Surg Am 89* (4), 758–764.

Lippincott, H.A. (1949) The Osteopathic Technique of Wm. G. Sutherland, D.O. In: W.G. Sutherland (1990) *Teachings in the Science of Osteopathy.* A.L. Wales (ed.). Fort Worth, TX: Sutherland Cranial Teaching Foundation, Inc./Rudra Press.

Lovse, L.J. & Getgood, A. (2021) Anterolateral rotational laxity: what is it, when to address it, and how? *Operative Techniques in Sports Medicine 29* (2), 10601872.

McCulloch, P.C., Bott, A.R., Ramkumar, P., *et al.* (2014) Strain within the native and reconstructed MPFL during knee flexion. *J Knee Surg 27* (2), 125–131.

Paulos, L., Swanson, S.C., Stoddard, G.J., Barber-Westin, S. (2009) Surgical correction of limb malalignment for stability of the patella: a comparison of 2 techniques. *Am J Sports Med 37* (7), 1288–1300.

Pekala, P.A., Rosa, M.A., Lazarz, D.A., *et al.* (2021) Clinical anatomy of the meniscofemoral ligament of Humphrey: an original MRI study, meta-analysis, and systematic review. *Orthop J Sports Med 9* (2), 325967120973192. https://doi.org/10.1177/2325967120973192.

Perdikakis, E. & Skiades, V. (2013) MRI characteristics of cysts and 'cyst-like' lesions in and around the knee: what the radiologist needs to know. *Insights into Imaging 4, 257–272.*

Pinskerova, V., Samuelson, K.M., Stammers, J. *et al.* (2009) The knee in full flexion: an anatomical study. *J Bone Joint Surg Br 91* (6), 830–834.

Provencher, M.T., Sanchez, G., Ferrari, M.B., *et al.* (2017) Arthroscopy-assisted fabella excision: surgical technique. *Arthroscopy Techniques 6* (2), e369–e374.

Rice, D.A. & McNair, P.J. (2010) Quadriceps arthrogenic muscle inhibition: neural mechanisms and treatment perspectives. *Seminars in Arthritis and Rheumatism 40* (3), 250–266.

Seitz, A.M., Schwer, J., de Roy, L., *et al.* (2022) Knee joint menisci are shock absorbers: a biomechanical in-vitro study on porcine stifle joints. *Front Bioeng Biotechnol 17*, 10, 837554.

Snow, M. (2021) Tibial torsion and patellofemoral pain and instability in the adult population: current concept review. *Curr Rev Musculoskelet Med 14* (1), 67–75.

Stevens, K.J., Albtoush, O.M., Lutz, A.M., *et al.* (2021) The Stieda fracture revisited. *Skeletal Radiology 50* (5), 945–953.

Tran, J., Peng, P.W.H., Chan, V.W.S., *et al.* (2021) Overview of innervation of knee joint. *Phys Med Rehabil Chin N Am 32*, 767–778.

Warren, L.F. & Marshall, J.L. (1979) The supporting structures and layers on the medial side of the knee: an anatomical analysis. *J Bone Joint Surg Am 61* (1), 56–62.

Wei, X., Wang, Z., Lu, Y., *et al.* (2021) Surgical treatment for avulsion fractures of the anterolateral ligament associated with periarticular fractures of the knee. *The J of Knee Surg 36* (4), 397–403.

Weng, S.P., Wu, T.M., Chien, C.S., *et al.* (2021) Treatment of fabella syndrome with arthroscopic fabellectomy: a case series and literature review. *BMC Musculoskeletal Disorders 22* (1), 748.

Widenfalk, B. & Wiberg, M. (1989) Origin of sympathetic and sensory innervation of the knee joint. A retrograde axonal tracing study in the rat. *Anatomy and Embryology 180*, 317–323.

Wong, J.S. & Lalam, R. (2019) Plicae: where do they come from and when are they relevant? *Seminars in Musculoskeletal Radiology 23* (5), 547–568.

Wroble, R.R., Grood, E.S., Cummings, J.S., *et al.* (1993) The role of the lateral extraarticular restraints in the anterior cruciate ligament-deficient knee. *Am J Sports Med 21* (2), 257–262.

CHAPTER 13

The Fibula and Interosseous Membrane

ZENNA ZWIERZCHOWSKA

This chapter explores the importance of realignment of the tibia and fibula by normalising reciprocal tension in their interosseous membrane (IoM).

Dr Sutherland tells the story of being a student, when one of his classmates had stepped on a rusty nail (Sutherland 1990, TSO p. 188). Despite appropriate management the wound would not heal. Dr Still was called in for advice. 'You damn fools,' he said, 'and so we were', says Dr Sutherland, for in paying attention to the wound, they had not considered what had actually happened at the moment of injury. As the patient stepped on the rusty nail, he had sharply drawn his leg away. This had caused the proximal tibiofibular joint to move posteriorly and the distal end of the fibula anteriorly, creating a strain through the IoM. Thus, a disturbance in the circulation and drainage of the foot was preventing proper healing of the wound.

This story illustrates the importance of taking aetiology into the picture, whether the cause be recent or distant. The body bears the tissue memory of the various forces it has absorbed over time. One of the beauties of the BLT approach is that, as we read the tissues at each phase of a therapeutic manoeuvre, the body often reveals the vectors of injury recorded in it, through the way our hands are invited to match them.

The importance of looking to strains in the tibiofibular relationship cannot be overstated, as these inevitably involve distortion of the IoM. As demonstrated in Sutherland's story, this is important for arterial flow and venous and lymphatic drainage of the ankle and foot (Arguello *et al.* 2016) as well as mechanical stability of the knee and ankle. The leg IoM spans the interosseous crests of the tibia and fibula, with its fibres mainly running obliquely inferomedially and a few running in the opposite direction. The tibiofibular syndesmosis below is continuous with it. A free border at both its upper and lower margin gives passage to the anterior tibial vessels. Between, the IoM provides a 'highway' for these major vessels on both sides, and also for the deep peroneal nerve. Smaller vessels also pass through its many perforations. It is thus possible that IoM strains may be a predisposing factor in varicose veins and deep vein thrombosis (DVT).

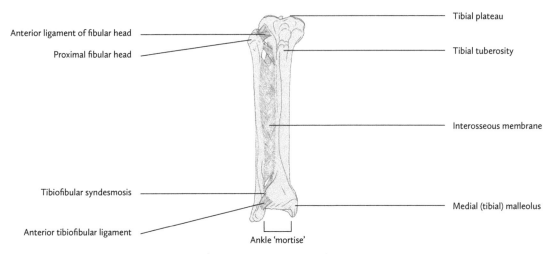

Figure 13.1 Tibiofibular interosseous membrane, anterior view.

The tibialis anterior, extensor digitorum longus, extensor hallucis longus and peroneus tertius muscles are in relation to the anterior surface of the IoM. The tibialis posterior attaches to 81 per cent of its posterior surface and extensor hallucis longus attaches to 62 per cent (Gray 1918). These muscles are key to the mechanical support and function of the arches of the foot in walking. Tibiofibular and IoM strains will tend to alter the relationship between origin and insertion of these muscles predisposing them to compromised function (see Figure 14.4).

The fibula is one of the three bones that may be addressed from both ends simultaneously, the clavicle and the radius being the other two (Wales 1995). All three have membranous or fascial bands attaching along their shafts. The radius and fibula are linked to their paired bone by the IoM, while the clavicle suspends the clavipectoral fascia. Sutherland described these as 'membranous articular mechanisms'. When working on these bones, use is made of balanced membranous tension (BMT), taking both ends of the bone and balancing along the full length.

There are three articulations of the fibula on the tibia. These are the proximal tibiofibular joint, the distal syndesmosis and the articulation through their length via the IoM. The proximal joint has a synovial capsule and can be considered a ligamentous articular mechanism. The distal joint is generally considered to be a syndesmosis with no capsule, tightly bound by anterior, posterior and inferior tibiofibular interosseous ligaments. The inferior ligament is an extension of the very strong posterior tibiofibular ligament which forms an articular labrum for the lateral edge of the trochlea of the talus. Dissection of the tibiofibular syndesmosis of 30 cadavers, however, showed two-thirds to have a small synovial component (Bartoníček 2003).

The fibula is not a weight-bearing bone, but it works by distributing weight in the manner of a shock absorber. Normal axial loading within the leg segment during walking involves a transfer of an average of 17 per cent of the axial compressive load from the tibia to the fibula through the distal interosseous ligament and membrane. The loading increases when the weight is shifted laterally or in dorsiflexion and decreases when the weight shifts medially or in plantar flexion (Wang *et al.* 1996).

THE FIBULA AND ANKLE/FOOT MECHANICS

At its distal end, the fibula helps to accommodate to the variation in width between the wider anterior part and narrower posterior part of the talus bone. The distance between the two malleoli is, correspondingly, approximately 1 mm wider anteriorly than posteriorly, ensuring a snug fit. This helps accommodation of the talus at the ankle mortise depending on whether it is in dorsiflexion or plantar flexion. Because the talus is wider anteriorly, the ankle mortise is at its most stable when the foot is dorsiflexed (Lin *et al.* 2006).

In plantar flexion the ankle joint is less stable as the narrower posterior part of the talus is held between the two malleoli. This requires the malleoli to be closer together posteriorly to enable them to hold the integrity of the joint. It is the interosseous ligament and membrane of the fibula that enable the space between the malleoli to accommodate to the varying widths on the superior surface of the talus in actions such as walking. In so doing, a stable and secure fit, both in dorsi- and plantar flexion, can normally be maintained. This is made possible by means of the dynamic change in direction of the fibres of the IoM, as it widens laterally and springs back, with the changing demands of the talus (Norkus and Floyd 2001).

A functional fulcrum of the IoM is normally found about one-third of the way up the fibula. It is the length of the fibula and its attachment to the tibia via the IoM that enables this long lever action to hold the talus.

If there is a strain, either in the ligaments at the distal joint or anywhere along this dynamic tibiofibular mechanism, there is a loss of responsiveness of the talocrural joint with consequent loss of stability at the ankle. The strained distal articulation leads to the lateral malleolus dropping distally and anteriorly together with the talus. The most usual strain within the interosseus membrane involves an anteriorisation at the distal end of the fibula and a consequent posteriorisation at the proximal head. When working with this long membrane, direct action, rather than exaggeration, often appears to produce effective therapeutic engagement with the fibres.

Ideally a well-aligned tibiofibular relationship, held in balance on the IoM, enables the distal tibia and fibula to function together like a mortise and tenon joint, holding the talus adaptively but securely (Gao *et al.* 2019). This stability between the talus and the malleoli should function primarily in flexion and extension like a hinge. However, as commonly happens, where the distal fibula has moved anteriorly, this widens the ankle mortise (Magan *et al.* 2014), allowing the talus to slip anteriorly, relative to a posteriorisation of the calcaneus. This creates ongoing instability because the hinge action of the joint is lost, causing it to function in an unprotected way as a universal joint. This leads to increasing loss of ligamentous support, not only for the ankle but for the whole foot (see Chapter 14).

It should also be borne in mind, however, that in certain severe or chronic injuries at the syndesmosis, the pathological mechanism can involve dorsiflexion and external rotation of the foot, causing the talus to move into external rotation, widening the syndesmosis. This will strain the anterior tibiofibular and deltoid ligaments, and can also result in a posterior positioning of the lower end of the fibula (De Albornoz and Monteagudo 2021; Hunt 2013; Wei *et al.* 2012; Yuen and Lui 2017).

The widening of the ankle mortise after an ankle sprain often leaves the bones in the same dysfunctional position they took on during the injury. Meanwhile the ligaments are left unable to create balance in relation to each other or to support the ankle. This predisposes the sufferer to repeated recurrence of the ankle injury. It is often cited that ligamentous injuries are slow to heal. However, the experience of the author suggests that restoration of a correct and balanced relationship of the involved bones and ligaments creates better conditions for healing and restoration of stability.

FIBULAR RELATIONSHIP TO THE KNEE

The lateral ('fibular') collateral ligament at the proximal fibular head connects the fibula with the femur. Its main function is stabilisation of the lateral side of the knee, protecting it from varus stress and lateral movement. It also stabilises anteroposterior translation when the cruciate ligaments are torn. The fibula, therefore, makes a significant contribution to knee stability (Branch and Anz 2015; Wroble *et al.* 1993) (see Chapter 12).

Realignment of the tibiofibular IoM is often an important first step in addressing problems, either with the knee or the foot and ankle.

THERAPEUTIC ENGAGEMENT

Engaging the tibiofibular IoM by direct action

The following approach uses direct action to challenge the IoM to dynamically seek a balance point, while encouraging both ends of the fibula to reverse the direction of the strain. This does not preclude simply supporting the fibula towards the direction of ease in relation to any strains in the IoM when appropriate.

1. TESTING
Sit in front of the patient who is seated on the couch with legs dangling. Examine each leg, holding the fibula at both ends to check its alignment with the IoM and tibia. If in strain, it is often anterior distally and posterior proximally.

2. HANDHOLD
Taking hold of the patient's right ankle with your left hand, wrap your fingers around the calcaneus from behind and your thenar eminence around the lateral malleolus in front.

With your right hand, cross over to take hold of the proximal fibular head with two fingers behind and the thumb in front and initially find the easy neutral position of the fibula.

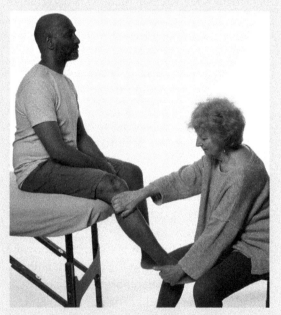

Figure 13.2 Seated hold of upper and lower ends of the fibula.

3. DIRECT ENGAGEMENT
This may feel slightly awkward as your upper hand reaches across your body, but *with the arms straightened, turn your whole body to introduce gentle proximal anteriorisation and distal posteriorisation. This direct action approach produces a*

powerful engagement and response through the length of the IoM.

The distal fibular joint is more fixed, so *it can be engaged with a slight squeezing action between your fingers and thenar eminence.* The proximal joint is freer, and *by gently pulling it anteriorly* the whole of the membrane is 'woken up' and challenged to seek a balance point.

4. RESOLUTION

As the membrane resolves the maintaining strain, the fibula will often be felt to reseat at both ends.

As mentioned above, the functional fulcrum of the IoM is normally found about two thirds of the way down the fibula. A strain may cause this fulcrum to shift either up or down. Checking for the fulcrum is a quick and easy way of diagnosing any disturbance in the movement of the tibiofibular articulation.

Supine IoM engagement

An activation of the IoM can also be achieved with the patient sitting as before, or supine, with the operator sitting to the side.

1. POSITION AND CONTACT

Lift up the patient's leg from the side and rest the heel on the lateral side of your knee OR simply have the patient supine on the treatment table.

Take up a contact with two fingers and thumb of each hand, holding the distal and proximal ends of the fibula.

2. FINDING AND SUPPORTING THE POSITION OF BALANCE

Test the movement and check for the functional fulcrum as in the previous approach. *Holding the fibula at both ends, suspend the IoM and balance.*

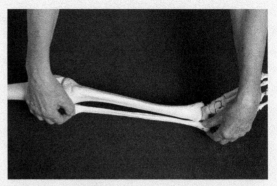

Figure 13.3 Supine fibula hold on skeleton.

Engaging the fluid field of the bone

Sometimes in treatment, holding an image in one's mind can help to make a deeper connection with the tissues under one's hands. *In this instance, engage the more delicate periosteum of the fibula and feel its blending with the tougher fibres of the IoM; follow right through to its blending with the periosteum around the tibia. This brings a more fluid field of operation.* A 'fluid fluctuation' is often felt through the different compartments as the whole mechanism shifts and rebalances.

BMT of tibiofibular IoM with active patient cooperation

This approach is very effective and quick for patients who are sufficiently flexible (Sutherland 1990, TSO p. 188).

1. PATIENT POSITION AND POSTURAL COOPERATION

The patient crosses the fibula of one leg over the other thigh, resting it at the fibula's natural fulcrum point, one-third of the way from its distal end.

Ask the patient to place both hands over the uppermost surface of the bent knee.

2. HANDHOLD

Sit facing the patient and hold each end of the patient's fibula between finger and thumb, gently allowing it to move towards an approximate position of ease and balance in relation to the IoM.

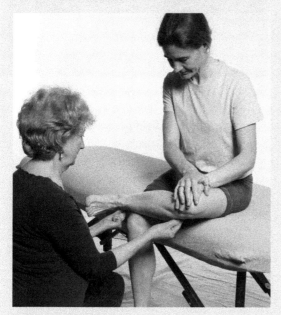

Figure 13.4 Hold for patient's active cooperation.

3. EMPOWERING THE PROCESS

Ask the patient to dorsiflex the foot while pressing down on the knee with the resting hands. This rotates the fibula around the fulcrum point and releases it at both ends from the tibia and talus. This often produces a dynamic response in the IoM, allowing it to reorganise and rebalance the fibula.

The role of the operator here is mainly one of *monitoring*, since the main drive comes from the patient's postural cooperation evoking a spontaneous corrective process in the fibular IoM. If necessary, however, once the IoM has been felt to reorganise, there is normally no resistance to gentle guidance of the fibula back towards realignment.

This last procedure can be taught to patients as a self-help treatment that can be used if unable to see an osteopath immediately, or if this procedure needs re-enforcing.

VIDEOS FOR CHAPTER 13

Scan the QR code or visit https://www.youtube.com/playlist?list=PL3j_YuMBqigH5TRqGCsDFUSDXFEBntizC to find a playlist of the video that accompany this chapter.

REFERENCES

Arguello, E., Stoddard, C., Liu, H., *et al.* (2016) Surface projection of interosseous foramen of the leg: cadaver study. *Anatomy Research International Vol. 2016,* Article ID 6312027. https://doi.org/10.1155/2016/6312027.

Bartonícek, J. (2003) Anatomy of the tibiofibular syndesmosis and its clinical relevance. *Surg Radiol Anat 25* (5–6), 379–386. https://doi.org/10.1007/s00276-003-0156-4.

Branch, E.A. & Anz, A.W. (2015) Distal insertions of the biceps femoris: a quantitative analysis. *Ortho J Sports Med 3* (9), 2325967115602255.

De Albornoz, P.M. & Monteagudo, M. (2021) Pathomechanics of syndesmotic injuries. *J Foot Ankle Surg (Asia Pacific) 8* (4), 162–167.

Gao, C., Chen, Z., Cheng, Y., *et al.* (2019) Comparative anatomy of the mouse and human ankle joint using micro-CT: utility of a mouse model to study human ankle sprains. *Mathematical Biosciences and Engineering 16* (4), 2959–2972.

Gray, H. (1918) *Gray's Anatomy,* 20th edition. Philadelphia, PA: Lea & Febiger; p. 348.

Hunt, K.J. (2013) Syndesmosis injuries. *Current Rev Musculo-skelet Med 6* (4), 304–312.

Lin, C.F., Gross, M.L., Weinhold, P. (2006) Ankle syndesmosis injuries: anatomy, biomechanics, mechanism of injury, and clinical guidelines for diagnosis and intervention. *The Journal of Orthopaedic and Sports Physical Therapy 36* (6), 372–384. https://doi.org/10.2519/jospt.2006.2195.

Magan, A., Golano, P., Maffulli, N., Khanduja, V. (2014) Evaluation and management of injuries of the tibiofibular syndesmosis. *British Medical Bulletin 111* (1), 101–115.

Norkus, S.A. & Floyd, R.T. (2001) The anatomy and mechanisms of syndesmotic ankle sprains. *J Athl Train 36* (1), 68–73.

Sutherland, W.G. (1990) *Teachings in the Science of Osteopathy*. A.L. Wales (ed.). Fort Worth, TX: Sutherland Cranial Teaching Foundation, Inc./Rudra Press; p. 188.

Wales, A.L. (1995) British tutorial group meeting. North Attleboro, MA, USA.

Wang, Q., Whittle, M., Cunningham, J., Kenwright, J. (1996) Fibula and its ligaments in load transmission and ankle joint stability. *Clin Orthop Relat* (330), 261–270. https://doi.org/10.1097/00003086-199609000-00034.

Wei, F., Post, J.M., Braman, J.E., Myter, E.G., *et al.* (2012) Eversion during external rotation of the human cadaver foot produces high ankle sprains. *J Orthopaedic Research 30* (9), 1423–1429.

Wroble, R.R., Grood, E.S., Cummins, J.S., *et al.* (1993) The role of the lateral extra-articular restraints in the anterior cruciate ligament-deficient knee. *Am J Sports Med 21* (2), 257–262.

Yuen, C.P. & Lui, T.H. (2017) Distal tibiofibular syndesmosis: anatomy, biomechanics, injury and management. *The Open Orthopaedics Journal 1* (Supplement 4), 670–677.

CHAPTER 14

The Ankle and Foot

ZENNA ZWIERZCHOWSKA

'The human foot is a masterpiece of engineering and a work of art.'

Leonardo da Vinci

Dr Wales liked to talk a lot about feet. As a young woman she had suffered with painful feet and was therefore keen to offer herself as a model for anyone demonstrating foot techniques during her college training. Some of the approaches she encountered were quite brutal and painful. The joy for her, of discovering Dr Sutherland's approach to working on the feet, was that 'it did not hurt' and 'it worked!' (Wales 1995, 1996).

She often described foot problems arising as a result of conflict between foot and shoe, decrying the fact that shoe salespersons were not sufficiently trained in recommending the right-shaped shoe for the different types of feet. An out-flared, in-flared or straight foot each require an appropriately shaped last to comfortably accommodate the foot with support for the tarsal arch.

In our practices we see many patients with a variety of foot problems. As a practitioner, one sometimes despairs when faced with a pair of totally misshapen feet. We may not always be able to produce any obvious aesthetic change but, by working in this way, we can reawaken the proprioceptive mechanisms, particularly located in the ligaments, and return a spring to the patient's step. The result is pain relief for which our patients are enormously grateful.

When thinking about diagnosis and treatment of the foot, it is helpful to take a systematic approach and therefore to divide the foot into its three component parts:

- The hindfoot, comprising the tibiofibular ankle 'mortise and tenon' joint and the talocalcaneal articulation.
- The midfoot forming the tarsal arch. This consists of the two tarsal bones (navicular and cuboid) and three cuneiforms. It articulates with the hindfoot by Chopart's ('transverse tarsal') joint. This is the composite curved articulation between the calcaneus and cuboid proximally and the head of the talus with the navicular distally (talonavicular and calcaneocuboid articulations).
- The forefoot consisting of the metatarsals and the phalanges. It is joined to the midfoot by the tarsometatarsal joints.

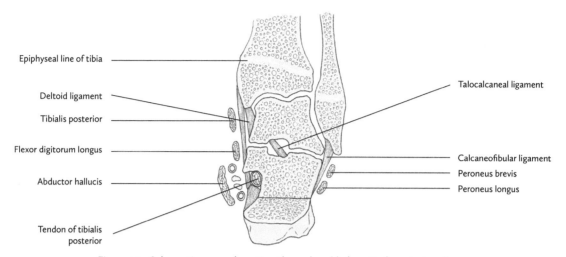

Figure 14.1 Schematic coronal section through ankle 'mortise', posterior view.

The main focus of treatment is to re-establish stability at the ankle and hindfoot and to restore the integrity of the arches of the foot.

The foot consists of three arches, one transverse and two longitudinal, at different heights.

The *transverse (tarsal) arch* is made up of the cuboid, navicular and cuneiform bones. It can be likened to a Roman arch with its keystone at the 2nd cuneiform.

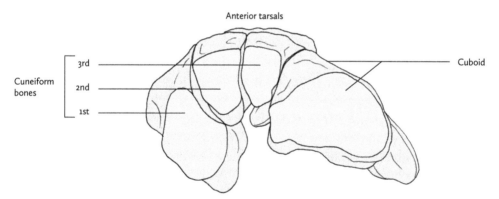

Figure 14.2 Distal row of tarsal arch, showing middle cuneiform as 'keystone'.

The *medial longitudinal (spring) arch* is made up of the calcaneus, talus, navicular, the three cuneiforms and the first, second and third metatarsals. Its apex is at the superior articular surface of the talus. In standing, this arch rests posteriorly on the tuberosity on the plantar surface of the calcaneus, and on the distal heads of the first, second and third metatarsal bones anteriorly. The medial arch is also known as the 'spring arch' as its main function is elasticity. Hence it is composed of more bones and more joints than the lateral arch.

The weakest part is at the talonavicular joint which is the highest point and where most of the compressive forces are absorbed. This point is braced by the plantar calcaneonavicular ligament, which is elastic and is able to spring back after the compressive forces are released. The ligament is strengthened medially by blending with the deltoid ligament of the ankle joint. It is supported inferiorly by the tendon of the tibialis posterior muscle, which spreads out in a fan-shaped insertion *as a key muscle in supporting the arch.* The arch is further supported by the plantar aponeurosis, the small muscles in the sole of the foot, the tendons of the tibialis anterior and posterior, peroneus longus and also by the ligaments of all the articulations involved.

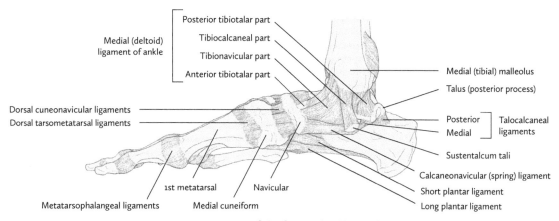

Figure 14.3 Ligaments of the foot and ankle, medial view.

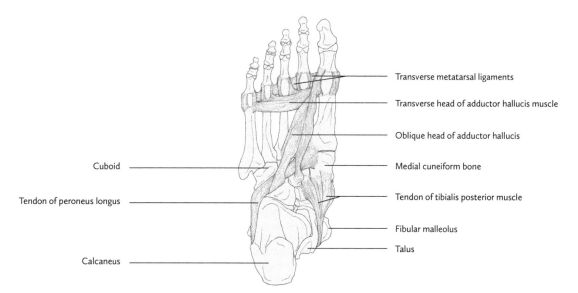

Figure 14.4 Muscles of the plantar surface of the foot.

The *lateral longitudinal (weight-bearing) arch* is composed of the calcaneus, the cuboid and the fourth and fifth metatarsals. Its apex is at the talocalcaneal articulation, and its chief joint is the calcaneocuboid. It is at a lower level than the medial arch and has fewer bones and fewer articulations, giving it greater solidity. The two strong ligaments that support it are the long plantar and plantar calcaneocuboid ligaments. These preserve its integrity, together with support from the extensor tendons and the short muscles of the little toe.

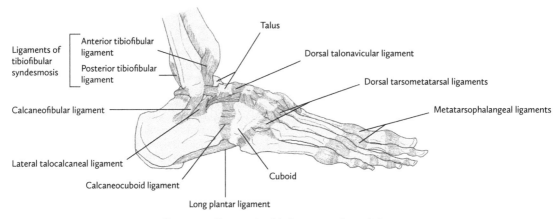

Figure 14.5 Foot and ankle ligaments, lateral view.

The two longitudinal arches are in the same plane but at different heights, providing first stability, then spring in our step. In standing and walking, the arches are crucial for proper distribution of body weight. *In walking, the bones of the arches guide the weight from the heel, along the lateral weight-bearing arch, to transfer to the medial side across the distal metatarsal heads to the base of the big toe.* From there, the big toe is used to propel the foot into the next step. During this process the arches 'collapse', especially the medial longitudinal spring arch. This collapsing is a normal and natural process for shock absorption. The elastic soft-tissue structures of the arch stretch and retain some of the load energy they experience (up to 20%) and then snap back on lift off, helping to propel the body forward. Hence weight bearing through the foot, when walking, starts with heel strike.

These arches should be viewed as suspension arches, dynamically held and suspended by ligaments, tendons and fascia, as illustrated in the tensegrity arch constructed by Graham Scarr and inspired by Kenneth Snelson's model.

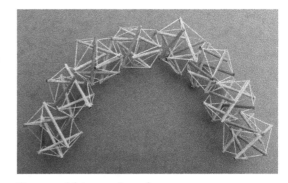

Figure 14.6 A tensegrity arch.
With permission, G. Scarr/Handspring Publishing.

The integrity of the arches is maintained architecturally by the relative positions of the bones, but supported predominantly by the ligaments. Working through BLT in the joints of the foot helps to re-establish this integrity through realigning the bones. Perhaps the most important effect, however, is through awakening the proprioceptive mechanisms of the ligaments to support the spring rebound in the arches.

FACTORS FOR ASSESSMENT

Examination and treatment of the ankle and foot is best approached with the patient sitting, as in this way, both gravity and the weight of the lower leg and foot can be used to provide the appropriate degree of traction needed to assist in the correction. With the patient sitting on the side of the couch and the osteopath sitting below at the feet, it is easy to also do a quick check of the hips and the knees for any imbalance which would affect weight bearing into the ankles and feet. External rotation of the leg, whether coming from the hip or the knee, tends to produce pronation in the foot, whereas internal rotation raises the tarsus and if extreme can produce a 'pigeon toed pattern' (Wales 1992).

Any treatment of the ankle always begins with looking at the tibiofibular articulations and the interosseous membrane (IoM) throughout its length. In particular, the distal tibiofibular articulation determines stability of the ankle 'mortise'.

All of the handholds and suggestions for treatment of the foot assume that the goal is to release and correct ligamentous articular strains through BLT. If the ankle and foot ligaments lose their integrity the action of muscles and tendons will be compromised. It is important to stabilise the ankle and hindfoot before working on the mid and forefoot, hence treatment generally begins at the ankle and works towards the toes.

For the part of the foot most used in weight bearing, such as the hindfoot, the principle of approximation often best activates the innate therapeutic potency in the ligaments. Where propulsion is the main function, as in the toes or metatarsals, distraction through suspension is normally most useful for activating the ligaments. The tarsals may need a combination of both methods.

THE HINDFOOT

The hindfoot consists of the ankle or talocrural joint and the subtalar articulation. The ankle mortise joint is a stable gliding hinge joint and should ideally permit only flexion and extension of the foot on the leg. Inversion and eversion of the foot should occur only at the subtalar joint.

The talocrural 'mortise' is formed by the articulation of the distal ends of the tibia and fibula on the talus. The superior surface and sides of the talus are articular. It has a large facet for the fibular malleolus and a smaller facet for the tibial malleolus. The talus has no muscle attachments and sits between the distal end of the tibial and fibular malleoli superiorly and laterally, and the calcaneus inferiorly. It is held in position by strong ligaments from all sides and by its articulation with the calcaneus inferiorly.

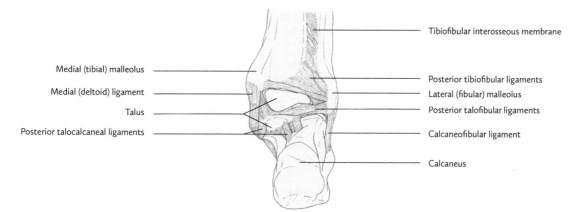

Figure 14.7 Foot and ankle ligaments, posterior view.

The talus is wider at its anterior end. In dorsi-flexion, this is accommodated for by a slight anterior widening of about 1 mm between the two malleoli at the IoM. This stabilises the hinge joint by maintaining a tight hold on the talus between the two malleoli. In plantar flexion the joint is less stable, as the narrower posterior part of the talus is held between the two malleoli. This risks forward slipping of the talus relative to the calcaneus when any anteriorisation of the distal fibula has caused a widening of the space between them, as described below.

The subtalar joint is a complex mechanism and is made up of posterior and anterior parts, divided by the talocalcaneal ligament. The posterior calcaneal facets are convex in relation to the concave facets on the talus; the smaller two anterior calcaneal facets are concave, meeting the convexity on the talus. This arrangement allows for a greater range of movement. There is some variability between individuals in the middle and anterior facets; these can vary in shape and even merge. The body of the talus is supported by the calcaneus at the posterior facets: the head of the talus is supported by the anterior facets on the sustentaculum tali, by the talonavicular articulation and by the spring ligament complex.

Movement at the subtalar joint is said to be flexion-supination-adduction or extension-pronation-abduction; in other words, eversion and inversion of the foot on the leg. This might also be described as the 'roly-poly' action of the foot to accommodate for rough and uneven surfaces.

Importance of the talus in foot stability

Stability of the whole hindfoot is dependent on the talus being held in position, both from above and from below. Problems arise when there is widening at the ankle mortise which does not spring back. This can happen in a traumatic torsion of the ankle or problems arising through stresses in the IoM. The tibiofibular syndesmosis, bound by anterior and posterior tibiofibular ligaments, is a stable joint, and although tears here are rare they can happen, particularly in sport injuries. In such a case it may require surgical intervention if there is a displacement of the two surfaces. More common injuries are strains of the ligaments of the syndesmosis. Lateral sprains of the ankle can affect the ligaments between the lateral malleolus (fibula), talus and calcaneus. This may lead to a widening of the mortise joint which turns it from a stable hinge joint into something more akin to a universal joint.

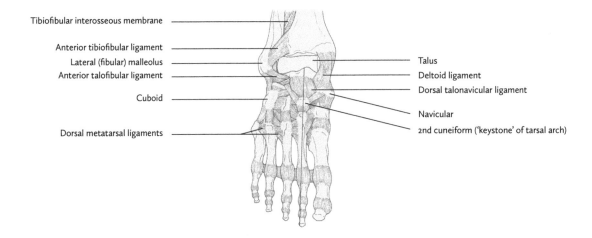

Tibiofibular interosseous membrane

Anterior tibiofibular ligament
Lateral (fibular) malleolus
Anterior talofibular ligament

Cuboid

Dorsal metatarsal ligaments

Talus
Deltoid ligament
Dorsal talonavicular ligament

Navicular
2nd cuneiform ('keystone' of tarsal arch)

Figure 14.8 Foot and ankle ligaments, anterior view.

This loss of integrity of the ankle joint's hinge action can have a profound effect, not only on the talus itself but on the mechanical balance of the whole foot. When weight is transmitted through the ankle, there is a natural tendency for the weight-bearing forces to direct the talus anteriorly and the calcaneus posteriorly because of the relative alignment of these two bones. Stability is normally maintained by the talus being held tightly between the malleoli from above, and by the subtalar ligaments and joints below. If, however, the ankle mortise joint is lax above, there is a loss of integrity of the whole complex and the head of the talus can slip anteriorly and inferiorly over the calcaneus. This takes the navicular and the cuneiforms with it while *the calcaneus moves posteriorly.* This puts an enormous strain on the ligamentous support of both longitudinal arches and may lead to a loss of integrity of all the arches. This also puts strain on the plantar fascia and the Achilles tendon; this pattern appears to be associated, in some cases, with Achilles tendinitis and plantar fasciitis.

If the talus slips anteriorly, relative to the calcaneus, it causes the navicular, which is carried with it, to drop medially, leading to a flattening of the transverse arch since the cuneiforms tend to follow the navicular. This domino effect causes an internal rotation of the first and second metatarsals, which Dr Wales found played a part in producing a hallux valgus. On the lateral side of the foot, the posteriorisation of the calcaneus produces a medial rotation of the cuboid which, in turn, leads to a medial rotation and crowding of the fourth and fifth metatarsals. Pain, as a result of this pinching between the two metatarsals, is often diagnosed as Morton's neuroma. Dr Wales believed that this was not always a neuroma, but that the pain was sometimes a result of mechanical strains originating in the loss of integrity of the ankle mortise and the hindfoot (Wales 1992).

THERAPEUTIC ENGAGEMENT

The ankle mortise or talocrural joint
A variation of all the following holds can be used, depending on the specific problems being addressed and the specific needs of each patient.

Addressing the distal tibiofibular articulation for the mortise of the talus is often the first step in working on the ankle and foot. It is common to find the distal fibular joint strained anteriorly, causing a widening of the ankle mortise and consequently a reduction of the stability of what should be purely a hinge joint. In diagnosis this is the first thing to check for.

1. DIAGNOSIS
Test the stability of the mortise joint, *particularly looking from behind to see whether there is a good alignment between the leg and the heel.*

A starting point is always to assess the IoM between the tibia and fibula.

2. PATIENT AND PRACTITIONER POSITION
With your patient seated on the side of the couch, sit on a stool in front at the feet. This position allows for greater control over the amount of traction required as it uses the assistance of gravity on the suspended leg and foot. This offers an advantage over treating the patient supine.

For greater stability, *bend forward at the hips and rest your elbows on your knees to create an elbow fulcrum for precise engagement.*

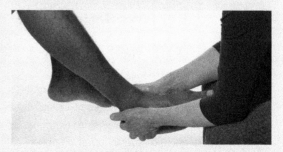

Figure 14.9 Talocrural hold.

3. HANDHOLD

Cradle the malleoli with the thenar eminences of both hands and your fingers wrapped around the heel.

The tibial and fibular malleoli have strong ligamentous attachments to both the calcaneus and the talus as well as to each other, all of which can be contacted with this hold.

Apply a slight medial compression with your thenar eminences from the sides on both malleoli, while at the same time approximating the heel from behind with the fingers wrapped firmly around it.

In this way, the talus is engaged at its articulation with the tibia through a contact on the calcaneus; it is not possible to contact the body of the talus directly as it lies nestled between the tibia above and the calcaneus below. With this hold, all the ligaments around the crural articulation can be engaged. Particular attention is given to the *distal tibiofibular syndesmosis* since the fibular head tends to slip anteriorly and inferiorly if there is any strain on the surrounding ligaments.

4. ENGAGEMENT

Maintain this hold until a release can be felt in the surrounding ligaments.

It is important to remember that, although the hold is firm, it is not achieved by gripping tightly with the muscular tension in the hands. Instead, it is made effective by engaging your whole body through the connective tissues from your back, shoulders, arms and (via the fulcra at the elbows resting on the knees) into the forearms and hands. In this way the hands are merely a contact point for a total body engagement of your proprioceptive mechanisms with those of the patient.

The 'bootjack' for the talocalcaneal joint

This approach is called the 'bootjack' as it recreates the action of a bootjack when used to lever a boot off the foot. Sutherland devised this technique as he noted that, despite spending all day on their feet, farmers did not appear to suffer problems with their feet. He concluded that this might have something to do with their use of a bootjack at the end of the day to remove their boots. The heel would be held firmly by the fork of the bootjack while the foot was being pulled out. At the same time, as the heel was tractioned from below, the front of the boot held and pushed the head of the talus posteriorly, thus helping to realign the subtalar articulation. In effect, Sutherland postulated that at the end of the day, the farmer was giving his hindfoot a little regular treatment which prevented the development of problems.

From his observation of the action of a bootjack, Sutherland devised a manual approach to rebalance the relationship between talus and calcaneus at the subtalar joint. A common strain pattern occurs when the calcaneus slips posteriorly, relative to the talus anteriorly, with the consequent strain on the plantar fascia, sometimes leading to plantar fasciitis and a loss of integrity of the arches of the foot.

This contact will follow from working on the ankle mortise joint. Again, having the patient sitting on the couch with the practitioner seated at the feet allows for the assistance of gravity in the manoeuvre.

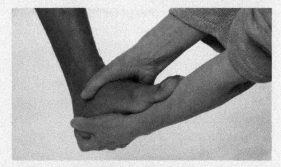

Figure 14.10 'Bootjack' handhold.

1. HANDHOLD

Cup the patient's heel with your hand from below, with the length of the plantar surface of the foot resting along your forearm. Using the web between the thumb and index finger of your other hand, wrap around the front of the ankle contacting the talus. The strong interosseous talocalcaneal ligament acts as the fulcrum for motion between these two bones. It is the developmental midpoint of the ankle and is therefore a useful reference for any assessment of alignment in the joint and is highly proprioceptive.

2. ENGAGEMENT AND BALANCE

With the forearm still along the sole of the patient's foot and the hand around the heel, dorsiflex the ankle slightly, while at the same time anteriorising the calcaneus. The web of the other hand is applying pressure to help posteriorise the talus. The focus is on the subtalar joint and the talocalcaneal ligament. It may require patience to find the point of balance and await a release. As the release begins to be felt, the 'story' of past inversion, eversion strains, etc., reveal themselves as the talus is encouraged posteriorly. A composite balance point emerges for all the vectors absorbed and held in the tissues.

3. RESOLUTION PHASE

In the resolution phase that follows, *the ligaments often retrace the pattern of the injury before realigning.* It is important to respect the idiosyncrasies of whatever 'return journey' the tissues choose as their path towards health. After the realignment, pressure is slowly released as the patient takes back postural control.

For added emphasis, it is possible to engage postural cooperation by *asking the patient to gently plantar flex the foot which is lying along the length of your forearm.* By resisting this action, you are introducing an additional amount of traction to disengage the calcaneus from the talus from above.

Chopart's joint

Chopart's joint or transverse tarsal joint is the composite plane of articulation of the head of the talus with the navicular, and the articulation of the calcaneus with the cuboid, i.e., talus and calcaneus proximally and navicular and cuboid distally. The main action at Chopart's joint is rotational, to help accommodate for uneven surfaces. This is the point of division of hindfoot from the midfoot.

When working on Chopart's joint, i.e., the relationship of the hindfoot with the midfoot, the functional fulcrum is through the cuboidonavicular ligament. This is a continuation of the interosseous talocalcaneal ligament which then extends to the middle metatarsal. It is the developmental midline of the ankle and foot and thus is a highly proprioceptive organising structure, key in the proprioceptive feedback of this self-correcting mechanism.

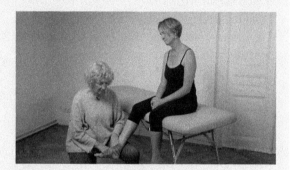

Figure 14.11 Chopart's joint hold.

1. HANDHOLD

Working from the patient's side, *contact the hindfoot by wrapping the web of your upper hand around the talus and calcaneus anteriorly, while contacting around the cuboid and navicular with the web of the other hand.*

The two hands are held close to each other in order to closely match the plane of Chopart's joint. It is important to remember that strong dorsiflexor tendons pass across this joint. These need to be in a relaxed position to allow the two hands to span the joints. The cuboid, laterally, gives a broad surface for contact, but the navicular is smaller, and a common mistake is to slip distally with the distal hand and contact the cuneiforms instead of the navicular.

2. TESTING AND ENGAGEMENT

Test for mobility in all the permissible directions of movement and, by going into the direction of ease, find a point of balance where all vectors feel in easy neutral.

In this composite joint which is more used to compressive forces of weight bearing, approximation will usually be of greater assistance than distraction in finding the point of ligamentous balance. To find the exact degree of approximation needed to match the compressive forces held in the joint, *lean your weight through your forearm fulcra on your thighs, to the degree that the ligaments seem to enliven and refine the position of balanced tension.*

3. REORGANISATION

Hold the point of balanced tension, allowing the ligaments to reorganise towards a more optimal position for resolution of any strain pattern.

This handhold in treatment will often show up more specific problems at either cuboid or navicular, which can then be addressed directly as described below. After rebalancing the cuboid and navicular, it is useful to return to Chopart's joint as a means of integrating the rotational balance of the hindfoot with the whole of the midfoot around its midline ligament.

Direct derotation of the cuboid with suspension

The cuboid and navicular may often need to be addressed individually.

It is common to find the cuboid twisted and dropping medially on its longitudinal axis, especially when the calcaneus has moved posteriorly in relation to the talus. As the cuboid articulates with the calcaneus, it is drawn back with it, leading it to its medial descent and rotation. This will take the 4th and 5th metatarsals with it as well as pulling the navicular or the lateral cuneiform down. In this way both the weight-bearing lateral longitudinal arch and the transverse arch become compromised.

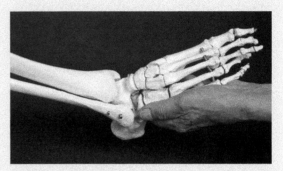

Figure 14.12 Cuboid hold on skeleton.

1. HANDHOLD

Suspension is used to float the cuboid within its ligamentous field. *Take a contact with the lateral aspect of your index finger on the cuboid from below and a thumb from above.*

2. DIRECT ACTION WITH SUSPENSION

Gently lift the medial side of the cuboid from beneath, within its articulations with the navicular medially, the calcaneus posteriorly, and the heads of the 4th and 5th metatarsals anteriorly. Allow it to balance with all the ligaments that surround it until you feel its medial aspect lifting.

If the patient is in a seated position, the weight of the leg and foot will often provide the degree of disengagement needed to assist the correction. *Placing the other hand under the heel can help to control the amount of distraction by subtly augmenting some of the weight of the foot.* It can also help to focus attention more specifically on the articulation between the cuboid and the calcaneus if required.

Navicular

The navicular can drop anteriorly and medially, especially if the head of the talus has moved forward. This has the effect of causing pressure on the spring ligament, resulting in the collapse of the spring arch as well as the transverse arch.

1. HANDHOLD

The navicular can be suspended in a similar way to the cuboid. It has a prominent tuberosity for contact but is narrower than the cuboid so needs to be *held between the middle finger below and the thumb above, floating it in the same way as the cuboid with assistance from gravity.*

Once the release is felt, *active turning of both navicular and cuboid may be needed to escort them directly back into position.*

Lift and spread of the 2nd cuneiform

The 2nd or middle cuneiform, which is the *keystone of the transverse arch,* may need individual attention.

A common sequence of events:

- If the hindfoot loses its integrity, allowing forward slippage of the talus on the calcaneus, this can cause an inversion of the cuboid and/or navicular.
- In turn, this can collapse the transverse arch so that the middle cuneiform is forced down and becomes wedged.
- This may take the proximal head of the metatarsal with it, collapsing the spring arch also. This collapse can also be caused by having the foot stepped on or having a heavy weight dropped on it.

The aim of the following manoeuvre is to open up the surrounding space to allow the middle cuneiform to lift back up into its position of keystone.

1. HANDHOLD

Place your middle fingers on the plantar surface of the foot, contacting the 2nd cuneiform from below and encouraging it to rise.

2. DIRECT ACTION LIFT AND SPREAD

In order to be able to lift the cuneiform back into position, you need to open up the space for it. This will require a composite action of *spreading and encouraging the arch from the sides and distracting the metatarsal heads from the front.*

Create a transverse spread with the thumbs from above. The pads of your index fingers lift the 2nd cuneiform from below as you wrap your hands around the transverse arch.

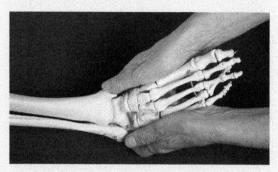

Figure 14.13 Simple cuneiform lift on skeleton.

At the same time, your thenar eminences are distracting the metatarsal heads, with the assistance of gravity on the suspended foot and by leaning your whole body slightly backwards. Wait with quiet steady insistence.

3. THE RESPONSE

As the ligaments start to let go, a space will open up and you may feel *the cuneiform lift back into its position.*

This procedure may at times produce results quickly, but often takes a little time and patience before the whole ligamentous complex wakes up and allows a change to take place. As with all these handholds, the hands around the foot are merely the point of contact; *activation occurs through your whole-body engagement with the proprioceptive fibres in the ligaments of the patient's foot.*

Tarsal arch lift with active patient cooperation

This is a more powerful approach for restoring the arches of the foot with resistance and the active postural cooperation of the patient; this can be used if simple lifting of the middle cuneiform, described above, has not produced sufficient resolution.

1. HANDHOLD AND POSTURAL COOPERATION

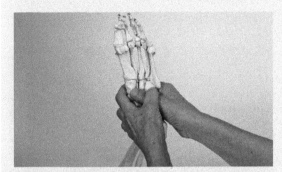

Figure 14.14 Handhold for active tarsal arch lift on skeleton.

Using a crossed thumb contact under the cuboid and 1st cuneiform, while wrapping your fingers around the dorsum of the transverse arch, ask the patient to dorsiflex the foot until you find a sense of balance in the ligaments. As this happens you may find that your thumbs move further apart as the foot is able to spread.

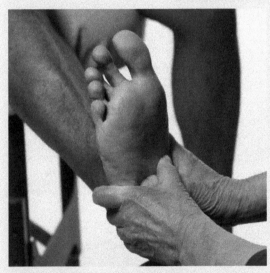

Figure 14.15 Tarsal arch lift, active patient dorsiflexion.

2. POSTURAL COOPERATION

Maintain the width you have gained as you ask the patient to slowly plantar flex against your resisting and spreading contact. The plantar flexion should begin with the toes, then the foot, and ankle. This is repeated two or three times if necessary. Each time the patient actively plantar flexes, the midtarsal bones are lifted into the space provided by your spread.

It is better to look for the beginnings of a release each time, before asking the patient to plantar flex gently. Your forces and the patient's should be comfortably matched rather than producing strain in your hands.

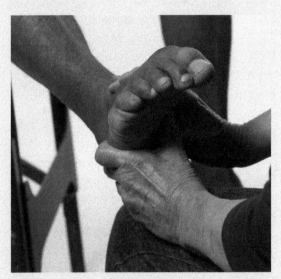

Figure 14.16 Tarsal arch lift, active patient plantar flexion.

Metatarsal lift using leverage with toe suspension

The metatarsals follow the transverse arch created by the cuboid and the cuneiforms. The proximal metatarsal heads may need assistance to lift, following the tarsal bone correction.

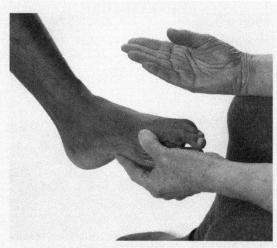

Figure 14.17 Proximal metatarsal head lift, leverage/suspension.

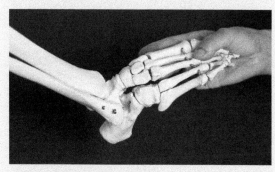

Figure 14.18 Proximal metatarsal head lift hold on skeleton.

1. POSITIONING

Sit in front of the patient who is seated on the couch with legs dangling.

2. HANDHOLD

Contact both ends of the metatarsal bone being addressed by placing your middle finger underneath the foot on the plantar surface of the proximal head. The thumb of the same hand contacts the dorsal surface of the distal head.

In this way the whole bone is suspended between finger and thumb, while the foot is positioned so as to take maximum advantage of the tractional weight of the ankle and leg behind it.

3. LEVERAGE WITH DISTRACTION

By introducing a slight upward leverage from under the proximal end, together with downward pressure on the distal end from above, the metatarsal can be encouraged to disengage at both ends and float out from the web of the other metatarsals surrounding it.

As with some of the other handholds it can be helpful to place the other hand under the heel in order to control the amount of weight needed to produce distraction.

Hallux valgus and Morton's neuroma

Common problems of the metatarsals are Morton's neuroma and hallux valgus. As mentioned previously, these have their origins in the destabilisation of the ankle joint, causing an anterior collapse of the talus on a posteriorised calcaneus.

Within the spring arch, if the navicular drops medially on the talar head, this causes a medial dropping of the cuneiforms also. This, in turn, can cause the 1st metatarsal to rotate internally at its proximal end and splay out at the distal end. In this way, the 1st metatarsophalangeal (MTP) joint is compromised, tending to form a bunion.

Likewise, within the weight-bearing arch, as the calcaneus moves posteriorly it leads to an internal rotation of the cuboid. This compromises the cuboid articulation with the 4th and 5th metatarsal heads and can sometimes lead to pinching of the interdigital nerve between the metatarsals, mimicking a Morton's neuroma (Wales 1992).

MTP and toe suspension for interphalangeal joints

Toes get twisted, bashed and bent. Each joint can be treated individually as required. *Contact is made by taking up the bone on each side of a joint between thumb and forefinger, bringing the whole joint to a point of balance and allowing the ligaments to bring about a resolution.*

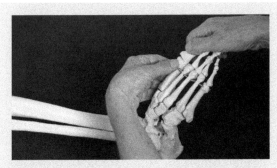

Figure 14.19 BLT hold for MTP of interphalangeal joint.

Toes can also be simply suspended with good effect; the ligaments will activate in response to the disengagement provided by the tractional

effect of suspension. As the joint fulcrum shifts, torsional strains will tend to exaggerate to their point of balanced tension and resolve.

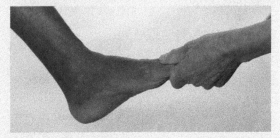

Figure 14.20 Toe suspension.

VIDEOS FOR CHAPTER 14

Scan the QR code or visit https://www.youtube.com/playlist?list=PL3j_YuMBqigGW6B4kHFmSJ_waN8Rq5_Xz to find a playlist of the videos that accompany this chapter.

REFERENCES

Wales, A.L. (1992) The living human foot: a viewpoint in osteopathy. Unpublished article.

Wales, A.L. (1995, 1996) British tutorial group meeting. North Attleboro, MA, USA.

For further sources, see bibliography.

CHAPTER 15

Supporting Lymphatic Flow

SUSAN TURNER

'The goal of an osteopathic treatment is to effect a more efficient interchange between all the fluids of the body across all tissue interfaces, extracellular and intracellular.'

(Wales 1995, quoting William Sutherland)

This was one of Dr Sutherland's last remarks to which Dr Wales would add 'And of course, that is physiology'. This refers to an interchange across the blood capillary membrane, interstitial fluid and cell membrane. It is with this 'connective tissue retort' (Wales 1988) that the osteopath engages in applying Dr Sutherland's lymphatic treatment sequence, described below. Its aim is to stimulate the production, flow and drainage of lymph from the interstitium through to the siphon action of its return into the venous system at the thoracic inlet.

The lymphatic system has been known since the time of Hippocrates yet, until relatively recently, it has received very little attention compared to its close associate, the cardiovascular system. It has always occupied an important place in osteopathic thinking, especially with reference to the treatment of febrile diseases.

It was the loss of Dr A.T. Still's children to meningitis in 1864 (Still 1908, pp. 87, 88) that inspired his resolution to find an effective way of treating infection, culminating in his realisation of the science of osteopathy on 22 June 1874 (Still 1908, pp. 258, 271, 339). An extraordinary rate of recovery from the 1918–19 Spanish flu was

recorded for people receiving osteopathic care, as compared with allopathic patients (Hulbert 1920). Having analysed both the medical and osteopathic records of the time, Arthur Hildreth noted a mortality rate of 50 deaths per 1000 (5%) for those under medicinal care, and 2.25 per 1000 (0.22%) in patients in osteopathic care (Hildreth 1942).

Alan Becker DO recounted how, when he and his brother Rollin were children, they did not see their father, Arthur Becker DO, for three months during the height of the epidemic. Like many others in the profession, he would leave home at 5am and return at 10pm treating his patients daily in their own homes (Becker 1998).

A.T. Still referred to the lymphatics as 'this fountain of life-saving water provided by nature to wash away impurities as they accumulate in our bodies' (Still 1899, p. 108). When he said 'We strike at the source of life and death when we go to the lymphatics' he was not exaggerating (Still 1899, p. 108). The lymphatics play a fundamental role in immunity and in the cleansing, maintenance and restoration of a healthy cellular environment throughout the body. The importance of their role in maintaining homoeostasis, controlling inflammation and in making nutrients and oxygen available to the cells and tissues cannot be overstated (Petrova and Koh 2020).

The study of the lymphatics draws our attention into the fluid microenvironment of the cells, capillary bed and interstitium. In the words of Still, once again, 'No space is so small that it is out of connection with the lymphatics, with their nerves, secretory and excretory ducts. The system of lymphatics is complete and universal in the whole body' (Still 1902, p. 65).

As a country doctor, it is likely that Dr Sutherland treated patients using these principles in the Spanish flu epidemic of 1918–19 along with many members of the osteopathic profession. His various accounts illustrate how treatment in the acute and convalescent phases of disease were a normal part of his osteopathic practice (Sutherland 1998, COT p. 35). In the experience of the author, this approach has proved invaluable in supporting the immune system and treating infection, e.g., colds, coughs, fevers. It is also useful for draining local areas of inflammation and congestion, as in sprained joints and fractures, to improve a self-healing tissue environment. Surprisingly, it often appears to have an unexpected benefit in the resolution of jet lag, where the tissues often show a congestive quality. Since almost all disease conditions are now understood to have an inflammatory component, improvement of lymphatic flow plays a crucial role in restoring health through normalising fluid interchange in the cellular environment (Zink 1970).

FUNCTIONS OF THE LYMPHATIC SYSTEM

- Drainage: The lymphatic system provides drainage of 10 per cent of body fluid from the interstitium into the venous system. This ensures optimum fluid balance in the cellular microenvironment, regulating the molecular composition of the extracellular matrix (ECM).
- Clearing of debris: This includes proteins and large molecules from the interstitial space which only the lymphatics can do. This is key in all inflammatory processes where increased capillary permeability causes proteins to leak into the interstitium producing stasis in the capillary network.
- Immune function: The production and distribution of lymphocytes is vital for protection against infection. The lymphatics also carry antigens to the lymph nodes where an immune response is initiated.
- Nutritive transport: Interstitial fluid and lymph flow ensure the availability of peptides, hormones, cytokines and oxygen etc. to the cells and tissues.
- Absorption and transport of lipids from the gut: It is also suggested that lymphatic vessels clear lipids from the walls of the large arteries, playing a role in the prevention of atherosclerotic plaque formation (Lemole 2016).

The lymphatic system consists of a network of capillaries (initial lymphatics), vessels, trunks and ducts, all draining unidirectionally to be returned to the venous system via the subclavian veins. The lymphatic vessels and interstitium together account for approximately 15 per cent of body fluids.

The immune function of the lymphatics works in concert with the encapsulated lymphoid organs, i.e., the nodes, spleen and thymus. In addition, non-encapsulated mucosal lymphatic tissue protects the interfaces with the external environment, e.g., tonsils, appendix and Peyer's patches. Through these interfaces, especially in early childhood, the mucosa-associated lymphatic tissue (MALT) response enables communication and simultaneous activation between all the mucous membranes of the body (Cesta 2006; Ruiz-Sanchez *et al.* 2017).

Lymphatic vessels are present in every tissue of the body except for avascular structures such as nails and cartilage. Their presence, even in bone, is now known to be significant in bone healing (Biswas, Chen and De Angelis 2023). They have been discovered to be present even in the venous sinuses of the cranium (Louveau *et al.* 2015, 2017) and these meningeal vessels have since been shown to be 'key regulators of neuroinflammation and neurodegeneration' (Petrova and Koh 2020).

The cerebrospinal fluid (CSF) fulfils an important cleansing function for the brain that is similar to action of the lymphatics for the rest of the body (Iliff *et al.* 2012). It has been postulated that the two intracranial fluid systems of lymph and CSF are crucial for clearing the brain of amyloid beta proteins found in high concentrations in sufferers from Alzheimer's disease (Louveau *et al.* 2017; Silva *et al.* 2021). Recent research has also shown that stress-induced brain inflammation is frequently present in depression and other psychiatric illnesses, suggesting the fundamental importance of efficient cerebral drainage (Lee and Giuliani 2019). A.T. Still's reference to the lymphatics consuming 'the finer fluids of the brain' (Still 1899, pp. 104–105) already acknowledges a significant relationship between the CSF and the lymphatics.

LYMPHATIC CIRCULATION

The natural flow of lymph circulation has three phases (Zink 1977):

- The *formation phase* consists of the movement of interstitial fluid into the lymphatic capillaries or *initial lymphatics.*
- In the *vascular phase* lymph is moved through the lymphatic vessels.

- In the *terminal phase*, 70 per cent of lymph drains via the thoracic ducts into the venous system at the subclavian veins. Thirty per cent drains directly into the venous system via the high endothelial venules, after being filtered in the lymph nodes (Mionnet *et al.* 2011).

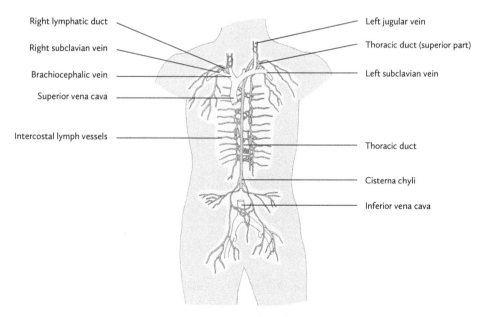

Figure 15.1 Lymphatic 'tree'.

Lymph originates as nutrient-rich blood plasma moving out of the vascular capillary bed into the interstitium. Here it becomes known as interstitial or extracellular fluid. The fluid then enters blind-ended tubes called initial lymphatics or capillaries where it becomes known as lymph. *To avoid confusion with the vascular capillaries, these will be referred by their alternative name, 'initial lymphatics'.*

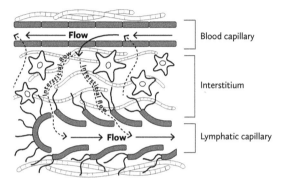

Figure 15.2 Fluid interchange between blood capillary, interstitium and lymphatic capillary.

The cyclic entry into the initial lymphatics is made possible because their walls consist simply of a single layer of endothelial cells overlap ping one another. The 'gaps', 'flaps' or 'button junctions' between these cells are open when the initial lymphatic is empty. This permits a cyclic influx of proteins and molecules that are too large to enter the capillary venules, to flow from the interstitium into the initial lymphatics.

For interstitial fluid to move into the initial lymphatics, a small uphill hydrostatic gradient must be overcome. This is made possible by normal extrinsic rhythmic tissue motion, such as thoracic pressure changes in respiration, cardiovascular pulse, gut peristalsis etc., all of which fluctuate the interstitial fluid. This explains why similarly small movements can be applied so effectively in osteopathic lymphatic treatment.

Lymph vessels tend to flow alongside arteries and veins and it has been shown that lymph flows faster where the vessel passes close to an artery (Moore and Bertram 2018). This is probably because pulsation of the vascular system transmits pressure and pulse to the lymphatic vessels. Conversely restrictions along the fascial planes, in which the lymphatic vessels are embedded, can in all likelihood impede flow and create congestion in the system. Twenty-five to 50% of lymph in the thoracic duct is produced in the liver (Tanaka and Iwakiri 2018).

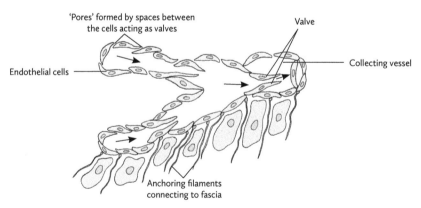

Figure 15.3 Lymph capillary, 'initial lymphatic'.

The endothelial cells in the walls of the initial lymphatics are each connected to the fascia by *anchoring filaments.* Because of this, they are responsive to every minute movement in the interstitium and wider tissue environment, especially the constant rhythmic motion of thoracic respiration. In response to the ebb and flow of interstitial fluctuation, fluid enters *non-selectively*, allowing in foreign antigens and large molecules. Their passage into the initial lymphatic increases the osmotic gradient within it, drawing in yet more fluid from the interstitium.

As the initial lymphatic fills with fluid, the gaps or button-like flaps close between the endothelial cells in the walls like valves. Once full, the fluid empties through a one-way valve in to a collecting lymphatic (Petrova and Koh 2020).

PERISTALSIS OF LYMPH VESSELS

The filling rate of the initial lymphatic for each cycle is somewhat inconclusive, and sources vary in their findings of between 5 and 10 seconds, i.e., between 6 and 12 contractions per minute (Margeris and Black 2012; Zawieja *et al.* 1993; McGeown, McHale and Thornbury 1987). The collecting lymphatics lead into vessels composed of a series of 2 mm-long chambers called *lymphangions.* These have smooth muscle walls lined by endothelial cells. One-way valves separate each lymphangion from the next one, ensuring unidirectional flow. The valves open and close in response to the pressure gradients on either side of them (Randolph *et al.* 2017).

The lymphangion units, comprising the lymph vessels, work in sequence as an *intrinsic lymphatic pump*, moving lymph by peristalsis. Stretch receptors in the smooth muscle wall,

on the downstream side of each valve, stimulate contractile waves to push a fluid bolus forward. The lymphangions also contain pacemaker cells for longitudinal continuity, further ensuring contraction in a specific direction. Lymphatic smooth muscle expresses ion channels that regulate the speed of contraction in a way that has been likened to the pacemaker system of the heart (Petrova and Koh 2020). Helden referred to lymphangions as 'tiny hearts' whose diastole and systole enable them to pump against increasing resistance (Van Helden 1993).

The lymphangions are self-propelling *so long as the path is clear with no tissue obstruction.* The implication of this, regarding osteopathic treatment, is that we only have to remove obstruction and get it moving for the flow to continue.

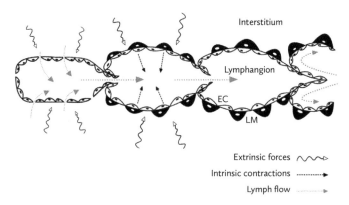

Figure 15.4 Lymphangion flow. EC, lymphatic endothelial cells; LM, lymphatic muscle cells.
Source: Solari, E., Marcozzi, C., Negrini, D., Moriondo, A. (2020) Lymphatic Vessels and Their Surroundings: How Local Physical Factors Affect Lymph Flow. Biology (Basel) 9 (12), 263. http://doi.org/10.3390/biology9120463.

DRAINAGE OF LYMPH INTO THE THORACIC DUCT

The lymphatic vessels coalesce to form larger lymphatic trunks named after the part of the body or organ they drain. Two main lumbar lymphatic trunks and one intestinal lymphatic trunk converge, normally forming the receptacle of the *cisterna chyli* which drains into the thoracic duct under the median arcuate ligament of the diaphragm. The median arcuate ligament acts as a fascial 'bridge' between the crura, forming a hiatus which the upward-flowing thoracic duct shares with the downward-flowing aorta. Sutherland was said to refer to the crura of the diaphragm as a 'central physiological plug for the body' with 'more effect on physiology than almost any other structure' (Wales 1988) (see Chapter 5). He emphasised the importance of freeing this portal to avoid the detrimental consequence of impeding aortic flow and lymphatic return (Sutherland 1990, TSO pp. 133–136).

The great lymphatic highway of the *thoracic duct* has randomly arranged valves and smooth muscle within the wall in the tunica media (Ilahi *et al.* 2021). It is only the width of a drinking straw and enters the thorax on the right side of the body of T12. It then crosses the front of the thoracic spine behind the aortic arch to drain into the left subclavian vein through a *lymphovenous valve* close to the junction with the left internal jugular vein. The lymph from the left side of the head, neck, arm and chest also enters the thoracic duct just before it enters the venous system.

A smaller right thoracic duct drains lymph from the right thorax, right side of the head, chest, neck and arm, and also the left ventricle of the heart, into the junction of the right subclavian and internal jugular vein (Feola *et al.* 1977). There are some variations in the structure of the thoracic ducts and their precise site of drainage. In a certain proportion of people, the cisterna chyli is absent as an anatomically distinct receptacle.

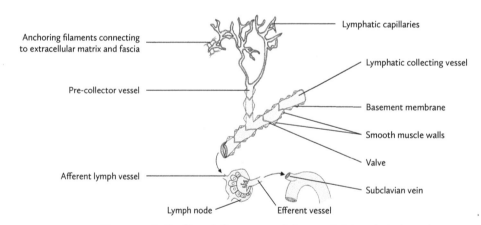

Figure 15.5 Path of lymph from extracellular matrix into subclavian vein.

Sutherland's thoughts on the thoracic duct

W.G. Sutherland likened the action of the major thoracic duct to a siphon, being a tube that takes fluid uphill before draining downhill. Once the fluid in a siphon is moving uphill it will continue its flow. With the diaphragm working as a pump at the lower end, and the suction flow in the duct as it ascends before descending into the subclavian vein, we see how apt this analogy is. The thoracic duct pierces the suprapleural membrane both on its ascent and descent, making it a perfect arrangement for the suction action of the siphon to benefit fully from the rhythmic movement of the thorax. The return of lymph in the thoracic duct is therefore naturally self-propelling. This explains Sutherland's statement that, in the absence of fascial drag, 'All that is involved is the goal of keeping things moving in their normal channels and through all the little lymph nodes' (Sutherland 1990, TSO p. 138).

THE DIAPHRAGM AS A 'LYMPHATIC SPONGE'

In addition to lymphatic return through the thoracic duct, the diaphragm contains tiny channels or 'lacunae' for the passage of lymph from the lower body into the thorax (Abu-Hijleh *et al.* 1995). Lymphatic vessels converge upon the lacunae from the peritoneum, gut, posterior body wall, pelvis and legs to drain mainly into the retrosternal nodes, before returning to the venous system via the thoracic duct. Free rhythmic respiratory movement of the diaphragm is essential to the pumping of these sponge-like channels.

Respiratory movement at both the diaphragmatic crura and the thoracic inlet are important for lymphatic flow through the thoracic duct. Thirty to sixty per cent of thoracic duct activity was found to be produced by pressure changes through the thorax and crura in respiration (Zink 1977).

THE OMENTUM

The omentum (Latin for 'apron') is the largest peritoneal fold, forming a thin, superficial covering over the intestines and lower abdomen. It is suspended from the greater curvature of the stomach and first part of the duodenum and encloses nerves, blood vessels, lymph channels, and connective and fatty tissue. It develops from the mesenteric root, connecting the stomach to the posterior abdominal wall. The lesser omentum is a double layer of peritoneum extending from the porta hepatis of the liver to the lesser curvature of the stomach.

This extraordinary organ contains angiogenic factors that stimulate the growth of new blood vessels as well as key neurotransmitters and nerve growth factors that enhance tissue growth. Because of this, it has been used for over a century to heal damaged organs and spinal cord injuries (Jurkiewicz and Arnold 1977). It moves by chemotaxis and has often been found wrapped around areas of infection and trauma, sealing off the area and limiting the spread of intraperitoneal infections. It also has the capacity to absorb fluid and reduce oedema (Forte *et al.* 2019; Wang *et al.* 2020).

Rich in lymphatic tissue, it is one of the body's main reserves of lymphocytes and macrophages which are activated as the first line of defence against foreign antigens (Meza-Perez and Randall 2017). Research on anaesthetised rats has re-examined some of the methods used by early osteopaths for treating infection, e.g., abdominal and upper thoracic lymph pump techniques. These simple manoeuvres resulted in a notable increase in immune cells in the circulation (Hodge *et al.* 2010). Oscillation or transmitted vibration of the omentum forms part of the lymphatic treatment sequence described below.

LYMPH NODES

The lymph nodes play a crucial role in immune surveillance. Lymph must be filtered in the lymph nodes before it re-enters the blood vascular circulation. Nodes are found predominantly in clusters in the areas of flexion in embryological development that form 'bottlenecks', i.e., the axillary and inguinal regions, pelvis, mediastinum and neck. These areas are especially prone to lymphatic congestion.

Afferent lymphatic vessels carry lymph into the nodes, enabling it to be filtered through the medullary sinuses and reticular network where immune cells move about 'sampling' antigens.

Thirty per cent of the lymph entering the lymph nodes is taken back into the bloodstream by the *high endothelial venules*, having passed the 'surveillance test' (Blanchard *et al.* 2021; Mionnet *et al.* 2011). The efferent lymphatics leaving the nodes carry the remaining, more concentrated lymph, together with circulating lymphocytes, back to the venous system at the thoracic inlet.

THE SPLEEN

The spleen filters the blood, phagocytising and removing old defective blood cells for the recycling of iron. It also plays a vital role in making and maturing B and T lymphocytes and blood cells. Every drop of blood entering the spleen is filtered for foreign particles by lymphocytes. It is a huge reservoir for monocytes which are released into the bloodstream whenever a crisis occurs such as coronary infarction, a wound or microbial invasion.

MUCOSA-ASSOCIATED LYMPHATIC TISSUE (MALT)

The greatest concentration of lymphatic tissue in the body is found at the mucosal interface of the internal and the external environments, e.g., at the mucous membranes of the respiratory, vaginal and gastrointestinal tracts (GITs). Together they are referred to as mucosa-associated lymphatic tissue (MALT). The MALT response initiates immediate communication between all mucosal tissues (Flynn *et al.* 2020). This explains why inflammation or irritation in one mucosal tissue can activate a response in another, e.g., nasal congestion in response to certain foods to which a person is intolerant. The MALT response is especially active in early childhood to allow the development of helpful microbiota (Zheng *et al.* 2020).

It is at the interfaces of MALT that the body's defence system needs to be most active. Gastrointestinal-associated lymphatic tissue (GALT) is estimated to comprise more immune cells than any other tissue. Another important site is Waldeyer's ring which protects the entry to the respiratory and GITs. This consists of adenoids and tubal, palatine and lingual tonsils. Peyer's patches provide immune surveillance and immune response in the gut.

THYMUS

The thymus is most active neonatally and up to the age of puberty. It does not filter lymph but matures, proliferates and activates the thymocytes produced in bone marrow to differentiate them into antigen specific T cells. The majority of these (i.e., any that produce a reaction when presented with self antigens) are destroyed in the process of negative selection. Only mature T cells that do *not react* to the body's own antigens are released for distribution in the lymphatic tissues of the body. In this way the thymus primes the immune system, teaching tolerance of self and avoidance of autoimmune reactions, i.e., discrimination between self and non-self. The position of the thymus behind the manubrium and body of the sternum merits consideration of the importance of free respiratory movement at the thoracic inlet (see manubrial lift, Chapter 5).

THE ROLE OF THE LYMPHATICS IN INFLAMMATION

Inflammation is a natural and important mechanism to control infection. However, when long-term, it is also a fundamental component of almost all disease processes. Chronic low-grade inflammation, for example, tends to be increasingly prevalent with ageing. Where inflammation becomes chronic, accumulation of protein in the interstitium leads to fibrosis, including scar tissue which can result in lymphoedema.

One of the dangers of inflammation is that it raises capillary permeability. This enables pro-inflammatory mediators to allow effector molecules (a molecule that binds to protein and regulates its activity) like complement and immunoglobulin into the interstitium. This increased influx of proteins and inflammatory mediators (e.g., cytokines) can only be drained by the initial lymphatics (capillaries) before they can be carried back to the systemic arterial circulation to be broken down. If an inflammatory response is too extreme, inflammation can cause the endothelial valve junctions of the initial lymphatics to close. This will prevent removal of inflammatory components from the interstitium. The maintenance of the osmotic gradient by which the initial lymphatics fill, and then drain, is dependent on their ability to constantly clear the interstitium of large effector molecules. Where this fails, inflammation can cause stasis of the local capillaries, so that the tissues become saturated with fluid, impeding the interstitial interchange necessary for cellular respiration (Randolph et al. 2017).

This static load is itself pro-inflammatory, which is why disturbance to lymphatic drainage is implicated in chronic inflammatory diseases. For resolution of inflammatory processes, interstitial clearance by the lymphatics is therefore essential. In such cases, the osteopathic application of gentle external forces can help to break the stasis, restimulate flow and ease obstruction.

To some extent, the proteoglycan filaments in the ECM counter compressibility and contribute to tissue hydration and resiliency. However, because the lymph channels are compressible, lymph flow can be obstructed anywhere that there is tissue tension. Fascial drag, torsion or compression through postural strains, scar tissue or ligamentous-articular strains appear to impede flow. It is this very delicacy and sensitivity of the lymphatic channels, though, that make them responsive to gentle osteopathic treatment.

THE VAGUS AND ITS SUPPORTING ROLE IN CONTROLLING INFLAMMATION

The immune system is in constant communication with the autonomic and central nervous systems and the vagus nerve is one of the important elements. The vagus provides internal surveillance to assist the lymphatics in protecting against the damaging effects of exaggerated inflammatory responses. It has an immunoregulatory function through its fast-acting efferent component. This can exert a specific cholinergic, anti-inflammatory response to calm or inhibit excessive cytokine production where necessary (Johnson and Webster 2009). In addition, its afferent component plays an important immunosensory role in detecting inflammation in the liver, spleen, visceral organs and reticuloendothelial system. This information is relayed back to the brain, enabling the efferent and afferent vagal pathways to coordinate immune response through the mediation of the hypothalamus and medullary vagal nuclei (Tracey 2009). With the vagus in mind, suboccipital muscle inhibition has been used since the earliest days of osteopathy when it was used in the calming of fevers.

PATHS OF LYMPH DRAINAGE

An important point for lymphatic drainage of the head is the jugulodigastric area between the transverse processes of the atlas and the mandible. This is a common area of tension, whether from emotional causes, dental malocclusion or neck tension, etc. Yawning may be nature's way of releasing obstruction here.

The arms and breasts drain below the axillary fold and then through the costoclavicular space before entering the thoracic duct. This is of special relevance when considering inflammatory conditions of the arms, hands and breasts and illustrates the importance of free movement of the clavicles and first ribs.

The femoral triangle and posterior knee are potential sites of impediment to drainage of lymph from the legs before passing through the abdominal lymph nodes on the posterior abdominal wall. Lymph from the gut drains through the root of the mesenteries, suggesting the potential risk imposed by fascial drag through visceroptosis and poor abdominal tone.

In normal function the lymphatic drainage from the heart at the junction of the atria and the ventricles is responsive to tensional changes in the pericardial fascia with each contraction. Cardiac lymph drains into the pericardium, through the mediastinal fascia and into the right thoracic duct (Miller 1982; Loukas, Abel and Tubbs 2011).

The transitional areas of the spine, i.e., occipito-atlantal (OA), cervico-thoracic, thoraco-lumbar and lumbo-sacral (LS) junctions, are key in global lymphatic flow but also particularly vulnerable to obstruction (see Chapter 2).

THE ROLE OF THE LYMPHATICS IN DISEASE PREVENTION AND HEALING

'Health represents the harmonious and undisturbed flow of fluid.'

(Still 1899)

A large body of research since the 1960s has illustrated the importance of lymphatic flow and drainage in relation to chronic, acute and inflammatory disease.

Cardiovascular disease
Many studies demonstrate the importance of the role played by the lymphatics in the prevention and healing of cardiovascular disease, including myocardial infarction and atherosclerosis. Chronic cardiac lymph obstruction has been shown to produce thickening and fibrotic changes of the coronary arterial wall. There is evidence that atherosclerosis is more of an inflammatory, proliferative disease than a degenerative one. This emphasises the importance of lymphatic clearance of the mediators that promote this disease process (Brakenheilm and Alitalo 2019).

Research using experimental animals with cardiac lymph drainage pathways either obstructed or removed showed resultant thickening and fibrotic changes in the mitral and tricuspid valves, as well as oedema, haemorrhage, ischaemia and fibrosis of the ventricular wall (Ullal *et al.* 1972).

Experiments with induced myocardial infarction on lymph-obstructed dogs showed delayed healing time, increased progression in seriousness of the infarct and degenerative changes, as compared with dogs in the control group with cardiac lymphatics intact (Kline *et al.* 1964; Miller 1963). Injection of hyaluronidase to open the lymphatics during an attack was shown, as early as the 1970s, to reduce the size of the infarction and preserve the ischaemic zone from further infarction (Marko *et al.* 1975; Yotsumoto *et al.* 1998; Huang, Lavine and Randolph 2017). This, again, is an indication of the importance of lymphatic clearance.

Tumours

It has been observed that the lymphatic drainage from cancerous tumours is greatly reduced (Steinskorg *et al.* 2016). This may suggest that healthy lymphatic drainage could provide some protection from the development of cancer in the organs and tissues concerned or render them more cancer-prone where lymph flow is obstructed or reduced. In 1902, A.T. Still wrote: 'Growths in the abdomen, such as tumors, only form when some channel of drainage is shut off' (Still 1902, p. 36).

Respiratory illness

'Pneumonia is too much dirt in the wheels of the lungs; if so we must wash it out. Nowhere can we go to a better place for water than the lymphatics.'

(Still 1899, p. 109)

Pneumonia and asthma both involve the smaller airways, e.g., terminal bronchioles and alveoli, where the mucociliary mechanism does not reach. For this reason, lymphatic clearance is crucial in the resolution of these acute conditions since, if they become chronic, this risks inflammation leading to the development of fibrosis (Ebina and Takahashi 2013). Healthy thoracic respiratory excursion enables lymph to be pumped by alternately opening and closing of the lymphatic capillaries.

Lymphatic support is diminished in most respiratory disease where thoracic excursion is frequently much reduced. This illustrates why rib raising has been so effectively used by osteopaths for the treatment of acute respiratory diseases since its earliest beginnings (Platt 1920). Hodge has shown that osteopathic lymphatic pump techniques, in experimental animals, can be used successfully to treat pneumonia (Hodge 2012).

Inflammatory bowel disease (IBD)

It has been suggested by a number of researchers that IBD is related to lymphatic dysfunction or obstruction (Bernier-Latmani and Petrova 2017). The tendency for gut inflammation to lead to fibrosis has its own consequence of increasing lymphatic obstruction. This, in turn, can result in yet more IBD. Where the intestinal lymphatics of experimental animals were removed, this was shown to produce bowel changes similar to IBD (Kalima *et al.* 1976; Witte and Witte 1984).

Histological studies have consistently revealed mesenteric lymphatic obstruction in Crohn's disease (Heatley *et al.* 1980). Hodge has again demonstrated that the use of traditional osteopathic lymphatic treatment procedures on experimental animals are effective in IBD (Hodge *et al.* 2010; Schander *et al.* 2020).

Pancreatitis

Lymph drainage has been shown to dramatically reduce the damaging effects of pancreatic enzymes on the pancreas in rats with acute oedematous pancreatitis (Hartwig *et al.* 2005). Obliteration of pancreatic lymph vessels can lead to fatal necrotic pancreatitis (Alexander *et al.* 2010); acute pancreatitis may develop following thoracic duct ligation through the resultant sudden stoppage of lymphatic flow (Bedat *et al.* 2017).

Post-surgery

In the post-surgical recovery phase, neither of the intrinsic lymph pumps of diaphragmatic respiratory excursion nor peristalsis tend to work efficiently. Restoration of lymph flow and respiratory excursion by very gentle osteopathic treatment has been found to be supportive of recovery (Ettlinger 2017).

CONTRAINDICATIONS TO THE LYMPHATIC TREATMENT SEQUENCE

There are certain contraindications and precautions to consider before stimulating lymph flow.

- An absolute contraindication is in patients with anuresis if they are not on dialysis. This is because this carries a risk of pulmonary oedema, leading to necrotising fasciitis in the area concerned.
- There is a relative risk for patients with congestive heart failure (CHF), as there is an inability to tolerate excessive preload, and residual volume may increase post-treatment.
- Care needs to be taken in applying the upper thoracic lymphatic 'siphon' in patients with a pacemaker so as not to disturb or put pressure on it.
- In patients with severe IBS and abdominal distension, the application of the omental lift needs to be very gently adapted to the sensitivity of the area.
- In cellulitis and its complication, necrotising fasciitis, the area needs to be rested/immobilised, avoiding vigorous exercise as too much movement risks spreading the infection. In such cases, necessary local decongestion and improvement of interstitial interchange can be achieved by simply holding the area to support any tissue movement naturally present. Stimulatory treatment however should be avoided.

In preliminary examination, it is advisable to check for supraclavicular oedema as an indication of lymphatic oedema, followed by palpation of Virchow's node which is a thoracic duct end node.

In patients receiving treatment for cancer, lymphatic treatment should be avoided.

There is no contraindication to using lymphatic techniques in febrile viral infection and post-infection recovery where it can be extremely helpful.

THERAPEUTIC ENGAGEMENT

Lymphatic sequence

'You realise that you are a mechanic of the fluids of the body as well as the osseous tissues, which are also fluid.'

(Sutherland 1990, TSO p. 192)

In the preliminary assessment of a patient, it is important to check the retroclavicular space for swelling, as a sign of lymphatic congestion. Check also for swollen lymph nodes in the neck, axillae and groin.

The following sequence should be adapted to the patient and pre-existing condition in terms of depth, speed, rate of the transmitted vibration and appropriateness of the manoeuvre. This consists essentially of the following areas of attention:

- Transmitted vibration to facilitate 'siphon' action for lymph flow from the thoracic duct into the left subclavian vein. Follow through with the right.

- Releasing restriction to the passage of lymph from the cisterna chyli into the thoracic duct as it passes under the median arcuate ligament between the diaphragmatic crura. The 12th rib provides a 'handle' to access and release the arcuate ligaments.
- Setting up an oscillatory frequency to stimulate the cisterna chyli and immune reservoir in the omentum.
- Oscillation of the lymphatic channels in the lower and upper extremities.

Before addressing the lymphatic system directly, it is advisable to release any areas of tissue tension or fascial drag, especially those affecting the thoracic inlet, diaphragm and pelvis.

The relationship between the clavicles, first rib and anterior cervical fascia is especially important for drainage into the subclavian veins. Fixed lumbar lordosis of pregnancy, involving tight crura, merits attention for the passage of lymph into the thoracic duct.

1. Restoring flow in the 'siphon' of the thoracic duct into the venous system

With regard to the following procedure, quoting Dr Sutherland, Dr Wales emphasised that this is not a 'lymphatic pump', but an activation of the inherent action of a 'siphon'. It is made more effective when the operator is well-grounded through the feet, synchronising breathing with that of the patient and in resonance with the tissues in hand, heart and mind.

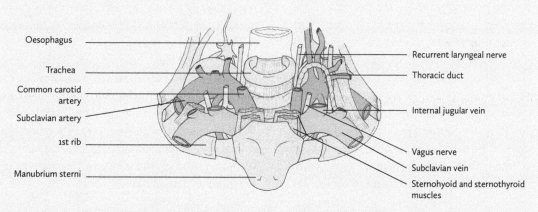

Figure 15.6 Thoracic inlet with thoracic duct, anterior view.

Caution: Anne Wales warned against putting weight into the patient's thorax during this manoeuvre. It should be only enough to transmit a vibratory impulse to the thoracic duct and fine channels within the fascia. 'We are admonished in all our treatments not to wound the lymphatics... It behooves us to handle them with care and tenderness' (Still 1899, p. 105).

The order in which this sequence is approached may vary.

1. CONTACT
Standing on the right side of the supine patient, with a gentle, plastic contact, place the fingers of one (passive, afferent) hand along the left second or third intercostal spaces. The contact is near the midclavicular line with fingers pointing towards the axilla. The other (active) hand is placed over the monitoring hand.

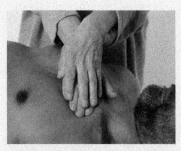

Figure 15.7 Lymphatic siphon manoeuvre.

2. SIPHON ACTION
Moving from the shoulder and with straight arms, transmit a vibration via the active (top) hand through to the sensory, monitoring hand beneath, to move the local fascia and fluid matrix.

The frequency of transmitted vibration is guided by the tissues themselves and their natural rhythmic resiliency so nothing is forced. *This induced fascial motion will be directed and received posteriorly, at the thoracic duct close to the spine.* The aim is to stimulate activity in its smooth muscle wall, to support the upward flow of lymph towards the subclavian vein. The activity of the axillary lymph nodes is also beneficially stimulated.

This is continued until a change is felt in the quality of the tissues beneath. There may be a sense of increased spaciousness, warmth or flow, sometimes with an impression of gentle upward movement. An enlivening effect can sometimes be observed throughout the fascia of the thorax and lung field. *Do not continue after this change is felt.*

This should be repeated for the junction of the right lymphatic trunk with the subclavian vein, standing on the left side of the patient.

2. Releasing tension around the cisterna chyli and posterior abdominal wall
Sit at the supine patient's right side with one sensory (monitoring) hand cradling the 12th rib. The other (motor) hand provides slight leverage under the monitoring hand.

1. FREEING THE 12TH RIB
Each time the patient exhales, lean back slightly to take up the slack as the rib relaxes laterally through several respiratory cycles. Resist the 'pull-back' on each inhalation until relaxation is felt at the costovertebral junction. The effectiveness of this is because the action is gentle enough to be below the level of tissue resistance.

2. FREEING THE FLOW INTO THE THORACIC DUCT
Once free, *the rib is used as a 'handle' to access the posterior abdominal wall via the lateral, medial and median arcuate ligaments.* These 'lumbocostal arches' are continuous with the suspension of the lateral arcuate ligaments from the 12th ribs (as described in Chapter 4).

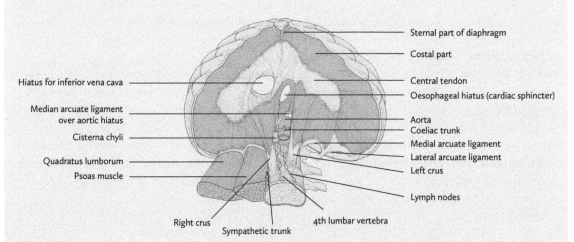

Figure 15.8 Posterior diaphragm showing the passage of the cisterna chyli under the median arcuate ligament.

Lean back slightly to create balanced tension in relation to the resistance in the tissues as the arches progressively relax laterally to medially each time the patient exhales.

Direct your awareness to within the cisterna chyli where it enters the thoracic duct under the median arcuate ligament, as the patient's breathing facilitates the flow of lymph.

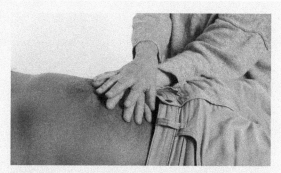

Figure 15.10 Omental oscillation manoeuvre.

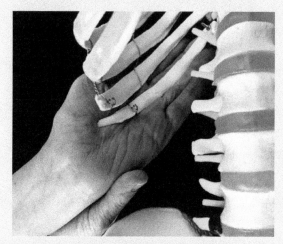

Figure 15.9 12th rib hand contact.

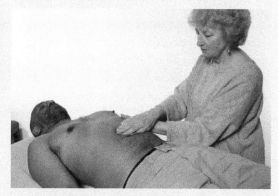

Figure 15.11 Cisterna chyli oscillation.

3. Abdominal lymphatic oscillation

1. CONTACT

For activation of the immune omental reservoir and abdominal lymphatics, *make a light plastic sensory contact over the patient's lower abdomen with one hand.*

Place the other (active) hand over it to gently engage the underlying lymphatic tissues through transmitted vibration and a slight cephalad lift. The endpoint is often signified by a sense of softening and unification of fluid activity in the abdomen.

4. Cisterna chyli simulation

2. TRANSMITTED VIBRATION

The flow through the cisterna chyli into the thoracic duct may be further enhanced by directing a transmitted vibration towards it from the upper abdomen.

5. Facilitating lymphatic flow through the lower extremity

This is useful both for re-establishing flow in local areas of congestion or inflammation and for integrating the flow of lymph with the body as a whole.

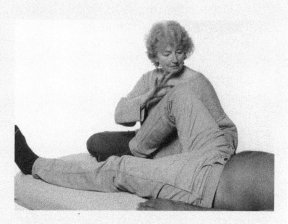

Figure 15.12 Leg lymphatic oscillation.

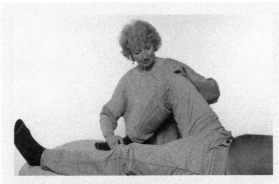

Figure 15.13 Alternative hand contact.

1. POSITION AND CONTACT

Stand facing the supine patient on the side to be addressed. The patient's knee is flexed with the foot flat on the table and the hip in a position of easy fascial neutral between internal and external rotation.

With one hand, hold the flexed knee, either between index finger and thumb or simply with one finger. The other hand monitors either from the foot or the hip.

2. INDUCING OSCILLATION

Induce a small medial/lateral oscillation of the knee, at a frequency which is taken up by the tissues themselves and is then self-perpetuating through the fascia of the whole limb. The intention is to fluctuate the extracellular fluid to facilitate flow in the lymphatic capillaries and vessels.

It is helpful to place your awareness within the ECM and minute lymphatic spaces. Continue until you sense fluid moving from the lower to the upper hand like a unified peristaltic wave through the limb.

The action of iliopsoas, responding to the oscillation of the hip, may stimulate the opening of the cisterna chyli. This manoeuvre may also be used simply for the purpose of balancing the fascia of an injured hip through the extracellular fluid.

6. Facilitating lymph flow in the upper extremity

1. CONTACT

Sit or stand beside the supine patient whose shoulder and arm should be relaxed, with the elbow at approximately 90 degrees, so that anterior and posterior fascial tone is balanced.

Hold the patient's hand in a 'shaking hands' position with one hand, the other hand monitoring his or her elbow. The patient's forearm should, initially, be in a fascial neutral position between pronation and supination and comfortably flexed at the elbow.

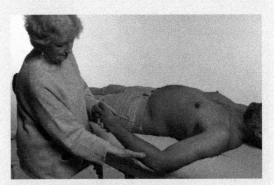

Figure 15.14 Lymphatic oscillation via the arm.

2. INDUCING OSCILLATION

Induce rhythmic oscillation in the patient's forearm fascia by slight alternate supination and pronation of your wrist to fluctuate the fine fluid channels and augment lymph flow. Continue until a tissue change or upward fluid wave is felt through the limb.

When successful, the end result is often a sense of the unified fluid field of the ECM in which the tissues of the whole body are softer, more perfused and more relaxed.

Pectoralis lift

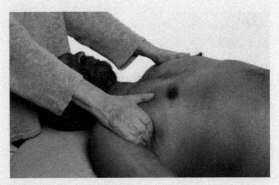

Figure 15.15 Pectoralis lift.

A simple lymphatic manoeuvre attributed to the 'lymphomaniac' Gordon Zink DO, but never recorded in print, involves standing behind the head of the supine patient and folding your fingers under the pectoralis major muscles on each side. *Lean back slightly, gaining a little more cephalad lift and relaxation of the muscle with each respiratory cycle.* If you place your awareness inside the thorax as if looking at its walls from the inside, it is possible to gain a sense of the whole thorax lifting as far down as the median arcuate ligament at the lower entry point of the thoracic duct.

VIDEOS FOR CHAPTER 15

Scan the QR code or visit https://www.youtube.com/playlist?list=PL3j_YuMBqigGrbJJ6jzk4LoBrZKhXQoXY to find a playlist of the videos that accompany this chapter.

REFERENCES

Abu-Hijleh, M.F., Habbal, O.A., Moqattash, S.T. (1995) The role of the diaphragm in lymphatic absorption from the peritoneal cavity. *J Anat 186* (Pt 3), 453–467.

Alexander, J.S., Ganta, V.C., Jordan, P.A., Witte, M.H. (2010) Gastrointestinal lymphatics in health and disease. *Pathophysiology 17* (4), 315–335.

Becker, A. (1998) Personal communication.

Bedat, B., Scarpa, C.R., Sadowski, S.M., Triponez, F., Karenovics, W. (2017) Acute pancreatitis after thoracic duct ligation for iatrogenic chylothorax. A case report. *BMC Surgery 17* (9). https://doi.org/10.1186/s12893-017-0204-3.

Bernier-Latmani, J. & Petrova, T.V. (2017) Intestinal lymphatic vasculature: structure, mechanisms and functions. *Nature Reviews Gastroenterology & Hepatology 14* (9). https://doi.org/10.1038/nrgastro.2017.79.

Biswas, L., Chen, J., De Angelis, J. (2023) Lymphatic Vessels in Bone Support Regeneration After Injury. *Cell 186* (2), 233–460.

Blanchard, L. & Girard J-P. (2021) High endothelial venules (HEVs) in immunity, inflammation and cancer. *Angiogenesis 24,* 719–753. https://doi.org/10.1007/s10456-021-09792-8.

Brakenhielm, E. & Alitalo, K. (2019) Cardiac lymphatics in health and disease. *Nat Rev Cardiol 16* (1), 56–68. https://doi.org/10.1038/s41569-018-0087-8.

Cesta, M.F. (2006) Normal structure, function and histology of mucosa-associated lymphoid tissue. *Toxicol Pathol 34* (5), 599–608.

Ebina, M. & Takahashi, T. (2013) Disruption of airway lymphatics as a novel cause of impairment of airway clearance in severe asthma. *Clin and Translational Allergy 3* (1), O5. https://doi.org/10.1186/2045-7022-3-S1-O5.

Ettlinger, H. (2017) Osteopathic Cranial Academy Conference. Minneapolis, MN.

Feola, M., Merklin, R., Cho, S., Brockman, S.K. (1977) The terminal pathway of the lymphatic system of the human heart. *Ann Thorac Surg. 24* (6), 531–536.

Flynn, S.M., Chen, C., Artan, M., *et al.* (2020) MALT-1 mediates IL-17 neural signalling to regulate *C. elegans* behaviour, immunity and longevity. *Nat Commun 11* (1), 2099.

Forte, A.J., Cinotto, G., Boczar, D., *et al.* (2019) Omental lymph node transfer for lymphedema patients: a systematic review. *Cureus 11* (11), e6227. https://doi.org/10.7759/cureus.6227.

Hartwig, W., Hackert, T., Schneider, L., *et al.* (2005) Lymphatic drainage in acute pancreatitis: its relevance in the pathogenesis of pancreatic and pulmonary injury. *Pancreas 31* (4), 445.

Heatley, R.V., Bolton, P.M., Hughes, L.E., *et al.* (1980) Mesenteric lymphatic obstruction in Crohn's disease. *Digestion 20,* 307–313.

Hildreth, A.G. (1942) *The Lengthening Shadow of Dr. Andrew Taylor Still,* 2nd edition. Paw Paw, MI: A.G. Hildreth & A.E. Van Vleck; p. 419.

Hodge, L.M. (2012) Osteopathic lymphatic pump techniques to enhance immunity and treat pneumonia. *Int J Osteopathy Med 15* (1), 13–21. https://doi.org/10.1016/j.ijosm.2011.11.004.

Hodge, L.M., Bearden, M.K., Schander, A., *et al.* (2010) Lymphatic pump treatment mobilises leukocytes from the gut associated tissue into lymph. *Lymphat Res Biol 8* (2), 103–110.

Huang, L.H., Lavine, K.J., Randolph, G.J. (2017) Cardiac Lymphatic Vessels, Transport, and Healing of the Infarcted Heart. *JACC Basic Transl Sci. 2* (4), 477–483.

Hulbert, R.G. (1920) The Influenza Epidemic. *Journal of Osteopathy*, March, Vol xxvii, No 3.

Ilahi, M., St Lucia, K., Ilahi, T.B. (2021) Anatomy, Thorax, Thoracic Duct [Updated Jul 31]. In: StatPearls [Internet]. Treasure Island (FL): StatPearls Publishing. Available from: https://www.ncbi.nlm.nih.gov/books/NBK513227.

Iliff, J., Wang, M., Liao, Y., *et al.* (2012) A paravascular pathway facilitates CSF flow through the brain parenchyma and the clearance of interstitial solutes, including amyloid β. *Sci Transl Med 15* (4), 147ra111. https://doi.org/10.1126/scitranslmed.3003748.

Johnston, G.R. & Webster, N.R. (2009) Cytokines and the immunoregulatory function of the vagus nerve. *British Journal of Anaesthesia 102* (4), 453–462.

Jurkiewicz, M.J. & Arnold, P.G. (1977) The omentum. *Annals of Surgery 185* (5), 548–554.

Kalima, T.V., Saloniemi, H., Rahko, T., *et al.* (1976) Experimental regional enteritis in pigs. *Scand J Gastroenterol 11* (4), 353–363.

Kline, I.K., Miller, A.J., Pick, R., *et al.* (1964) The effects of chronic impairment of cardiac lymph flow on myocardial reactions after coronary artery ligation in dogs. *Am Heart J 68*, 515–523. https://doi.org/10.1016/0002-8703(64)90153-x.

Lee, C-H. & Giuliani, F. (2019) The role of inflammation in depression and fatigue. *Front Immunol 10*, 1696.

Lemole, G.M. (2016) The importance of the lymphatic system in vascular disease. *J Integr Cardiol 2*. https://doi.org/10.15761/JIC.1000188.

Loukas, M., Abel, N., Tubbs, R.S. (2011) The Cardiac Lymphatic System. *Clinical Anatomy 24*, 684–691.

Louveau, A., Plog, B.A., Antila, S., *et al.* (2017) Understanding the functions and relationships of the glymphatic system and meningeal lymphatics. *J Clin Invest Sept 127* (9), 3210–3219.

Louveau, A., Smirnov, I., Keyes, T.J., *et al.* (2015) Structural and functional features of the central nervous system lymphatic vessels. *Nature 523*, 337–341. https://doi.org/10.1038/nature14432.

Margeris, K.N. & Black, R.A. (2012) Modelling the lymphatic system: challenges and opportunities. *J R Soc Interface 9*, 601–612. https://doi.org/10.1098/rsif.2011.0751.

Marko, P.R., Davidson, D.M., Libby, P., *et al.* (1975) Effects of hyaluronidase administration on myocardial ischaemic injury in acute infarction. A preliminary study in 24 patients. *Ann Intern Med 82* (4), 516–520. https//doi.org/10.7326/0003-4819-82-4-516.

McGeown, J.G., McHale, N.G., Thornbury, K.D. (1987) The Role of External Compression and Movement in Lymph Propulsion in the Sheep Hind Limb. *J. Physiol. 387*, 83–93.

Meza-Perez, S. & Randall, T.D. (2017) Immunological functions of the omentum. *Trends in Immunology, 38* (7), 526–536. https://doi.org/10.1016/j.it.2017.03.002.

Miller, A.J. (1963) The lymphatics of the heart. *Arch Intern Med 112* (4), 501–511. https//doi.org/10.1001/archinte.1963.03860040097008.

Miller, A.J. (1982) *Lymphatics of the Heart*. New York, NY: Raven Press Books; p. 117.

Mionnet, C., Sanos, S., Mondor, I., *et al.* (2011) High endothelial venules as traffic control points maintaining lymphocyte population homoeostasis in lymph nodes. *Blood 118* (23), 6115–6122. https://doi.org/10.1182/blood-2011-07-367409.

Moore, J.E. & Bertram, C.D. (2018) Lymphatic system flows. *Ann Rev Fluid Mech 50*, 459–482.

Petrova, T.V. & Koh, G.Y. (2020) Biological functions of lymphatic vessels. *Science 369* (6500), eaax4063. https://doi.org/10.1126/.eaax4063.

Platt, R. (1920) As I find the flu this year. *The Journal of Osteopathy*, Vol xxvii, No 3. p. 153.

Randolph, G.J., Stoyan, I., Zinselmeyer, B.H., *et al.* (2017) The lymphatic system: integral roles in immunity. *Annu Rev Immunol 26*, (35), 31–52. https://doi.org/10.1146/annurev-immunol-041015-055354.

Ruiz-Sanchez, B.P., Cruz-Zarate, D., Estrada-Garcia, I., *et al.* (2017) Innate lymphoid cells and their role in immune response regulation. *Revista Alergia Mexico 64* (3), 347–363.

Schander, A., Castillo, R., Pareredes, D. & Hodge, L.M. (2020) Effect of abdominal lymphatic pump treatment on disease activity in a rat model of inflammatory bowel disease. *J Am Osteopath Assoc 120* (5), 337–344. https://doi.org/10.7556/jaoa.2020.052.

Silva, I., Silva, J., Ferreira, R., *et al.* (2021) Glymphatic system, AQP4, and their implications in Alzheimer's disease. *Neurol Res Pract 3* (1), 5. https://doi.org/10.1186/s42466-021-00102-7.

Solari, E., Marcozzi, C., Negrini, D., Moriondo, A. (2020) Lymphatic Vessels and Their Surroundings: How Local Physical Factors Affect Lymph Flow. *Biology (Basel) 9* (12), 263. http://doi.org/10.3390/biology9120463

Steinskorg, E.S.S., Sagstad, S.J., Wagner, M., *et al.* (2016) Impaired lymphatic function accelerates cancer growth. *Oncotarget 7* (29), 45789–45802. https://doi.org/10.18632/oncotarget.9953.

Still, A.T. (1899) *Philosophy of Osteopathy*. Kirksville, MO: A.T. Still; pp. 104–105, 108, 109.

Still, A.T. (1902) *Philosophy & Mechanical Principles*. Kansas City, MO: Hudson Kimberley Co.; pp. 36, 65.

Still, A. T. (1908) *Autobiography*. Kirksville, MO: A.T. Still; pp. 87, 88, 258, 271 & 339.

Sutherland, W.G. (1990) *Teachings in the Science of Osteopathy*. A.L. Wales (ed.). Fort Worth, TX: Sutherland Cranial Teaching Foundation, Inc./Rudra Press; pp. 127, 133–136, 138, 192.

Sutherland, W.G. (1998) *Contributions of Thought*, 2nd edition. A.L. Wales and A.S. Sutherland (eds). Fort Worth, TX: Sutherland Cranial Teaching Foundation, Inc.; p. 35.

Tanaka, M. & Iwakiri, Y. (2018) Lymphatics in the liver. *Curr Opin Immunol 53*, 137–142.

Tracey, K. (2009) Reflex control of immunity. *Nat Rev Immunol 9*, 418–428.

Ullal, S.R., Kluge, T.H., Gerbode, F., *et al.* (1972) Functional and pathologic changes in the heart following chronic cardiac lymphatic obstruction. *Surgery 71* (3), 328–334.

Van Helden, D.F. (1993) Pacemaker potentials in lymphatic smooth muscle of the guinea pig mesentery. *J Physiol* 465–479. https//doi.org/10.1113/jpyysiol.1993.sp019910.

Wales, A. (1988, 1995) Personal communication.

Wang, A.W., Prieto, J.M., Cauvi, D.M., *et al.* (2020) The greater omentum – a vibrant and enigmatic immunologic organ involved in injury and infection resolution. *Shock (Augusta, Ga)* 53 (4), 384–390.

Witte, C.L. & Witte, M.H. (1984) Lymphatics in the pathophysiology of edema. In: *Experimental Biology of the Lymphatic Circulation*. M.G. Johnston (ed.). New York: Elsevier; pp. 167–188.

Yotsumoto, G., Moriyama, Y., Yamaoka, A., *et al.* (1998) Experimental study of cardiac lymph dynamics and edema formation in ischemia/reperfusion injury – with reference to the effect of hyaluronidase. *Angiology 49* (4), 299–305.

Zawieja, D.C., Davis, K.L., Schuster, R., *et al.* (1993) Distribution, propagation and coordination of contractile activity in lymphatics. *Am J Physiol 264* (4 Pt 2), H1283–1291. https//doi.org/10.1152/ajpheart.1993.264.4.H1283.

Zheng, D., Liwinski, T., Elinav, E. (2020) Interaction between microbiota and immunity in health and disease. *Cell Research 30*, 492–506.

Zink, G. (1970) *The Osteopathic Holistic Approach to Homeoostasis*. AAO Yearbook. Indianapolis, IN: American Academy of Osteopathy.

Zink, G. (1977) Respiratory and circulatory care: the conceptual model. *Osteopathic Annals,* p.11.

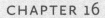

CHAPTER 16

Engaging with Traction and Addressing Specific Muscles

KOK WENG LIM

PART 1: THE USE OF TRACTION

CERVICAL TRACTION

This gentle, unhurried procedure can be deeply relaxing. It is useful for integrating the therapeutic changes that have taken place during a treatment and can also be a simple calming approach in itself.

CONTRAINDICATIONS

Cervical traction may be helpful in small disc protrusions but is contraindicated in many clinical situations such as acute whiplash injury, cervical spinal stenosis, Chiari malformation, syringomyelia, vertebral artery disease and Down's syndrome. Be aware that congenital conditions such as Chiari malformation may be symptom free and undiagnosed. It should also be avoided in patients with rheumatoid arthritis because of the fragility of the apical ligament between the odontoid peg and basiocciput.

THERAPEUTIC ENGAGEMENT

Cervical traction

BLT of the neck and spine can be engaged by traction. It is interesting to note that the writings of A.T. Still's student, Edythe Ashmore, referred to Dr Still's indirect 'tractional method' (Ashmore 1915). Sensitively applied traction may alert the vertebrae within the ligamentous spinal stocking to explore, express and release any inherent strain patterns such as torsion, sidebending, shear or even axial compression. Using the handhold suggested below, these can become apparent in the neck, thoracic and lumbar spine, down to the sacrum and pelvis via the core-link.

Engagement

To engage with the involuntary self-correcting action of the ligamentous-articular mechanism, *it is more effective for the operator to match the forces within the patient by leaning back slightly, using body weight rather than any active muscular pulling with hands and arms.* The reason for this is that the application of voluntary muscular effort will tend to engage only with the patient's voluntary musculoskeletal system.

To engage this intelligent mechanism through traction and enable the patient to surrender to the inherent therapeutic forces, *our contact needs to be safe, supportive and comfortable.* The sense of traction, tissue engagement and release unfold progressively on different levels. There should never be any sense of hurry since it is the inherent forces that set the tempo for the treatment.

1. HANDHOLD
Standing behind the head of the supine patient, place the palms of both hands under the neck, one resting over the other.

The ulnar borders of the two hands are placed horizontally along the supraocciput just above the occipito-atlantal (OA) junction. This is to avoid disturbing the temporal bones or occipitomastoid sutures.

The palms cradle the neck while the thumbs hold each side of the spinous processes of T1/T2. In this way the tractional forces are well distributed through the neck without any risk of destabilising the cranio-cervical or cervico-thoracic junctions which are fully supported.

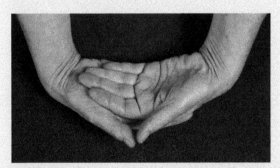

Figure 16.1 Hand position for cervical traction.

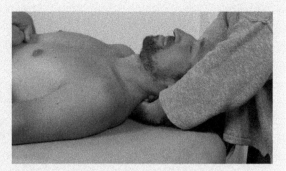

Figure 16.2 Hand position for cervical traction on live model.

2. ACTION
Lift the patient's head very slightly into cervical flexion by sinking your own weight, and gradually introduce the merest traction by shifting your weight backwards onto your heels. Your stance should be broad-based.

3. ENGAGEMENT
The direction of traction is in an arc along the long axis of the neck and spine, sweeping upwards towards the vertex of the patient's head. *Listen for the first hint of ligamentous engagement which often occurs as the first moment of tissue resistance is perceived.*

4. READING TISSUE RESPONSE
Subtle twists and sidebending patterns may become apparent, as the ligamentous spinal stocking expresses previously undiagnosed positional strains held in the tissues. *With your still hands, quietly maintain the same steady degree of subtle traction as you observe one vertebral segment after another seeking its position of BLT, releasing and realigning.*

5. SIMPLY MATCHING RESISTANCE
If you meet resistance at any level, resist pulling against it. If you wait at the barrier, simply matching the forces present, the patient's thoracic respiration normally resolves the strain.

6. PROGRESSIVE ENGAGEMENT OF THE WHOLE SPINE

As the segment releases you may find yourself engaging with the next area seeking attention further down the spine. *You may progressively find each level releasing until there is an impression that even the lowest spinal levels and sacrum are yielding to the offer of more spaciousness.*

Further considerations to keep in mind

Sense the suspension of the cervical vertebral bodies within the ligamentous stocking of the anterior and posterior longitudinal ligaments and allow it to seek a balance point. Tension of the anterior, lateral and posterior muscles may be apparent; wait for these muscles to relax.

This engagement also includes the superficial and deep fascias of the neck, including the prevertebral fascia (PVF) and the neck flexors, the longus colli (LC) and longus capitis muscles beneath the PVF. Tension in these neck flexor muscles can adversely affect cervical proprioception (Ha and Sung 2020). This can occur from increased use of electronic devices and after whiplash injury.

Acknowledge the myodural bridges at C1 and C2 which contribute to the suspension of the cervical cord within the bony spinal canal, in conjunction with the fibrous suspensory ligaments within the vertebral canal (Enix *et al.* 2014).

The tension of the reciprocal tension membrane (RTM) can also be engaged with this hold. Note any feeling of tightness or desiccation and *appreciate how the head, neck and the whole spine suspend from the fulcrum at the junction of the falx and the tentorium* (Sutherland 1990, TSO p. 42).

The suspension of the spinal cord within the spinal canal can also be appreciated. The denticulate ligaments are lateral expansions of pia mater and are thickest in the cervical spine, anchoring the cord to the dura mater (Ceylan *et al.* 2012). They suspend the cord in cerebrospinal fluid (CSF) in the subarachnoid space. Sense this fluid suspension of the CNS: brainstem and cervical spinal cord.

The cervical spinal cord and its dural covering adapts to the length of the spinal canal, so that when the cervical spinal column is flexed the cord is stretched and lengthened (Breig 1978; Breig *et al.* 1966). *Sense the relationship between the cervical spine and the spinal cord within:* poor alignment of the vertebrae may lead to perceivable tension and abnormal stretching of the cord. This is a possible factor in scoliosis or reduced cervical lordosis, with hypertonic LC.

Is there a sense that the spinal cord is suspended centrally in the spinal canal by its fibrous suspensory ligaments (Klinge et al. 2021)?

Allow these different interfaces to integrate: bony, ligamentous, muscular, dural, CNS floating within the subarachnoid space, CNS and its myodural bridges and fibrous suspension ligaments.

It may also be helpful to keep the myodural bridges in mind. These are epidural connections to the cervical dura from the fascia of the suboccipital muscles. They extend from the rectus capitis posterior minor, rectus capitis posterior major and obliquus capitis inferior muscles. These connections are between the occiput, C1 and C2 vertebrae.

The myodural bridges cross the epidural space and anchor and stabilise the spinal dura and spinal cord during head and neck movements. There may be central control of the tone of these suboccipital muscles to regulate dural tension. These muscles are often implicated in cervicogenic headaches (Wonho 2021) and following whiplash.

PSOAS TRACTION

This approach bilaterally engages with the fascial envelopes of the lower extremity muscles towards the psoas and fascia of the posterior abdominal wall. From here, attention is paid to any related structures including the diaphragm and fascias above and below it. The use of minimal traction from the feet enables our proprioception to progressively feel and engage structures that are more distal. If a psoas muscle is tight or contracted, it may cause one half of the pelvis to rotate around the other, leading to a short leg and sacroiliac, hip and lumbar spine problems.

RELEVANT ANATOMY

Engagement of the muscles and fascia of the posterior abdominal wall may include:

- Iliacus: taking origin from the iliac wing.
- Psoas major: this takes origin from the transverse processes, vertebral bodies and intervertebral discs of T12 to L5 and the tendinous arches. The psoas has a bilateral circular shape on cross-section on each side of the vertebral body.
- Psoas minor: from T12 and L1.
- Quadratus lumborum: this is a continuation of the transverse abdominal muscle and is an integral part of the thoracolumbar fascia (TLF), acting as a crossroad of forces exerted by the surrounding muscles. The TLF encloses the quadratus lumborum muscle and the deep back muscles, covering the latissimus dorsi. Superiorly the TLF condenses to form the lateral arcuate ligament on the anterior surface of rib 12.
- Diaphragm: posteriorly from the lumbar vertebrae and arcuate ligaments. The posterior attachments on the lumbar spine are the tendinous right and left crura (the median arcuate ligament between them).

The psoas is posterior to the peritoneum and is therefore posterior to retroperitoneal structures such as the kidneys, ureters, aorta and pancreas.

The sympathetic chain passes into the abdomen under the medial arcuate ligament and it is helpful to acknowledge this during this procedure. The cervical sympathetic chain is posterior to the PVF and posteromedial to the carotid sheath.

The root of the mesentery suspends the small and large intestine from the posterior abdominal wall, from the duodenojejunal flexure at the level of L1/L2 on the left, descending diagonally at 45° to the iliocaecal junction at the level of the right sacroiliac (SI) joint. It crosses the aorta and right psoas muscle along this diagonal. Cadaveric dissections by Kumar *et al.* (2019) demonstrated that mesentery is continuous from the duodenojejunal flexure to the anorectal junction.

THERAPEUTIC ENGAGEMENT

Psoas traction

The principle of allowing the patient's mechanism to surrender to the inherent forces is supported by *the operator shifting his or her body weight* *posteriorly and using gravity rather than muscular effort. This is key to success in this tractional approach.*

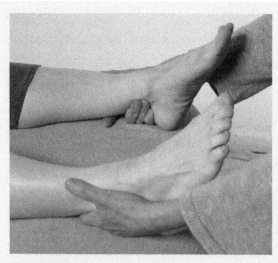

Figure 16.3 Psoas traction.

1. HANDHOLD

With the patient supine on the treatment table, stand with a broad base at the feet. Cup your hands under the heels of the patient with your thenar eminences on the lateral malleoli. It is advisable to make sure the patient is not lying with the lumbar spine in a hyperextended position.

2. SHIFTING YOUR WEIGHT

Wait for the hip capsule to relax. Then minutely lean back, shifting your body weight posteriorly onto your heels. This will engage the tissues under your hands into traction. Listen for the first hint of fascial engagement.

3. READING THE TISSUES

Sense your traction acting on the straight legs, through the femurs and psoas muscles, where they originate on the lumbar spine. Is the response to traction symmetrical?

Sense the fascial compartments of the leg, the interosseous membrane (IoM) between the fibula and tibia, and up through to the fascial compartments of the thigh and hamstrings.

Sense the insertion of the psoas major and iliacus on the lesser trochanter bilaterally and the insertion of the psoas minor on the pectineal line.

Maintain and refine the traction through the feet and feel the tension of the psoas and its fascia, right up to the medial and lateral arcuate ligaments and 12th ribs. Acknowledge that the psoas fascia is continuous with the TLF laterally and with the iliac fascia inferiorly.

The posterior layer of the TLF integrates the legs, pelvis, spine and arms via the conduction of forces or load transfer (Vleeming *et al.* 1995). *This function may be appreciated under your hands.*

4. END POINT

As you continue to observe with your weight slightly shifted back on your heels, you may find that as the psoas muscles release through their length the legs also lengthen, giving the impression of elasticity. This is often the end point. However, you may also find the following pointers rewarding to take this journey deeper.

Further considerations

Acknowledge that developmentally the lower extremities develop from limb buds opposite L5 and the lower extremities 'suspend' from L5. The neurophysiological origin of the lower extremities is the thoracolumbar junction, and this represents the biodynamic fulcrum of the lower extremities (Carreiro 2009).

Allow your attention to sense the crura of the diaphragm and the median arcuate ligament where the two crura join near the 12th thoracic vertebra. The median arcuate ligament forms the boundary of the aortic arch transmitting the aorta, thoracic duct and azygos vein. Sense these vessels and sense for any congestion in this area.

Sense the vertebral and costal attachments of the diaphragm, the central tendon and the doming of the diaphragm. Acknowledge its origins, three-dimensional shape, change and tone. Watch the breathing as the tone and excursion of the diaphragm changes. The breathing may change in depth and rate. Does the patient breathe in an ideal pattern, right down to the pubic symphysis

(Zink and Lawson 1979)? Hypertrophy, or tension or shortening of the psoas, will affect the excursion of the diaphragm.

Place your attention posteriorly on the ligamentous stocking (anterior longitudinal spinal ligament, ALSL) of the whole spine, then the root of the mesentery and the suspension of the gut.

Compare the abdominal and negative mediastinal pressures (Milanesi and Caregnato 2016).

Acknowledge the continuity of the diaphragm, fibrous pericardium, pretracheal fascia (PTF) and the fascial tubes of the anterior cervical fascias to their attachments to the hyoid bone, thyroid cartilage, mandible, pterygoid plates, base of the skull and ligamentum nuchae.

Acknowledge these inferior fascial and muscular influences on the sphenobasilar symphysis.

This fascial continuity extends to the anterior dural girdle attached to the lesser wings of the sphenoid. Sense the shape and the suspension of the five-pointed star of the dural membrane: falx cerebri, tentorium cerebelli and anterior transverse dural girdles.

How does the RTM suspend from the fulcrum where the falx cerebri adjoins the tentorium cerebelli?

How does the whole body, right down to the legs and feet, suspend from the Sutherland fulcrum? (Close to where the falx cerebri adjoins the tentorium cerebelli towards the anterior end of the straight sinus; see Key Terms.)

Allow the whole body to re-integrate while maintaining a sense of spacious attention.

This approach allows the patient to sense wholeness, in terms of structural, visceral and functional integrity, normalising the autonomic tone. This sets the stage for the self-corrective process to continue its work.

PART 2: SPECIFIC MUSCLES

Although the primary emphasis of this book is on the ligaments, their reciprocal interaction with the muscles sometimes means that these also require attention. The following two procedures have particular relevance to articular balance of the hip joint and were taught by Anne Wales as demonstrated to her by William Sutherland (Wales 1997) (see also Chapter 11).

THERAPEUTIC ENGAGEMENT

Iliopsoas tendon release

This approach can be very useful in femoroacetabular impingement and can positively shift the ligamentous-articular and muscular relationships of the hip. Lippincott (1949) suggested that iliopsoas release is helpful in cases of excessive lordosis, kidney stones and sciatic scoliosis. Chronic psoas tension has also been reported secondary to kidney stones (Lurz *et al.* 2018).

1. HANDHOLD
Stand to the side of the supine patient. Place the heel of your hand on the anterior superior iliac spine (ASIS) so that your fingers are pointing towards the feet. Your middle finger rests firmly, just lateral to the iliopsoas tendon. The fingertip should be just below the rim of the pelvis, where the tendon crosses over it before inserting into the lesser trochanter. This iliopsoas tendon contact serves as a firm fulcrum throughout the procedure. *Place the other hand under the patient's heel or calf.*

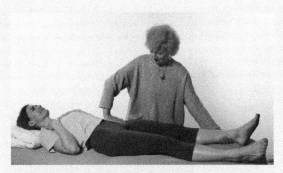
Figure 16.4 Iliopsoas tendon release (1).

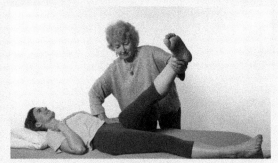
Figure 16.6 Iliopsoas tendon release (3).

2. FOCUSSING THE FULCRUM

Lift up the patient's straight leg vertically into hip flexion to relax the psoas tendon, as you maintain the firmness of your finger fulcrum.

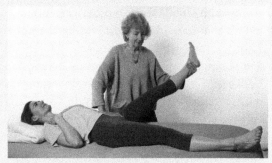
Figure 16.7 Iliopsoas tendon release (4).

The leg is then carried laterally around the fulcrum of your finger and lowered in a smooth arc down onto the table.

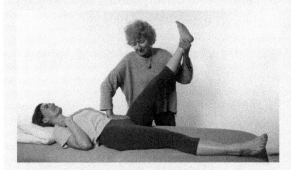
Figure 16.5 Iliopsoas tendon release (2).

3. STRETCHING THE PSOAS TENDON OVER YOUR FINGER

Then bring the straight leg medially, crossing it over your finger into adduction. This carries your finger slightly beneath the tendon.

Keeping your hand in this position, carry the leg laterally and into external rotation. This tenses the tendon, stretching it slightly over your finger fulcrum.

4. REPLACING THE LEG

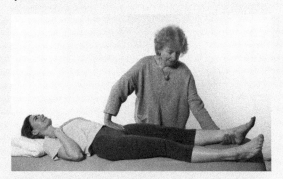
Figure 16.8 Iliopsoas tendon release (5).

5. REASSESSMENT
Recheck the tone of the iliopsoas.

Obturator internus release

This follows naturally as a continuation from the sidelying pelvic floor lift described in Chapter 5. Like the iliopsoas, the obturator internus muscle is often implicated in hip dysfunction.

When there is tension in the obturator membrane, the patient may complain of discomfort when sitting. This is often associated with a contracted obturator internus muscle. The obturator membrane is an IoM, almost closing the obturator foramen, which lies between the ischium and pubis. The membrane balances the tension between the obturator internus and externus muscles, attached to it on either side. Sutherland commented that unequal tension between these two muscles can produce strain in the membrane. This potentially compromises the passage of arterial vessels and a small branch of the sciatic nerve, where they pass through a small hiatus towards the acetabulum (Sutherland 1998, COT p. 251).

1. POSITIONING
Standing behind the patient who is sidelying with hips flexed, check if there is tenderness behind the greater trochanter.

2. CONTACT
The pelvic floor will have already relaxed through the pelvic lift manoeuvre and your hand will then be in position to release the obturator membrane. *Your two finger contact (second and third fingers) is immediately medial to the ischial tuberosity. The other hand initially rests on the ilium. Your action is directed along the medial surface of the ischial tuberosity into the ischiorectal fossa so as to contact the obturator membrane and obturator internus muscle.*

3. ADVANCING WITH RESPIRATION
As in the pelvic lift, *when the patient exhales, advance your contact gently as the area may be tender. Maintain your advance each time the patient inhales. This is repeated until you come into contact with the obturator membrane where your laterally facing fingertips establish a fulcrum for the release of obturator internus.*

4. ABDUCTION
Maintaining your finger fulcrum, reach over the patient's body with the other hand, to grasp and support the patient's bent knee from beneath. Lift the knee into abduction and external rotation towards you.

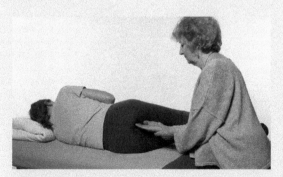

Figure 16.9 Obturator internus manoeuvre (1).

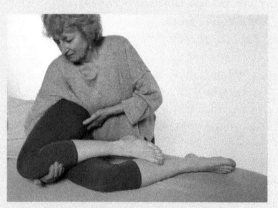

Figure 16.10 Obturator internus manoeuvre (2).

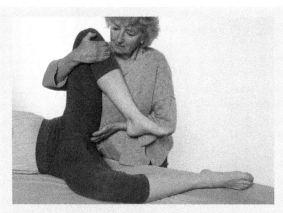

Figure 16.11 Obturator internus manoeuvre (3).

5. COMPLETION
When you feel a change in the tension of the muscle and membrane under your finger fulcrum, adduct, lower and straighten the leg.

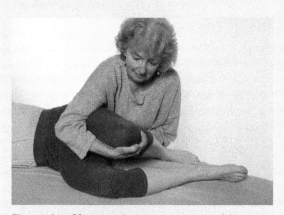

Figure 16.12 Obturator internus manoeuvre (4).

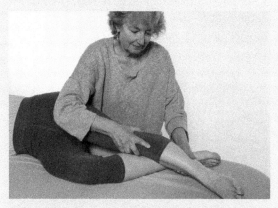

Figure 16.13 Obturator internus manoeuvre (5).

Repeat on the other side.

LC muscle
Like the psoas muscle, the LC spans a transitional area between vertebral curves on the interior surface of the body. The LC is vulnerable to hypertonicity, especially after whiplash injury. This may result in stiffness and loss of cervical lordosis.

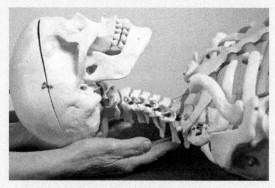

Figure 16.14 Handhold for longus colli approximation on skeleton.

A simple manoeuvre may relax the LC, enabling the neck to regain its natural curve:

Contact the upper neck of the supine patient with one hand on the articular pillars of C2, and the other on the transverse processes of T1 or T2. Directing your forces towards the anterior surface of the vertebral bodies, approximate your two hands, drawing the tissues together slightly. The aim is to change the relationship between origin and insertion. This may alter the fulcrum around which the LC and ligaments are organised, beneficially relaxing tension in the muscle. See Figure 2.4.

Transversus thoracis muscle
Yet another muscle which exerts its influence from the interior surface of the trunk is the transverse thoracis. This fan-shaped muscle which lies behind the sternum originates on the posterior surface of the xiphoid process, lower sternum and costal cartilages. It attaches to the interior surfaces of the costal cartilages of ribs 2–6. Because

it contracts strongly in the action of coughing, it is often found to remain slightly hypertonic following a respiratory infection. This anterior contractile influence can adversely affect the thoracic curve, respiratory excursion and lymph flow. An approach for releasing the transversus thoracis and restoring anteroposterior thoracic balance is described in Chapter 5. This may also be helpful when this pattern is being maintained by emotional stress. See Figure 4.3.

Suboccipital muscle inhibition

This approach was frequently used by A.T. Still and the early osteopaths, including J.M. Littlejohn, for releasing the OA joint and in the treatment of fevers etc. (Wernham 1975–1979). It appears to have a distinctly calming and balancing effect on the autonomic nervous system which may, in part, in osteopathic terms, be associated with improvement of brainstem circulation and beneficial effects on the vagal nuclei (Roberts *et al.* 2021).

1. HANDHOLD
Sit behind the head of the supine patient, bilaterally cupping the fingers of both hands under the occiput and suboccipital muscles. As one of the aims is to give more space to the OA relationship (OA), care should be taken to avoid compressing the atlas onto the occiput (see Chapter 2, Part 2: Transitional areas).

2. ACTION
Each time the patient exhales, gently take up the slack in the suboccipital muscles by drawing the occiput towards you very slightly. On the patient's inhalation, resist the tendency of the muscles to pull the occiput away from you. On each exhalation, continue to take up the slack in the muscles, maintaining this advance on inhalation, until you sense softening and greater spaciousness between the occiput and atlas. This may be accompanied by warmth in the tissues as the circulatory perfusion of the area improves.

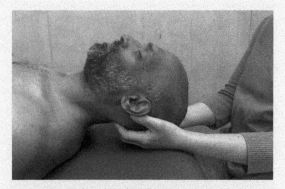

Figure 16.15 Suboccipital inhibition.

Paraspinal muscle inhibition

Paraspinal inhibition was used frequently by A.T. Still (Hildreth 1942) and by the early osteopaths, e.g., J.M. Littlejohn (Wernham 1975–1979). The aim, through relaxing the spinal muscles, is to beneficially affect facilitated segmental reflexes through its effectiveness in calming sympathetic activity. It is often surprisingly effective in freeing intersegmental movement in stubbornly rigid spines.

While engaging with the paraspinal muscles, keep in mind the viscerosomatic and somaticovisceral reflex relationships of the area under your hands, and also between the muscle spindles and the spinal cord (see Chapter 2).

1. HANDHOLD
Very simply, with the patient prone, stand on the opposite side to the muscle group being addressed. Place your soft thenar eminence receptively (afferently) between the spinous processes and the paraspinal muscles. Place the other (active) hand over the sensory hand.

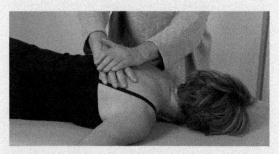

Figure 16.16 Paraspinal inhibition.

2. ENGAGEMENT

Lean towards the muscles slightly to take advantage of their relaxation on each outbreath. Gently and slowly take up the slack on each outbreath, to ease the muscles away from the spine. Maintain the progress gained on each inhalation, as each exhalation increasingly yields, until the muscles relax and lengthen.

On re-examination check for any improvement in local spinal mobility and tissue rehydration.

VIDEOS FOR CHAPTER 16

Scan the QR code or visit https://www.youtube.com/playlist?list=PL3j_YuMBqigFldhawr0_598nA_AsuxMss to find a playlist of the videos that accompany this chapter.

REFERENCES

Ashmore, E. (1915) *Osteopathic Mechanics: A Textbook.* Kirksville, MO: Journal Printing Company; p. 72.

Breig, A. (1978) *Adverse Mechanical Tension in the Central Nervous System: An Analysis of Cause and Effect: Relief by Functional Neurosurgery.* Almqvist & Wiksell International, New York, NY: John Wiley & Sons Inc.

Breig, A., Turnbull, I., Hassler, O. (1966) Effects of mechanical stresses on the spinal cord in cervical spondylosis. *J of Neurosurgery 25* (10), 45.

Carreiro, J.E. (2009) *An Osteopathic Approach to Children,* 2nd edition. London: Churchill Livingstone Elsevier; Chapter 2.

Ceylan, D., Tatarli, N., Abdullaev, T., *et al.* (2012) The denticulate ligament: anatomical properties, functional and clinical significance. *Acta Neurochir (Wien) 154* (7), 1229–1234.

Enix, D.E., Scali, F., Pontell, M.E. (2014) The cervical myodural bridge, a review of literature and clinical implications. *J Can Chiropr Assoc 58* (2), 184–192.

Ha, S-Y. & Sung, Y-H. (2020) A temporary forward head posture decreases function of cervical proprioception. *J of Exercise Rehab 16* (2), 168–174.

Hildreth, A.G. (1942) *The Lengthening Shadow of Dr. Andrew Taylor Still,* 2nd edition. Paw Paw, MI: A.G. Hildreth & A.E. Van Vleck; p. 194.

Klinge, P.M., McElroy, A., Donahue, J.E., *et al.* (2021) Abnormal spinal cord motion at the craniocervical junction in hyper mobile Ehlers-Danlos patients. *J Neurosurg Spine 21,* 1–7.

Kumar, A., Faiq, M.A., Krishna, H., *et al.* (2019) Development of a novel technique to dissect the mesentery that preserves mesenteric continuity and enables characterisation of the ex vivo mesentery. *Frontiers in Surgery 6,* 80.

Lippincott, H.A. (1949) The Osteopathic Technique of Wm. G. Sutherland, D.O. In: W.G. Sutherland (1990) *Teachings in the Science of Osteopathy.* A.L. Wales (ed.). Fort Worth, TX: Sutherland Cranial Teaching Foundation, Inc./Rudra Press.

Lurz, K.L., Dawish, A.D., Treffer, K.D. (2018) Recurrent psoas syndrome secondary to urolithiasis and indwelling ureteral stent. *Osteopathic Family Physician 10* (6), 36–38.

Milanesi, R. & Caregnato, R.C.A. (2016) Intra-abdominal pressure: an integrative review. *Einstein (Sao Paulo) 14* (3), 423–430.

Roberts, B., Makar, A.E., Canaan, R., Pazdernik, V., Kondrashova, T. (2021) Effect of occipitoatlantal decompression on cerebral blood flow dynamics as evaluated by Doppler ultrasonography. *J Osteopath Med 121* (2), 171–179. https://doi.org/10.1515/jom-2020-0100.

Sutherland, W.G. (1990) *Teachings in the Science of Osteopathy.* A.L. Wales (ed.). Fort Worth, TX: Sutherland Cranial Teaching Foundation, Inc./Rudra Press; p. 42.

Sutherland, W.G. (1998) *Contributions of Thought,* 2nd edition. A.L. Wales and A.S. Sutherland (eds). Fort Worth, TX: Sutherland Cranial Teaching Foundation, Inc.; p. 251.

Vleeming, A., Pool-Goudzwaard, A.L., Stoeckart, R., van Wingerden, J-P., Snijders, C.J. (1995) The posterior layer of the thoracolumbar fascia. Its function in load transfer from spine to legs. *Spine 20* (7), 753–758.

Wales, A.L. (1997) British tutorial group meeting. North Attleboro, MA, USA.

Wernham, J. (1975-1979) Lectures given at the European School of Osteopathy, UK.

Wonho, C. (2021) Effect of 4 weeks of cervical deep muscle flexion exercise on headache and sleep disorder in patients with tension headache and forward head posture. *International J of Environmental Research and Public Health 18* (7), 3410.

Zink, G.J. & Lawson, W.B. (1979) An osteopathic structural examination and functional interpretation of soma. *Osteopathic Annals 7,* 12–19.

CHAPTER 17

Intraosseous Engagement

KOK WENG LIM AND SUSAN TURNER

'Work with the forces within the patient that manifest the healing process.'

W.G. Sutherland

The impression of spontaneous intraosseous reorganisation, following ligamentous or membranous-articular release, has been referred to in the treatment of the clavicle, fibula, radius, sacrum, occiput and ribs, especially rib 1. The potential for internal remodelling is present in all bones especially when their articular relationships are free.

When a bone has been subject to strong impact and has either fractured or simply absorbed injurious forces, it often appears to retain a degree of strain intraosseously. This lack of intraosseous integration may explain an occasional difficulty in achieving stable harmonisation of its articular relationships, since a joint can only be as balanced as the bones that comprise it.

Bone is in a continuous state of internal reconstruction, according to the daily forces absorbed by its trabeculae and fluid matrix. It is helpful to think of even these densest of living structures as *evolving processes*. Sutherland goes further in thinking of bone as fluid in a perpetual process of creation:

'What are bones but fluid, a different form of fluid?

What is that little hailstone that comes down from Heaven but fluid?
What is the earth out here, this world that we walk on, but fluid?
It is all a material manifestation and, back of that, fluid,
When we learn to think with Dr Andrew Taylor Still.
He lived closer to his maker than mere material breathing.
Do you get the thought?'

(Sutherland 1990, TSO p. 31)

This passage is a call to make a shift in the way bone is perceived and engaged with, beginning with a consideration of its microscopic fluid spaces. The connective tissue framework of bone consists of collagen which is hydrophilic, enabling it to attract and hold water. This is infiltrated by calcium phosphate and other biominerals which provide it with strength, some flexibility and the capacity to accommodate mechanical stresses.

Theodore Schwenk describes bone as 'a monument in "stone" to the flowing movement from which it originates; indeed one might say that the liquid has "expressed itself" in the bone' (Schwenk 1965). The cortex could be said to 'float' in a very fine layer of subperiosteal metabolic water. Cortical bone contains approximately 20 per cent free water within its pore system, and bone water concentration is the new metric for bone quality for cortical bone in vivo (Techawi-boonwong *et al.* 2008).

The cortex contains a microvascular network of capillaries within its anastomosed functional units (osteons). These contain blood vessels which penetrate the Haversian (longitudinal) canals and Volkmann's (transverse) perforating canals. Fluid interchange within the cortex is crucial for nutrition and information transmission through the anastomosed capillary network within the Haversian and Volkmann's canals. Skeletal muscle contractions and response to gravitational forces stimulate the drainage of these capillary systems into the central venous sinus, nutrient veins and venous sinus complexes.

Osteocytes (the most long-lived of bone cells), residing in the fluid-filled lacunar spaces in the extracellular matrix (ECM), enable intercellular communication via their long processes which extend through the ECM. This extensive communication network through the Haversian system enables the sensing of changes in the interstitial fluid, registering and responding to mechanical signals (Bonewald 2010; Knothe Tate 2003; Palumbo and Ferretti 2021).

Winet (2003) described a connective capillary filtration-based interstitial flow through the bone matrix, stimulating and nourishing bone cells. This enables the capillaries to and from the bone cells to exchange nutrients for waste products. Pre-lymphatic (initial lymphatic) channels in cortical bone drain interstitial fluid, aided by body movements, weight bearing, and muscle pump actions which all augment interstitial flow.

Bone is a dynamic metabolic organ, constantly remodelling in response to movement and gravity. The trabecular lines reveal the gravitational and weight-bearing stresses impressed upon the bone on a daily basis. The double-spiral arrangement of the trabeculae enables cortical bone to be 'spring-loaded' and allow some resiliency in response to movement and gravity. This trabecular formation, together with the hydrated state, are essential to the viscoelastic properties of bone.

Healthy bones should 'breathe'. On palpation, inherent physiological motion expresses itself through long bones as a subtle rhythmic lengthening/narrowing and shortening/widening. This motion may appear to be absent where there is a state of intraosseous compression, either because of dehydration, general depletion or sustaining strong compressive impact. More commonly though, a long bone in intraosseous strain will give the impression of 'breathing', not as one bone, but as two individual parts whose motion is not synchronised, especially following a fracture, even after its healing.

Bones with a more complex shape each have their characteristic expression. Where the sacrum has sustained a compression pattern through the whole bone, it may feel hard and brittle on palpation. Childhood and adolescence provide plenty of opportunity for traumatic or compressive forces to be absorbed and retained in one or more of the five unfused sacral segments. This may feel as if the segments' inherent breathing movements are out of alignment with one another.

THERAPEUTIC ENGAGEMENT

Intraosseous integration in a long bone

The following way of engaging with the resolution of intraosseous strains is an interpretation of what was shown to James Jealous DO by his mentor, Ruby Day DO, who was a student of William Sutherland.

This approach is especially useful when fractures fail to fully unite and also for the integration of the whole bone after healing. It is useful where a bone has sustained vectorial or compressive impact and absorbed that force without dispersing it through a fracture. It is also applicable to the absorption of slow sustained forces, such as through intrauterine moulding in the treatment of infants.

This involves engagement with the fluid component of bone, and to do this, it is helpful to acknowledge the minute spaces of the bone's internal fluid world. As mentioned in Chapter 1, looking at a miniature painting allows the brain to amplify the tiny image into a vast landscape. In a similar way, sensing such potential spaces as the subperiosteal layer of metabolic water in which the cortex 'floats' may enhance the operator's perceptual experience of bone as a 'fluid'. Within this fluid dimension there is optimum capacity for positive change and remodelling; this could be seen as a realignment with the innate geometry of the formative embryonic matrix (Blechschmidt 1904) or the organising field of the biosphere. A fixed idea of bone as solid, on the part of the operator, may limit its potential for change.

When practising BLT, it can make it easier to engage with the ligaments as the 'power agents' in the process, if the extracellular and fluid dimension of bone is perceptually included in the operator's engagement.

It can be surprising to feel a bone remoulding when its ligamentous articular relationship releases and realigns. There are also times, though, when a specific intraosseous strain needs to be addressed directly as follows. This is always easier when the articular ends are first freed from restriction.

1. CENTRING
When engaging with the fluid nature of bone, it helps to be present to the fluid held within the fascial matrix of one's own body.

2. HANDHOLD
Contact the epiphyseal plates at each end of a long bone with index fingers and thumbs only. The epiphyses are where the growth centres of a long bone are found, making them potent points of contact to engage with the piezoelectric quality between the hands. When referring to 'fluid' this does not only mean liquid, but probably includes a bioelectrical field phenomenon.

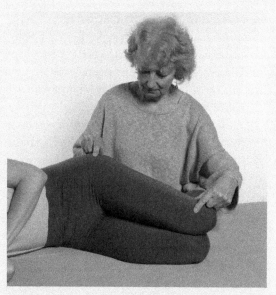

Figure 17.1 Femur, intraosseous contact.

3. ENGAGEMENT
Sense the fluid bone's connective tissue network and observe what is happening in the space between your hands.

Sense the gradients of fluid density between compact and cortical bone and the spacious matrix of cancellous bone.

To access the fluid life of the bone, acknowledge the very fine subperiosteal space of metabolic water in which the cortex is suspended.

Invite the fluid-filled micro-spaces of the bone to come to your awareness.

Be open to a sense of inherent physiological motion as a tidal breathing, expressed as rhythmic shape change between your hands. If present, does it rhythmically shorten and widen and then lengthen and narrow in an organised and fluid way?

Or is rhythmic shape change only perceivable at one end?

Maybe the two ends move as if independent of one another? If so, where is the break in that continuity?

Does the bone feel dry or 'juicy'?

4. AWAKENING THERAPEUTIC ACTIVITY

It may be enough to simply hold the two epiphysial plates and acknowledge the pattern and shape of fluid expression between them, 'listening' and *trusting the self-organising potency of the fluid as a formative force within the bone.*

As you spaciously support and observe, there is sometimes a sense of the fluid flow being naturally attracted to the area of compression or strain where its motion becomes still.

5. RESOLUTION

When it emerges from stillness, intraosseous motion expresses a unified quality of homogeneous and rhythmic inherent motion.

Sometimes, simply noting the peak of the swelling (inhalation) phase of tidal motion within the bone will diagnostically reveal the shape and quality of a distortion. When this moment is observed and honoured, there is often a pause in inherent motion, followed by resolution on the receding (exhalation) phase as the fluid reorganises.

INERTIA

Where there is a state of inertia or compression within the bone, the fluid flow within it may need to be activated directly. This can be achieved by *setting up an alternating longitudinal fluctuation as if 'pushing fluid' backwards and forwards between the two ends.* Once this sense of alternating flow is set up, *simply observe and be receptive to where that tidal flow directs itself. It will seek the area where therapeutic change is needed. Stay present as the system goes to work in the stillness and accept whatever way it resolves towards homogeneity of fluid expression within the bone.*

Similar principles can be applied to complex bones as follows below.

Sidelying intraosseous release of the hip joint

This is particularly helpful when a gentle approach is required, such as in the case of an acutely painful hip to calm the shock in the tissues. Also, following an old trauma, such as from a fall on the side of the hip, the inertia within the tissues sometimes requires the matching of absorbed vectorial forces by compression or approximation of the joint. With the patient sidelying, the uppermost, injured hip can be approximated by shifting your weight gently and precisely downwards into the table.

1. POSITIONING

Stand behind the sidelying patient whose hips and knees are flexed on the table. Stand in line with, and facing towards, the long axis of the patient's femur.

2. HANDHOLD

Place your crossed or connected thumbs over the patient's greater trochanter. This serves as a fulcrum for the patient's tissues to seek and refine the point of balance and for the tissue release.

Place the rest of your finger contacts over the three parts of the innominate: ilium, pubis and ischium.

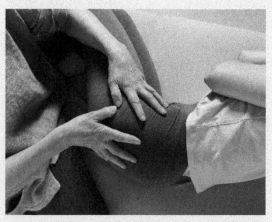

Figure 17.2 Hip intraosseous hold.

3. ENGAGEMENT

Allow your attention to appreciate the alignment of the greater trochanter, neck of femur and head of femur from your connected thumb contact. Femoral anteversion or antetorsion can often be appreciated. The degree of the femoral neck-shaft angle and the position of the femoral head on the neck of the femur may also be apparent.

The relationship of ligamentum teres to the fovea capitis can be sensed and this may be considered as a functional fulcrum for the joint in treatment. *Inwardly ask the question: 'How does the head of the femur sit in the acetabulum?'*

The intraosseous relationship between the three parts of the innominate can be appreciated for quality, three-dimensional shape and shape change through its subtle intraosseous tidal breathing motion. *Appreciate the three component bony parts of the innominate that make up the acetabulum.* Shears may be felt in these embryological 'seams', which perceptually are not just as bony parts, but are also in reality embryological fluid fields coming together during development. Listening in this way, with centred observation and palpation, a precise palpatory diagnosis may be made.

4. WATCH THE INHALATION PHASE OF PRIMARY RESPIRATORY MOTION

The strain pattern is expressed most clearly at the peak of the primary inhalation phase, which is the maximal point of expansion and disengagement. *The sensing of this tidal motion through the tissues, therefore, is an aid to diagnosis.*

5. OBSERVATION

Observe the treatment process that unfolds from the peak of primary respiratory inhalation. Watch the inherent fluctuation of the fluids, as the intelligence of the Tide goes to work (see Key Terms). Sense the inherent treatment principle that the body itself is using to bring the tissues to a point of balanced tension in the self-corrective process.

Sense the overall three-dimensional shape under the hands come into a balanced state. James Jealous DO spoke of the resolution happening on the exhalation phase of the Tide to be 'like seaweed' under the hands (Jealous 1988).

Include the thoracolumbar junction in your awareness and acknowledge this biodynamic fulcrum for the lower extremity. While the treatment unfolds, a still point, and/or stillness, may be reached before the return of inherent involuntary breathing of the tissues, the Tide.

6. RESOLUTION

The end point of the treatment is a greater sense of intraosseous breathing of the parts of the innominate, a harmonising change in shape of the acetabulum and in the relationship between the femoral head and the acetabulum.

Application to DDH in infancy

In infants with clicky hips or developmental hip dysplasia (DDH), this approach can be adapted to any position, including sitting. It can be done with the infant in a Pavlik harness, or even in a short leg 'Frog' cast.

Tension in the psoas muscle also needs to be relaxed to allow the femoral head to come up into the acetabulum (see Chapter 16, psoas traction and psoas tendon release). This is because tension in the iliopsoas tendon, sitting over the empty acetabulum, causes an 'hourglass' constriction of the capsule from front to back. The hourglass shape of the capsule then has one cavity containing the head of the femur and the other covering the acetabulum; the iliopsoas tendon acts to constrict it in the middle. The important ligamentum teres passes through this narrow channel.

During treatment, attention may be drawn to this *capsular constriction* and also to the *ligamentum teres* which is often thickened, as is the *transverse acetabular ligament*. There are often *fibro-fatty deposits in the acetabulum* (pulvinar) and an *inverted or everted labrum* which constrict the reduction of the femoral head in the acetabulum. All these factors are considered as intracapsular and extracapsular soft tissue obstacles to obtaining a closed reduction of DDH (Studer *et al.* 2017).

In infants or children presenting with a packaging disorder of in-toeing and femoral anteversion (increased internal and decreased external rotation of the hip joint), the femoral shaft often compensates by an intraosseous rotation within itself (Harris 2013). This may be apparent under the hands.

Intraosseous release of the atlas

This approach can be helpful where intraosseous strains have been sustained by the atlas, in the process of birth and childhood, especially before the component parts are ossified. Intraosseous strains can also happen even in adult life, through the impact sustained in head injuries.

A typical vertebra has three primary ossification centres: one for the body and one for each half of the neural arch. These appear in the 7th and 8th week in utero, and the centrum and neural processes fuse around 3 to 6 years of age (Skorzweska *et al.* 2013). Secondary ossification centres appear by puberty and fuse between 25 and 30 years of age (Byrd and Comiskey 2007).

The atlas, similarly, has three ossification centres:

- One for the anterior arch which develops towards the end of the first year. It is connected to the posterior neural arches by a neurocentral synchondrosis on each side. These fuse around 5–8 years of age.
- Two bilaterally, for the posterior neural arches. These are present at birth and are separated by the posterior synchondrosis which fuses around 3–5 years of age.

The anterior arch is therefore usually cartilaginous at birth. While a single ossification centre of the anterior arch is commonly described, variations exist, such as two symmetric anterior arch ossification centres. Such multiple ossification centres of the anterior (and posterior arches) may be seen in over 25 per cent of children younger than 8 years old (Junewick *et al.* 2011).

The atlas ring is therefore incompletely ossified for most of childhood and the split ring of the atlas may serve to accommodate the birth forces on the cranium, together with the four parts of the occiput, temporals and parietals. Shears can occur between the parts of the ring, and midline shears may be apparent on palpation if there are two symmetrical anterior arch ossification centres.

1. EXAMINATION
Assess for motion and resiliency at the cranio-cervical junction.

2. HANDHOLD
Contact the atlas by placing your index fingers on the lateral masses on each side, with third or ring fingers on the posterior arches of the atlas. It is such a small space that your fingers will span the whole posterior arch. *Support the occiput and temporal bones with the rest of your hands in a cradle hold.*

3. PALPATION AND SENSING
Acknowledging the fluid dimension of the bone within its periosteum, sense the three or more parts of the atlas for strains in the adult or child along the ossification unions. There may be a sense of left-right asymmetry or shear which may have been present since birth. Superimposed on this may be forces or strains from trauma after birth.

4. THE WIDER FIELD
As the strain between the parts of the atlas becomes clear, sense this in the context of the four parts of the occiput, temporals and parietals and the entire posterior cranial fossa.

5. BALANCE POINT
Allow the atlas within itself, and in the context of the whole cranio-cervical junction, to come to a point of balanced membranous tension (BMT). This is achieved by listening, paying attention to the underlying fluid forces and being receptive to their inherent action.

Following internal resolution of the atlas, recheck and rebalance the cranio-cervical junction (see Chapter 2).

Intraosseous release of the sacrum

The sacrum ossifies from five segments with five primary sacral ossification centres present at each level: a centrum, two posterior neural arches and two costal processes lateral to the centrum (S5 lacks costal processes). By 32 weeks of gestation or a birth weight of 1800 g, the vertebral body ossification centres are present followed by the costal element ossification centres (Cloete *et al.* 2013; Jian *et al.* 2019; Moradi *et al.* 2019). These appear in a cranial to caudal direction.

When considering intraosseous strains, it is helpful to know that these five primary ossification centres at each sacral level do not fuse until about 7 years of age (Broome *et al.* 1998).

The sacral segments begin fusion from 18 years of age over the next two decades from a caudal to cranial direction. Complete fusion of the sacrum may occur between 25 and 33 years of age (Cheng and Song 2003).

It is therefore possible for intraosseous strains to be present within each sacral segment between the five primary ossification centres, and also between each sacral vertebra. This can lead to a palpable sense of shear, torsion or compression.

Intraosseous dysfunction in the sacrum can also occur as a result of physical or emotional trauma. This may lead to a loss of the natural flexibility of the fibrous components of the bone tissue matrix or locking of the fluid fluctuation within the bone (Sergueef 2007). This can give a palpable quality of density and hardness. In emotional trauma, the lack of 'intraosseous breathing' has a palpatory sense of the osseous fluid and its inherent potency being 'locked away'.

The area between the S2 segment and the coccyx is derived from the caudal eminence (tail bud) during secondary neurulation. This caudal cell mass also forms the caudal notochord as well as the caudal neural cord and hindgut. The palpatory sensation of the sacrum and its relations include an integrated function and expression of primary (weeks 3–4 of gestation) and secondary neurulation (from week 5 of gestation).

1. HANDHOLD AND POSITIONING
The patient may be treated in the sitting, supine or sidelying positions, *and the operator's hands are placed over the sacrum with the finger pads contacting the spinous tubercles or median sacral crest of the sacrum as well as L5 and the coccygeal segments.* The first coccygeal segment may be identified by the vertical cornua and transverse processes on each side.

2. PALPATION OF INHERENT MOTION
Diagnostic sensing of the quality of the sacrum and the ability of the sacrum to change shape (shortening along its long axis and broadening transversely alternating with lengthening and narrowing transversely) is key to identifying intraosseous strain or compression. In health the sacrum has a floating and rocking quality with a sense of an alternating lift and descent axially.

Acknowledge the primary respiratory axis of the sacrum as you find it. It should ideally breathe around a transverse axis at the lamina of S2. Be alert to the possibility of sacral sag.

3. ENGAGEMENT
To engage with the inherent forces of correction, it may be necessary to match the intraosseous compression or strain precisely by the use of your forearm fulcrum. The tissues may require you to match the forces within.

4. Anatomical considerations

Sense the suspension of the sacral segments within the anterior and posterior longitudinal ligaments. The dura is attached to the posterior longitudinal ligament via the sacrodural ligament which strengthens caudally from L4/L5 to S5 (Sakka 2020; van Dun and Girardin 2006).

Note the relationship of S2 to the dural 'cul-de-sac'.

Acknowledge the sacral segments as floating within their periosteal envelope. This floating quality is fluid in nature.

Sense the relation of the parts of the sacrum to the notochordal midline.

Take into your attention the first coccygeal segment as the filum terminale attaches to the periosteum on its dorsal aspect.

5. Resolution

The end point of the treatment is *a change of quality and movement, with a sense of breathing within the bone.*

For sensing and treating strains within the sacral segments, it is also possible to contact the sacrum using *a bilateral hold with the finger pads on the lateral sacral crests.*

VIDEO FOR CHAPTER 17

Scan the QR code or visit https://www.youtube.com/playlist?list=PL3j_YuMBqigGJglwqHqsYnoVyZwYz4Luk to find a playlist of the video that accompanies this chapter.

REFERENCES

Blechschmidt, E. (1904) *The Ontogenetic Basis of Human Anatomy: A Biodynamic Approach to Development from Conception to Adulthood.* Edited and translated by B. Freeman. Berkeley, CA: North Atlantic Books (2004); p. 61.

Bonewald, L. (2010) The osteocyte network as a source reservoir of signalling factors. *Endocrinology & Metabolism 25* (3), 161.

Broome, D.R., Hayman, L.A., Herrick, R.C., *et al.* (1998) Postnatal maturation of the sacrum and coccyx: MR imaging, helical CT and conventional radiography. *Am Roentgen Ray Society 170,* 1061-1066.

Byrd, S.E. & Comiskey, E.M. (2007) Postnatal maturation and radiology of the growing spine. *Neurosurg Clin N Am 18,* 431-461.

Cheng, J.S. & Song, J.K. (2003) Anatomy of the sacrum. *Neurosurg Focus 15* (2), E3.

Cloete, E., Battin, M.R., Farhad, B.I., Teele, R.L. (2013) Ossification of sacral vertebral bodies in neonates born 24–38 weeks' gestational age and its relevance to spinal ultrasonography. *Am J Perinatal 30* (6), 519-522.

Harris, E. (2013) The intoeing child aetiology, prognosis and current treatment options. *Clinics in Podiatric Medicine and Surgery 30* (4), 531-565.

Jealous, J.S. (1988) Personal communication.

Jian, N., Lin, N., Tian, M-M., *et al.* (2019) Normal development of costal element ossification centres of sacral vertebrae in the fetal spine: a postmortem magnetic resonance imaging study. *Paediatric Neuroradiology 61,* 183-193.

Junewick, J.J., Chin, M.S., Meesa, I.R., *et al.* (2011) Ossification patterns of the atlas vertebra. *Am J of Roentgenology 197* (5), 1229-1234.

Knothe Tate, M.L. (2003) 'Whither flows the fluid in bone?' An osteocyte's perspective. *J Biotech 36* (10), 1409-1424.

Moradi, B., Ghanbari, A., Rahmani, M., *et al.* (2019) Evaluation of bi-iliac distance and timing of ossification of sacrum by sonography in the second trimester of pregnancy. *Iran J Radio 16* (2), e79940.

Palumbo, C. & Ferretti, M. (2021) The osteocyte: from 'prisoner' to 'orchestrator'. *J Funct Morphol Kinesiol 6* (1), 28. https://doi.org/10.3390/jfmk6010028

Sakka, L. (2020) Anatomy of the spinal meninges. In: J.M. Vital and D.T. Cawley (eds) *Spinal Anatomy: Modern Concepts.* Berlin: Springer; p. 407.

Schwenk, T. (1965) *Sensitive Chaos.* London: Rudolf Steiner Press; p. 25.

Sergueef, N. (2007) *Cranial Osteopathy for Infants, Children and Adolescents: A Practical Handbook.* Amsterdam: Churchill Livingstone; p. 86.

Skorzewska, A., Grzymisławska, M., Bruska, M., *et al.* (2013) Ossification of the vertebral column in human foetuses: histological and computed tomography studies. *Folia Morphol 72* (3), 230–238.

Studer, K., Williams, N., Studer, P., *et al.* (2017) Obstacles to reduction in infantile developmental dysplasia of the hip. *J Child Orthop 11* (5), 355–366.

Sutherland, W.G. (1990) *Teachings in the Science of Osteopathy.* A.L. Wales (ed.). Fort Worth, TX: Sutherland Cranial Teaching Foundation, Inc./Rudra Press; p. 31.

Techawiboonwong, A., Song, H.K., Leonard, M.B., Wehrli, F.W. (2008) Cortical bone water: in vivo quantification with ultrashort echo-time MR imaging. *Radiology 248* (3), 824–833.

van Dun, P.L.S. & Girardin, M.R.G. (2006) Embryological study of the spinal dura and its attachment into the vertebral canal. *Int J of Osteopathic Medicine 9* (3), 85–93.

Winet, H. (2003) A bone fluid flow hypothesis for muscle pump-driven capillary filtration: II Proposed role for exercise in erodible scaffold implant incorporation. *European Cells and Material 6,* 1–11.

CHAPTER 18

The Body-Mind Interface

SUSAN TURNER

'If one is truly to succeed in leading a person to a specific place, one must first and foremost take care to find him where he is and begin there. This is the secret in the entire art of helping.'

(Kierkegaard 1998)

BEING PRESENT TO THE WHOLE PERSON

A fundamental aim of osteopathic treatment is to restore the harmonious function of the physical vehicle and the aim of this, in turn, is to support wellbeing, as a state where body, mind, emotions and spirit are in balance. This may facilitate a person's capacity to live his or her potential, both inwardly and as expressed in the world.

A.T. Still's definition of what constitutes health, wholeness, 'complete-ness' is far from limited to anatomy and physiology alone:

*'Man is Triune **when complete**.
First there is the material body;
Second, the spiritual body;
Third, a being of mind which is far superior to all vital motion and material forms, whose duty is to wisely manage this great engine of life...
To obtain good results, we must blend ourselves with and travel in harmony with Nature's truths.'*

(Still 1902, p. 16)

Still's vision of man 'when complete' was one of alignment, not just of the physical body but harmony between all levels, which he saw as rooted in the universal wisdom of Being. There is a material and a non-material aspect to osteopathy, encompassing a spectrum between the mechanical laws of physical structure and the subtle frequencies of a person's being and deeper context.

In engaging balanced tension, we seek to meet the body as we find it, in acceptance rather than judgement, where the strain pattern is perceived, matched, supported and acknowledged. In a state of balanced ligamentous, membranous or fascial tension, all the forces, present and historic, that have contributed to the state of strain converge at a neutral point from which a spontaneous resolution is made possible. The psyche, as inseparable from the body, partakes in this process.

Healing can come from being seen and listened to deeply, especially when the awareness of the listener is in resonance with what is being expressed and with the person expressing it.

Edward Whitmont, a Jungian analyst and homoeopathic doctor, noted that the principles of healing are similar on all levels, in that they involve meeting, matching, acceptance and resonance. In this, he likened the rebalancing action of the homoeopathic remedy that matches the patient's symptom picture to the empathic understanding of the psychotherapist (Whitmont 1993).

In osteopathy, through the indirect or functional approaches especially, in matching the vectorial story and mechanical forces held within the physical strain pattern, the operator is practising a manual approach based on the same principle. It is possible, likewise, to match the emotional, mental, spiritual or viscerosomatic forces held in the 'lesion', to enable them to release the life potency locked in the pattern and become available to the total vitality of the patient. In this process, the patient's body and inner being knows when the pattern has been recognised.

For the patient, the experience of receiving empathetic and non-judgemental attention on a physical level can be one of relief, emotionally as well as physically. This is especially so when the area of the body being attended to has been subject to trauma or shock. Accidents often happen at times of chaos in a person's life situation. Painful emotions, associated with the time of injury, may lie hidden in the tissues for many years after the sufferer has forgotten them on a conscious level. In a treatment session, the state of balanced tissue tension sometimes brings such associated feelings into focus. When they surface, the release of an emotional fulcrum maintaining an acute or chronic strain pattern may be the key to its healing. The tissues of the body clearly hold memory through the interweaving of body, psyche and spirit.

The body's metaphors

Everyday language reveals how commonly the body is experienced as a metaphor for a person's inner state. Expressions such as 'light-hearted', 'heart in my boots', being 'beside myself', having a 'gut feeling', 'I couldn't stomach it', or 'the bottom has fallen out of my world' coinciding with a sudden attack of haemorrhoids, are but a few.

The language of posture is also revealing. In a person who feels 'deflated', the lungs and ribcage often tend towards respiratory exhalation. Someone feeling 'braced to face the world' may give the impression of the front of the chest being held like an armoured breastplate. An internally rotated left shoulder may express a person's need to protect the vulnerable feelings of the heart.

The fascia has its own language for the mental and emotional nuances imprinted in its patterns (Michalak 2021). A palpable sense of the permeation of the psyche through the body is communicated by Still when he states: 'The soul of man with all the streams of pure living water seems to dwell within the fascia of the body' (Still 1902, p. 61). It often appears, on palpation, that the body does not always differentiate between emotional and physical blows. The metaphors of feeling 'kicked in the guts', 'stabbed in the heart' or 'hit between the eyes' etc. often seem to be recorded in tissue memory as if they were experienced as actual physical impacts.

Embodiment

There are times when, on palpation, a specific part of the body feels 'uninhabited', as if its owner had psychically withdrawn from it. This commonly happens after a fracture or in an area of debilitating pain. Similarly, when a woman has had a difficult or traumatic birth, there may be a sense of 'no-one at home' in the sacrum. An area of the body from which there is a psychic withdrawal will frequently be resistant to healing, making it difficult to engage the tissues therapeutically. If this quality of absence is quietly supported and acknowledged by the operator with hands, heart and mind, the area may begin to feel 'lived in' again.

Occasionally it can be helpful to feed these impressions back to a patient, who may confirm a sensation subjectively and express relief at having it acknowledged. It is often enough though to simply stay present, supporting and acknowledging the situation as it is, while engaging with that person's innate potential for health. It is as if consciousness itself is a substance so that the silent act of presence, acceptance and holding, on the part of the operator, may enable the patient's system to perceive itself, allowing the pattern of conflict to come to rest.

Alteration of rhythmic expression

Thoracic respiration has its own language also. A quiver in the surface pattern of the breathing can suggest fear. Tentativeness, love or peace all have their characteristic respiratory expression. Subtle variations of inherent body rhythm, tissue density, alignment, energy flow etc. may inform us, from the edges of awareness, of feelings that are familiar from our own life experience. A developing 'sensory vocabulary' can make it possible to read and recognise what the patient's system requires the practitioner to encompass in the field of the treatment.

Where there is old shock, internalised anger, anxiety or simply heightened adrenal/sympathetic drive, a very fine vibration is sometimes perceived permeating the tissues. On palpation this can feel like an inner tremble. In such a case it may be necessary to calm sympathetic tone before addressing specific areas and there are many ways to do this. The thoracic spine with its paraspinal muscles is one of the many points of access (see Chapter 16, paraspinal inhibition). An approach often used by Dr Wales to such states of high sympathetic tone was to release the costo-vertebral junctions in the supine patient (see Chapter 4). Her intent here was the 're-setting' of the sympathetic chain ganglia on the anterior surface of the rib heads to defacilitate the spinal reflex arcs (see Chapter 2).

RECIPROCITY OF PSYCHE AND SOMA

Much is now being published and practised, that acknowledges the interweaving of psyche and soma by writers such as Peter Levine, Susan Aposhyan, Bessel Van der Kolk, Robert Scaer, Paul Pearsall, Ewa Robertson, Bonnie Bainbridge Cohen and others. The research of Candace Pert has shown that the chemicals that are running our body and our brain are the same chemicals that are involved in emotion, and that these have a significant influence on health. The field of psycho-neuro-immunology is revealing how the brain is integrated into the body at a molecular level (Pert 1997).

Just as each transient or recurrent emotional state is reflected in its unique way on the body's tissues, the resulting pattern, in turn, may inform the psyche. An example is where a downward drag on the pericardial attachments, from an emotionally heavy heart, tends to pull the thoracic spine into a kyphosis. This posture itself may, in turn, signal to the person's brain a sense of the burden of grief or weariness that further reinforces the emotional state.

Encouragingly, meditation and mindfulness practice have been shown, within a short time, to diminish the size of the amygdala (the 'stress organ' within the brain), but increase the vascularisation and size of the hippocampus which is associated with pleasure (Sanabria-Mazo et al. 2020). Knowing that something as simple as this can have such an effect on the circuitry of the brain is empowering to many people. In light of this, touching an experience of peace in an osteopathic treatment may do more than we realise.

SOMA-PSYCHE IN EARLY OSTEOPATHY

A study of early osteopathy reveals that an understanding of the somatico-psychic connection was part of what Still imparted to his students. Littlejohn referred to the body-mind as an integral unit, with the mind present throughout the body, and therefore accessible through it (Littlejohn 1899). According to the following account by an osteopathic patient of Henry Lee DO, Littlejohn treated shell-shocked soldiers and civilians in a state of mental collapse in London during and after the First World War.

'My mother, Elsie Goddard, was born in 1897 and her osteopathic treatment must have commenced after she started working at Roehampton Post Office when she was 16. She became very stressed due to her manning a very large Post Office, often on her own, with crowds of people pressing up against the counters coming to collect news of their loved ones in the trenches in the First World War. There were machines behind the counters and she would be collecting and deciphering the messages and giving the telegrams to grieving relatives. She would be collecting messages in Morse code and presumably transmitting them too. It was a very distressing and responsible job for a 16 year old and she often forgot to eat her lunch. I think that she may have had a nervous breakdown. She became so tense that she sought the help of a new treatment: Osteopathy and found it amazingly helpful. The caring osteopath was Dr Littlejohn, who she said had the kindest eyes. He restored my mother to full health and she took up a job as a statistician working for the Prudential Insurance company. He even massaged her eyeballs and she talked about the other patients she saw in his waiting room waiting for their treatment, some of them she told me had 'sleeping sickness' and she would see them restored to health and walking upright again.' (Institute of Classical Osteopathy 2010; permission to print given by Henry Lee DO and The Institute of Classical Oseteopathy)

It is clear that Sutherland was no stranger to the reciprocity of psyche and soma. His rationale for seeing a post-partum sagged sacrum as a contributary factor in disturbed brain physiology is described in Chapter 3, anterior approach to the sacral alae (Sutherland 1998, COT p. 286). Charlotte Weaver, a student of Still and contemporary of Sutherland, is known to have treated hospitalised patients with psychiatric illness in Paris through her own cranial osteopathic approach (Sorrel 2010).

One of the first osteopathic hospitals, founded in 1914, was the Still Hildreth Sanatorium, a psychiatric hospital, which recorded treating patients with a high rate of success. Hildreth describes a calming approach to the nervous system through manual relaxation of the suboccipital and thoracic paraspinal muscles (see Chapter 16). The programme also included supportive company, hydrotherapy, walks in nature and nourishing food (Hildreth 1942). On 12 December 1917, a week before he died, Dr Still wrote to his son, Charles, expressing his delight at the successful work of the sanatorium, and affirming the importance to him of the mental dimension in osteopathy (Lewis 2012, p. 354).

On 24 May 1912, Still wrote that he saw life in the body as an incubator 'developing the spiritual man to take the step from mortality to immortality', so that at death the spiritual nature being breaks free like a chick from the egg into a higher existence (Lewis 2012, p. 342). Likewise in another context, he referred to the body as 'the second placenta'. This suggests that he saw the purpose of osteopathic treatment to be, not only physical health, but harmony of the body as a vehicle for the maturation of a person's essential being. In a similar vein, in 1819, the poet John Keats (1795–1821) referred to this world, in a letter, as 'the vale of soul making' (Johns 2014).

IMPRESSIONABILITY OF THE BODY TO MENTAL SUGGESTION

The body is noticeably imprinted, moment-to-moment, by the thoughts of its owner. In an osteopathic treatment session, the 'closing down of vital force', in response to a patient's self-criticism, is immediately palpable. Conversely, a sense of energetic flow in the tissues frequently follows a happy thought.

Dr Still impressed on his students the great responsibility that the osteopath bears through his or her words:

'What you say is weighty beyond your concept. Should you find any hope for his recovery and make that your report, like a thrill of lightning dipped in a sea of love, his vitality dances for joy. But if you should be indiscrete enough in your report to remove every ray of hope, you have chilled the vital energy, you have silenced it... More patients suffer and die from such imprudence and fright than the world ever dreamed of.' (Lewis 2012, p. 266)

This raises the question as to how a patient's problems can be acknowledged without leaving that person with a negative expectation or view of his or her own health. Without denying a patient's difficulties, they can be placed in the context of the truth that, in the living body, the life principle constantly seeks solutions to re-establish physiological and mechanical balance. Because of this, it is always worth a person making any small lifestyle, dietary, spiritual and relational changes that are possible. Even small changes can sometimes 'shift the fulcrum' of a physiological and psychological status quo, towards greater progress to follow.

There is a non-verbal meta-conversation in any therapeutic or interpersonal interaction. A sense of being in a safe space of 'unconditional positive regard' (a phrase first coined by Carl Rogers in 1959 (Bozarth 2007)), where there is an energetic meeting point, can enable a person to feel free to be his or her natural self, emotionally and physically. The relaxation this brings may allow a patient to open to an innate therapeutic potency that is perpetually present.

Some patients need a greater sense of space in the way we approach them in palpation, while others need to be met more closely since each person has an individual natural boundary. In order to find the meeting point, it can be helpful to inwardly ask: 'How do I need to be in myself for you to feel free to be yourself, natural, relaxed and safe?' This can enable an entrainment and resonance between osteopath and patient, opening a conduit to an awareness and understanding that guides the treatment.

PARTICIPATION AND EMPATHY

Rollin Becker communicates a sense of working alongside the patient in a spirit of common humanity:

'Literally what you are doing is sharing the experience of a living being with the experience of another living being...They have a problem and I have to experience that problem. I can't experience it if I am being a teacher; I have to experience it as a student.' (Becker 2000)

In a similar way, A.T. Still before him participated in what he sought to understand or treat (Lewis 2012, p. 268).

'He studied Nature always from the inside, the heart, and as a subject, not an object.' (Tucker 1918)

'He made himself en rapport with the body he studied, he tried to be that bone; he thought as a measle, he put himself inside of the spleen, or the trochanter major, to feel its operation as part of the great unity of action and of logic and of life that was the body.' (Charles E. Still Collection 1997)

INNER DEVELOPMENT

The scientific method of Wolfgang Von Goethe has much in common with the inner discipline of osteopathic practice. Goethe saw the necessity for true and objective scientific insight to include an empathetic and intuitive faculty. In this he viewed science as a path of inner development for the scientist, as well of a way of gaining objective knowledge (Naydler 1996). To Dr Still also, it was understood that it was not just knowledge of anatomy, physiology and skilled hands that were important, but the development of latent mental and intuitive faculties.

In a lecture that Rollin Becker was giving to course participants who were just beginning their study of osteopathy, he shared these words:

Did you think you came...to acquire information? To develop palpatory skills? To become knowledgeable in services to give to your patients and their problems? No, you have come to *be* the work you are going to understand and use in your service to your patients. (Becker 1997)

REFERENCES

Becker, R.E. (1997) *Life in Motion: The Osteopathic Vision of Rollin E. Becker, DO.* R.E. Brooks MD (ed.). Portland, OR: Stillness Press; p. 11.

Becker, R.E. (2000) *The Stillness of Life: The Osteopathic Philosophy of Rollin E. Becker, DO.* R.E. Brooks MD (ed.). Portland, OR: Stillness Press; p. 16.

Bozarth, J. (2007) Unconditional positive regard. In: M. Cooper, M. O'Hara, P.F. Schmid, and G. Wyatt (eds.) *The handbook of person-centred psychotherapy and counselling.* Palgrave Macmillan/Springer Nature; pp. 182 -193

Charles E. Still Collection (1997) Kirksville Museum of Osteopathy, 1997.04.119, p. 94.

Hildreth, A.G. (1942) *The Lengthening Shadow of Dr. Andrew Taylor Still,* 2nd edition. Paw Paw, MI: A.G. Hildreth & A.E. Van Vleck; Ch.19.

Institute of Classical Osteopathy (2010, winter). J.M. Littlejohn's Treatment: A Personal Osteopathic History. *The Institute of Classical Osteopathy Newsletter.*

Johns, J.C. (2014) The Vale of Soul-Making. *The Paris Review,* July.

Kirkegaard, S. (1998) *The Point of View for My Work as An Author.* Trans. Hong and Hong. Princeton, NJ: Princeton University Press; p. 45.

Lewis, J. (2012) *A.T. Still, From Dry Bone to Living Man.* Blanau Ffestiniog: Dry Bone Press; pp. 266, 268, 342, 354.

Littlejohn, J.M. (1899) *Lectures on Psycho-Physiology.* Kirksville, MO: EG Kinney.

Michalak, J., Aranmolate, L., Bonn, A., *et al.* (2021) Myofascial tissue and depression. *Cognitive Therapy and Research 46,* 560–572. https://link.springer.com/article/10.1007/s10608-021-10282-w.

Naydler, J. (1996) *Goethe on Science, An Anthology of Goethe's Scientific Writings.* Edinburgh: Floris Books.

Pert, C. (1997) *Molecules of Emotion.* London: Simon & Schuster UK Ltd.

Sanabria-Mazo, J.P., Montero-Marin, J., Feliu-Soler, A., *et al.* (2020) Mindfulness-Based Program Plus Amygdala and Insula Retraining (MAIR) for the treatment of women with fibromyalgia: a pilot randomized controlled trial. *Journal of Clinical Medicine 9* (10), 3246.

Sorrel, M. (2010) *Charlotte Weaver: Pioneer in Cranial Osteopathy.* Indianapolis, IN: The Cranial Academy.

Still, A.T. (1902) *Philosophy and Mechanical Principles.* Kansas City, MO: Hudson-Kimberly Pub Co.; pp. 16, 61.

Sutherland, W.G. (1998) *Contributions of Thought,* 2nd edition. A.L. Wales and A.S. Sutherland (eds). Fort Worth, TX: Sutherland Cranial Teaching Foundation, Inc.; p. 286.

Tucker, E. (1918) *Journal of the American Osteopathic Association,* p. 247.

Whitmont, E.C. (1993) *Psyche and Substance.* Berkeley, CA: North Atlantic Books.

CHAPTER 19

Engagement with the Living System

SUSAN TURNER

'The Breath of Life is the fundamental principle in the science of osteopathy.'

(W.G. Sutherland in Becker 1997, p. 37)

These words, written by William Sutherland in a letter to Rollin Becker, make a definitive statement about the essence of osteopathy. Fundamental to this art and science is a recognition of the power and intelligence of the Life principle that breathes and continuously forms and maintains physical structure. Engaging with the structure of the living body would be incomplete without interacting, first and foremost, with the quality of aliveness that permeates and animates it.

The living body functions as a unified whole, where each part is interrelated on every level from the gross structure to the most minute movement of molecules, atoms and bioelectrical field phenomena. Every part is a differentiation of the first cell at fertilisation, still united by the fluid extracellular matrix (ECM) and the ubiquity of the myofascial, nervous, vascular and lymphatic fields. Every part is in a constant dynamic dance of self-organising readjustment in relation to every other part.

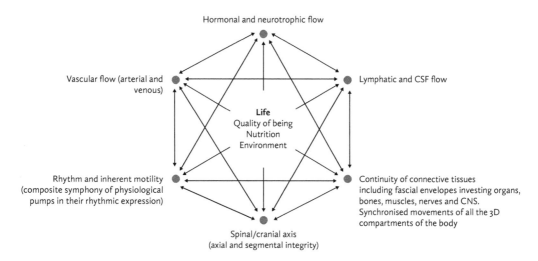

Figure 19.1 Interconnectedness of the living system.

Figure 19.1 illustrates the interconnectedness of each system with every other one, with a person's expression of Life at the centre. In diagnosis, it can be helpful to take all these aspects into the picture: essential vitality, alignment of the neurospinal axis, efficiency of fluid interchange, rhythmic flow and free reciprocal movement of the fascial 'containers' large, small and microscopic. These have been considered in the previous chapters.

LIFE

The *living action* within anatomical form is the most essential and informative element accessible in osteopathic palpation. When the listening hands and heart-mind are quiet, a sense of the essential person and the rhythmic expression of life may be perceived permeating the tissues of the whole body.

No-one has ever successfully defined what life is. We can describe its attributes, observe its expression and feel its vibrancy in the living body and natural world, but it remains a mystery. One attribute of life is its transformational nature. Living systems constantly regenerate and renew themselves to promote life and health. The bacterial action and moisture in the earth cause the roots of a dead tree to rot and return to their basic constituents, whereas a living healthy tree uses those same earth elements to transmute them into growth and fruition.

One of the ways that vitality is perceived through palpating hands is through motion. The living body is in constant rhythmic motion from conception to the final breath. Stasis in any tissue or organ signifies dysfunction. The coexisting rhythms of the cardiovascular and respiratory systems, lymphatics and gut peristalsis, the central nervous system and cerebrospinal fluid fluctuation are harmonically interdependent in a quantum biological symphony. This interplay of perpetual rhythmic motion interacts with the movement of the fascial continuum to ensure fluid interchange.

Cellular nutrition, oxygenation and waste clearance in every organ and tissue depend on the physiological pumps, provided by three-dimensional rhythmic shape change, from the gross structures to the most minute spaces. If stasis is the enemy of health, one of the aims of osteopathic treatment is 'giving body's lost rhythm back to itself' (Wernham 1976).

Another expression of aliveness, perceivable to listening hands, is a sense of fluid flow and interchange. Cellular nutrition and waste clearance are dependent on the interchange of fluids through their ebb and flow in the ECM. The ECM represents the original embryonic circulatory system within which vascular and lymphatic channels gradually develop as the body differentiates. It continues to form the fluid environment throughout life, for cells, nerves and vessels. Where there is excessive tissue tension, expressed in torsion or compression of an articulation or fascial boundary, there is loss of extracellular space; this implies restriction of blood and lymphatic flow, resulting in a poor cellular environment (Sutherland 1990, TSO p. 31).

There is a palpable impression of expansion, warmth and aliveness that accompanies the resolution of osteopathic strain patterns. This may be partly explained by the alteration of spatial relationships that permit fluid interchange and rhythmic flow in the interstitium and all channels, as an expression of the life permeating them.

A brief glimpse into osteopathic history reveals how central an awareness of the Life principle has been from the beginning. In the words of Carl McConnell DO, a student of A.T. Still and teacher of Anne Wales, 'In clinical practice it is helpful to hold the view that the life impulse is not created, for it is of an eternal nature' (Becker 2000, p. 184). Rollin Becker echoed this in a letter to William Sutherland: 'The Breath of Life is the same as the Space that shapes the Universe' (Becker 2000, p. 200). We see this creative force expressed throughout the ecosystems of Nature and in the healing powers at work within the living body.

What Sutherland called the 'breath of life', J.M. Littlejohn referred to as 'vital force' as the union of spirit and matter within the body. To him, also, engagement with the life within the body was fundamental to osteopathy as expressed in his words, 'the system pulsates with the rhythm of life' (Wernham 1999). In the words of his student, John Wernham, 'It never fails to delight me when I feel the vital force returning to the tissues under my fingers.'

Still saw life as primary to everything. In saying 'Life is a substance that fills all the space of the whole universe' (Truhlar 1950), he communicates a sense that we are embedded in an alive Cosmic field. He saw life as preexisting and underlying physical form: 'His (man's) existence in form is the effect of Life; The cause antedates him in mind and deed. His life or spirit must be the cause of his form' (Still 1898).

The way we frame our world view and context inevitably influences the way we engage with palpation and treatment and our openness to sustenance from the environment for both ourselves and the patient. Ilya Prirogone, a Nobel prize laureate and professor of physical chemistry, described the living system as a 'dissipative structure': 'A living system is both open and closed; structurally open for energy and matter to continually flow through it, but organisationally closed, maintaining stable form autonomously through stable organisation' (Capra 1997). If this is so, we clearly do not stop at our skin surface.

This is reflected in Rollin Becker's reference to the universal life field through which we are interwoven and permeated:

'The bioenergy of Wellness is the most powerful force in the world. It is dynamic. It is rhythmic… It is in constant interchange with its external environment physically, mentally and emotionally. This external environment extends from a person's immediate surroundings to the farthest reaches of the universe…Instead of the terminology, "man and his environment", these can be joined in one term, "the biosphere".' (Becker 1997, p. 203)

Expressing her awareness of the interconnectedness of the human field with that of the earth and its atmosphere, Anne Wales commented that 'a fluctuating body of fluid within a closed container within an electromagnetic field constitutes a battery'. The neurospinal axis and whole living body is 'a fluctuating body of fluid within a closed container within the electromagnetic field of planet earth' (Wales 1996).

In the words of Harrison Fryette DO:

'Osteopathy is as simple as the human organism; and that is as simple as the Universe, for in the human organism are embraced the physical, mental and spiritual laws of the Universe. To perfectly understand the human organism then, it would be necessary to possess an infinite mind.' (Fryette 1938)

These thoughts of our osteopathic ancestors suggest that an awareness of interchange with the creative life field of the cosmos, and the sustenance that this perpetually offers to both practitioner and patient, are an essential part of the original vision of Still's osteopathy.

Rollin Becker's saying that 'The Breath of Life is the same as the Space that shapes the Universe' (Becker 2000, p. 200) calls for deep reflection. It sheds light on what Sutherland may have meant when he said to Anne Wales, 'I can't get him (a student on a course) to understand that we are not so much treating the structure as the Space' (Wales 1988). When asked if Dr Sutherland meant the space defined by the large body cavities, the spaces containing the organs, the space between the cells or the space between the atoms, Dr Wales replied 'all of that'. Perhaps, in the light of Dr Becker's statement, she was also saying 'more than that'.

REFERENCES

Becker, R.E. (1997) *Life in Motion: The Osteopathic Vision of Rollin E. Becker, DO.* R.E. Brooks MD (ed.). Portland, OR: Stillness Press; pp. 37, 203.

Becker, R.E. (2000) *The Stillness of Life: The Osteopathic Philosophy of Rollin E. Becker, DO.* R.E. Brooks MD (ed.). Portland, OR: Stillness Press; pp. 184, 200.

Capra, F. (1997) *The Web of Life.* Flamingo.

Fryette, H.H. (1938) Simplicity in Osteopathy. AAO Convention lecture. AAO Yearbook 1938.

Still, A.T. (1898) *Journal of Osteopathy,* Vol 5, No 4, September 1898, p. 163.

Sutherland, W.G. (1990) *Teachings in the Science of Osteopathy.* A.L. Wales (ed.). Fort Worth, TX: Sutherland Cranial Teaching Foundation, Inc./Rudra Press; p. 31.

Truhlar, R.E. (1950) *Dr A.T. Still in the Living.* Cleveland, OH; p. 83.

Wales, A.L. (1988) Personal communication.

Wales, A.L. (1996) British tutorial group meeting. North Attleboro, MA, USA.

Wernham, J. (1976) ESO, personal communication.

Wernham, J. (1999) *The Life and Times of John Martin Littlejohn.* Maidstone, Kent: John Wernham College of Classical Osteopathy.

Bibliography

Agur, A.M.R. & Dalley, A.F. (eds) (2005) *Grant's Atlas of Anatomy*, 11th edition. Baltimore: Lippincott Williams and Wilkins.

Agur, A.M.R. & Lee, M.J. (eds) (1999) *Grant's Atlas of Anatomy*, 10th edition. Baltimore: Lippincott Williams and Wilkins.

Basmajian, J.V. (1982) *Primary Anatomy*, 8th edition. Baltimore: Williams and Wilkins.

Basmajian, J.V. & Slonecker, C.E. (eds) (1989) *Grant's Method of Anatomy*, 11th edition. Baltimore: Williams and Wilkins.

Bhatia, M. & Thomson, L. (2020) Morton's neuroma – current concepts review. *J Clin Orthop Trauma 11* (3), 406–409. https://doi.org/10.1016/j.jcot.2020.03.024.

Brockett, C.L. & Chapman, G.L. (2016) Biomechanics of the ankle. *Orthop Trauma 30* (3), 232–238. https://doi.org/10.1016/j.mporth.2016.04.015.

Crow, W.T., King, H.H., Patterson, R.M., Giuliano, V. (2009) Assessment of calvarial structure motion by MRI. *Osteopath Med Prim Care 3*, 8.

Elftman, H. (1969) Dynamic structure of the human foot. *O&P Library Artificial Limbs 13*, 1, 49–58.

Grietz, D., Wirestam, R., Franck, A., *et al.* (1992) Pulsatile brain movement and associated hydrodynamics studied by magnetic resonance phase imaging: the Monro-Kellie doctrine revisited. *Neuroradiology 34*, 370–380.

Kashyap, S., Brazdzionis, J., Savla, P., *et al.* (2021) Osteopathic manipulative treatment to optimize the glymphatic environment in severe traumatic brain injury measured with optic nerve sheath diameter, intracranial pressure monitoring, and neurological pupil index. *Cureus 13* (3), e13823. https://doi.org/10.7759/cureus.13823.

Krähenbühl, N., Horn-Lang, T., Hintermann, B., Knupp, M. (2017) The subtalar joint: a complex mechanism. *EFORT Open Reviews 2* (7), 309–316. https://doi.org/10.1302/2058-5241.2.160050.

Lin, C.F., Gross, M.L., Weinhold, P. (2006) Ankle syndesmosis injuries: anatomy, biomechanics, mechanism of injury, and clinical guidelines for diagnosis and intervention. *The Journal of Orthopaedic and Sports Physical Therapy 36* (6), 372–384. https://doi.org/10.2519/jospt.2006.2195.

Magoun, H.I. (1966) *Osteopathy in the Cranial Field*, 2nd edition. Kirksville, MI: The Journal Printing Company.

Moskalenko, Y.E., Kravchenko, T.I., Gaidar, B.V., *et al.* (1999) Periodic mobility of cranial bones in humans. *Human Physiology 25* (1), 51–58.

NCT (2018) Pregnancy hormones: progesterone, oestrogen and the mood swings. Accessed September 2023 at: https://www.nct.org.uk/pregnancy/how-you-might-be-feeling/pregnancy-hormones-progesterone-oestrogen-and-mood-swings.

Sarrafian, S.K. (1993) Biomechanics of the subtalar joint complex. *Clin Orthop Relat Res 290*, 17–26.

Standring, S. (ed.) (2016) *Gray's Anatomy: The Anatomical Basis of Clinical Practice*, 41st edition. Amsterdam: Elsevier.

Stolarczyk, A., Stepinski, P., Sasinowski, L., *et al.* (2021) Peripartum pubic symphysis diastasis: practical guidelines. *J Clin Med 10* (11), 2443. https://doi.org/10.3390/jcm10112443.

Tamburella, F., Piras, F., Piras, F., *et al.* (2019) Cerebral perfusion changes after osteopathic manipulative treatment: a randomized manual placebo-controlled trial. *Front Physiol 10*, 1–9.

Ueno, T., Ballard, R.E., Macias, B.R., *et al.* (2003) Cranial diameter pulsation measured by non-invasive ultrasound decrease with tilt. *Aviation, Space and Environmental Medicine 74* (8), 882–885.

Venkadesan, M., Yawar, A., Eng, C.M., *et al.* (2020) Stiffness of the human foot and evolution of the transverse arch. *Nature 579*, 97–100. https://doi.org/10.1038/s41586-020-2053-y.

Williams, P.L. & Warwick, R. (eds) (1980) *Gray's Anatomy*, 36th edition. Edinburgh: Churchill Livingstone.

Subject Index

Sub-headings in *italics* indicate figures.

Author Index